Bodies for Battle

Bodies for Battle

US Army Physical Culture and Systematic Training, 1885–1957

GARRETT GATZEMEYER

UNIVERSITY PRESS OF KANSAS

Published by the University Press of Kansas (Lawrence, Kansas 66045), which was organized by the Kansas Board of Regents and is operated and funded by Emporia State University, Fort Hays State University, Kansas State University, Pittsburg State University, the University of Kansas, and Wichita State University.

Library of Congress Cataloging-in-Publication Data

Names: Gatzemeyer, Garrett, author.
Title: Bodies for battle : US Army physical culture and systematic training, 1885–1957 / Garrett Gatzemeyer.
Other titles: US Army physical culture and systematic training, 1885–1957
Description: Lawrence, Kansas: University Press of Kansas, 2021. | Series: Modern war studies | Includes bibliographical references and index.
Identifiers: LCCN 2021018726
ISBN 9780700632589 (cloth)
ISBN 9780700632596 (ebook)
Subjects: LCSH: United States. Army—Physical training—History—19th century. | Physical education and training, Military—United States—History—19th century. | United States. Army—Physical training—History—20th century. | Physical education and training, Military—United States—History—20th century. | Physical fitness—United States—History.
Classification: LCC U323 .G38 2021 | DDC 355.5—dc23
LC record available at https://lccn.loc.gov/2021018726.

British Library Cataloguing-in-Publication Data is available.

Printed in the United States of America

10 9 8 7 6 5 4 3 2 1

The paper used in this publication is acid free and meets the minimum requirements of the American National Standard for Permanence of Paper for Printed Library Materials Z39.48-1992.

CONTENTS

ACKNOWLEDGMENTS

This book is the product of time, sweat, and tears, not all of which were mine. Much of the research and writing was shoehorned into late nights, lunch breaks, weekends, and family vacations over the past six years. Many people sacrificed their time, shared their talents, and lent encouragement during these odds hours and over the long haul. Without them I could not have completed this project.

Some of my supporters may not even know that their names are going into print. I am indebted to the librarians and archivists who helped me access obscure documents and offered insights from their own areas of expertise. I think especially of Benjamin Gross from the Linda Hall Library, Mary Brutzloff from the Eisenhower Presidential Library, and Alicia Mauldin and Mark Danley from the United States Military Academy's Special Collections and Library. Bethany Davis and David McCartney of the University of Iowa libraries graciously packaged and sent digitized copies of the Charles McCloy papers, saving me thousands of dollars and days of leave. Rebekka Bernotat of the Donovan Research Library found Fort Benning physical training conference reports, the existence of which I only suspected, and then located even more and digitized the whole lot.

A corps of readers and commentators provided a circle of support. Cliff Rogers and Sam Watson, brilliant historians with whom I have had the honor to work, both read and commented on multiple drafts. My manuscript benefited from their insights, and I found their friendship and mentorship to be invaluable. I am also indebted to members of the USMA History Department's informal junior faculty dissertation working group. I thank especially Ben Brands, Jim Villanueva, Mark Askew, John Fahey, and Brendan Griswold for their feedback and for sharing their projects with me. I would be remiss if I did not thank my former division chief, Col. Bryan Gibby, whose encouragement and advice were vital. I doubt that I would have been able to sustain this project had I not belonged to the culture of respect, excellence, and care he cultivated in our division. I am also deeply grateful to readers outside of USMA, especially John Dzwonczyk, Brett Beneke, and Trent Gatzemeyer. Finally, I thank my advisers at the University of Kansas: Adrian Lewis, Jennifer Weber, Sheyda Jahanbani, and Beth Bailey. Professor Lewis asked hard questions and kept me on track. Professor Weber challenged me to be a better writer and more critical thinker. Professor Jahanbani offered her wisdom in this project's earliest stages, probably without even realizing it. Professor Bailey's insightful feedback, curiosity, and expertise helped me take this project to a new level.

I am most obliged to my immediate family. My father, Steve Gatzemeyer, listened to me when I was at a low point and encouraged me to drive on. He is a model of dependability and solid character. Amy, my incredible wife, deserves an entire book to detail her contributions. Amy believed in my work from the beginning, sacrificed our time together, accepted periods in which I was mentally or physically distant during the writing process, and actively labored to keep me energized and balanced. She also read every draft, which is a remarkable accomplishment. Finally, I thank my children: Quenby Anne and Theodore Rex. They did not always understand why I had to hide somewhere to write, or why we went on family vacations to archives, but they were always ready with a hug or word of encouragement. Like Amy, they sacrificed our time together to bring this project to completion. It is to them that I dedicate this manuscript and a lesson I learned while writing—nearly anything is possible given planning, determination, dedication, and the support of those whom you love.

INTRODUCTION
MODERN WAR, MODERN FITNESS

The US government "selected" Ely J. Kahn for service in the US Army in 1941, relabeled him Private Kahn, and dispatched him to training. Before long, Kahn found himself sweating in a field in South Carolina, sharing in an early morning combat-preparation ritual common to the experiences of millions of American soldiers that began with a "brisk dose of calisthenics." During those physical drill sessions, Kahn remembered his officers exclaiming that every exercise "would develop some especially useful muscle," warning their charges "not to bend those knees as we strove earnestly to touch our toes," and urging the troops on "by announcing that every uncomfortable position we got ourselves into was for our own good." That was one of Kahn's great lessons: "You don't have to be in the Army long to learn, from some superior or other, that everything you do, or that is done to you, is for your own good."[1] What Kahn and his peers may not have realized is that their officers had more in mind than muscular strength and cardiovascular endurance when they spoke of exercises doing soldiers good. In truth, the workouts were part of an uplift project intended to produce better men in a holistic sense: more disciplined, more resilient in the face of adversity, and more morally upstanding. While some elements of that uplift project could claim a general heritage from warrior cultures stretching back through millennia, the particulars of Kahn's exercise ritual were less than a century old.

Kahn's enforced early morning routines were grounded in an eternal fact: war is physical. In combat, fortune favors the soldier in better condition. Superior conditioning enables troops to fight longer and harder, to move farther and faster, to carry heavier loads and endure greater hardship. These relative advantages can be the difference between life and death, victory and defeat. The Prussian philosopher of war Carl von Clausewitz once observed that "War is the realm of physical exertion and suffering. These will destroy us unless we can make ourselves indifferent to them, and for this birth or training must provide us with a certain strength of body and soul."[2] So long as humans make war, this will be an enduring truth. Thus, physical training in some form has always been a part of the preparation for war. Western traditions locate the origins of martial physical training, and often the ideal male body type, in ancient

Greece and Rome. Whether in the broader educational approach of the Athenians or the utilitarian version of the Spartans and Romans, physical training shaped bodies for war. The humanist impetus behind physical training faded in the medieval period, but warrior castes in feudal systems sustained utilitarian physical training. Militaries in the early modern period had little need of individual warriors, but elaborate drill regulations fitted soldiers' bodies to a new sort of combat and battlefield. Later, nationalism brought with it more widespread demands on citizenries for military service. Whole populations needed to be made healthy and strong in the name of war.[3]

Kahn's particular experience also reflected the heritage of a new political, cultural, military, and intellectual juncture that emerged in the twentieth century's dawning years. Military leaders and thinkers in the United States at the time believed that war—as it always had—demanded bodily preparation. However, physical training assumed increased importance and new characteristics that reflected a modern confidence in man's ability to manipulate nature and society.[4] Progressive educators such as John Dewey, and members of the new physical education profession such as Thomas Wood, Luther Gulick, and Clark Hetherington, endorsed an organic unity of mind and body. They argued that learning a physical act was not just physical but also mental and social. Play and exercise could therefore develop the whole individual, even societies.[5] Some military officers recognized the potential power of this new physical education philosophy and others like it in popular fitness movements. The rational application of modern, scientific training methods seemingly created opportunities to shape both physical and non-physical qualities. Militaries around the world developed and promoted gymnastics systems and sport to take advantage of these perceived opportunities. The US military followed suit, anxious about entering a competitive imperial world where embodied nations battled for survival in the framework of social Darwinism.[6]

What follows is an exploration of the specific heritage that informed Kahn's exercise experience—those philosophies and practices that guided the US Army's efforts to shape soldiers' bodies between 1885 and 1957. Taken together, these philosophies and practices formed a physical culture, here defined as a constellation of ideas about the nature and value of fitness, and of the means by which one should achieve it. While multiple physical cultures could and did exist simultaneously, this study traces the official culture promulgated in policy and doctrine, the one top US Army leaders intended to be dominant. That culture's foundation was systematic exercise. Its producers posited that physical training should be a distinct activity instead of an incidental byproduct of other activities, and that it should be rationally structured and applied to maximize its intended effects. Four key questions impel analysis of this culture. In whose interests were bodies shaped? To what ends were they shaped? How did the philosophy and practice of shaping those bodies change over time? How did the shaping of bodies contribute to projects of man-, soldier-, and citizen-making? Answers to these questions reveal more than just simple exercise preferences. Martial physical training advocates aspired to more than utilitarian benefits. The systems and practices they advocated therefore also opened windows onto how they conceived of the future battlefield, the ideal soldier, the relationship between man and machine, and the nature of American citizenship. In short, these exercise systems were cultural expressions. Exploring the official physical culture's development over time yields insights into military culture in general, and into relationships and interactions between the US Army and wider society in the first half of the twentieth century.

At every stage of its development, the Army's physical culture reflected unique contexts informed by perceived military demands, the state of exercise science and physical education, popular culture, and its own accumulating tradition. Modern war's demands were particularly influential and largely justified systematic exercise. At the turn of the twentieth century, new technologies rendered battlefields simultaneously deadlier and emptier while mechanizing and industrializing the act of killing.[7] Individuals paradoxically seemed to become more important on apparently empty battlefields—devoid of mass troop formations and the concomitant reassuring "elbow-touch"—even as the individual soldier's relative significance ostensibly declined in inverse proportion to battle's growing spatial and temporal scope.[8] In the 1950s, another possible technology-driven battlefield revolution appeared to be afoot, this time driven by nuclear weapons. Tactics and organizational structures adapted to the imagined battlefield of the future, again seemingly reducing the individual's relative significance. Yet in both these periods and all the years between, military theorists and leaders in Europe and in the United States emphasized moral forces as a key to the offensive and victory. Theorists and military leaders often conceived of war before World War I as a contest of wills that hinged on the human element's performance, both en masse and individually. "The true strength of an army," wrote Britain's Col. Frederic Maude, an influential commentator on military tactics and affairs before World

War I, "lies essentially in the power of each, or any, of its constituent fractions to stand up to punishment, even to the verge of annihilation when necessary."[9] Men required moral and muscle fiber to withstand the terrifying effects of devastating weapons while advancing in isolation from others, to bear increasingly heavy physical and psychic loads, and finally to close with and kill the enemy—sometimes by bayonet or bare hand.[10] More than fifty years later, US Army leaders such as Gen. Maxwell Taylor likewise emphasized the human element in war. Scoffing at the idea of a "push-button war," Taylor and others doubled down on the need for fit, resilient troops to prosecute war on a nuclear battlefield. Leaders in both eras and in the intervening years looked to systematic exercise as a way of sculpting the sort of soldier they needed.

Broader cultural, political, social, and intellectual contexts informed and constrained the imaginations of those seeking to improve the Army's human material and the tools at their disposal. Early in the official physical culture's development, for instance, Social Darwinism and neo-Lamarckianism fixed attention on bodies and stressed race. Under these theories, physical appearance revealed internal qualities, and physical struggle shaped character or even strengthened offspring.[11] Concerns voiced mainly by white, male Americans about racial and masculine decline at the turn of the century fueled intense anxieties that translated into worry over national strength and vigor.[12] Perhaps the modern world's "overcivilized" men were not ready for the modern battlefield's challenges.[13] But the "crisis in masculinity" opened avenues for improving soldiers, too. If bodies could degenerate, they could also regenerate. A popular physical culture grew up in America around sport and bodybuilding. With the right diet and exercise, men could cultivate corporeal proportions like the world's "perfect man," Eugen Sandow. And if people could improve themselves, then the military might also engineer men's bodies for martial purposes.[14] Officers drew on the language and practices of popular physical cultures in developing solutions to battlefield problems, and they continued to do so throughout the twentieth century.

Martial physical training resonated with movements applying scientific knowledge and methods, and occasionally pseudoscience such as eugenics, to improve the human body and thereby improve society. Nutritional science, which arose in the first two decades of the twentieth century, is one example. Nutritionists revolutionized the way Americans approached eating by breaking food down into its component parts, such as calories and vitamins, and reimagining food as fuel. This approach theoretically enabled efficient and economic consumption, all while improving the health of individuals and the nation. Physical training advocates moralized exercise in much the same way as nutritionists moralized food consumption. Physical educators, belonging to a field that professionalized alongside the emergence and evolution of the Army's physical culture, also sought to apply scientific knowledge and methods to improve bodies and society. Trends in physical education and in US Army physical training typically moved in similar directions, and in several cases educators decisively influenced developments in the Army's physical culture.

A final contextual factor is that making soldiers and making citizens overlapped in an age of nationalism and conscription. All male citizens were potential soldiers. Military service seemed to some a way of inculcating discipline, health, and patriotism in the public. Soldiering could be a means of elevating humanity, and certainly of bettering manhood. Yet physically fit, patriotic, and courageous soldiers could not be made in a few weeks of training. Such soldiers were the products of a culture, a people, and a society. Consequently, politicians, educators, and Army leaders also deployed the ideals and tools of martial physical training in spaces outside the military: schools, preparedness camps, paramilitary programs, and more. Through these deployments, martial physical training abetted the efforts of elites seeking to define the nature of citizenship in terms of obligations, and to leverage military service as a positive good for society. In general, the Army's physical culture supported an obligation-based model of citizenship that privileged certain bodies, namely, those of healthy, white, military-aged males. It also often framed the soldier and his body as interchangeable parts in a larger machine. These models did not always sit well with American society.

In addition to broader contextual factors, persistent tensions within the Army's physical culture also shaped its development over time. The relative influence over the culture enjoyed by institutional outsiders and insiders at any given time was one such tension. Only when outsiders exercised decisive influence did the Army's physical culture change significantly. This was the case at the very beginning, when West Point hired young Herman Koehler to take charge of its physical training program, and at major points of inflection during both World Wars, when massive and rapid end-strength growth brought civilian physical educators into positions of authority. Whereas institutional insiders tended to preserve the values, assumptions, and practices they inherited, outsiders tended to inject the latest trends from civilian physical education and popular culture. Ironically, these outsiders usually placed greater emphasis on practical combat preparation than did insiders, whose goals typically aligned more with visual sculpting and discipline. This observation points to another tension commonly found in studies of military culture: the paradoxical pulls of tradition and innovation. Only in times of major dislocation and upheaval did the Army's physical culture bend toward innovation. Other, smaller tensions also played their parts. For instance, recreational athletics consistently competed against systematic exercise for time and attention. While producers of the Army's physical culture emphasized the latter, soldiers and their immediate superiors often preferred the former. Of the tensions explored in this work, only one dissipated by 1957—debate among senior leaders about the value of and real need for physical training. At the end of the nineteenth century, many of the Army's top officers questioned whether units should spend time exercising instead of training soldier skills through marching, digging, and drilling. By 1957, top officers assumed that systematic exercise was an inherently necessary activity, and that physical fitness was a trait to be valued over most others in their subordinates.

Three punctuated periods are apparent in the evolution of the Army's physical culture between 1885 and 1957: Koehler's disciplinary era, the combat-readiness interregnum of 1917–1919, and the scientific measurement school's rise after 1942. Because understanding the particular context in which the Army's physical culture originated is crucial to understanding its nature and subsequent development in these three periods, an analysis of military problems and proposed solutions at the turn of the twentieth century makes a good point of departure. Most solutions involved improving an army's and nation's human material. This concept drew on popular fitness cultures, evolutionary science, and racial pseudoscience while echoing impulses toward order, systems, control, and moralizing in Progressivism and industrial management. From the beginning, the Army's physical culture was about much more than a soldier's physical efficiency. It was also about cultivating desirable qualities, especially discipline; promoting an idealized warrior masculinity; and improving the moral fiber of individuals and units. The soldier's body existed at the intersection between the battlefield, Progressive culture, physical education philosophy and pedagogy, transnational influences, and the period's "crisis in masculinity." Training philosophies and practices emerged from this context that coalesced into the Army's official physical culture. Politicians, physical educators, Army officers, and other elites deployed this emergent physical culture to support arguments for improving American citizens' bodies as a matter of national security in an age of American imperialism.

The Army's official physical culture underwent its first major change between 1917 and 1920. West Point's Master of the Sword, Herman Koehler, and his disciplinary gymnastics largely defined US Army physical training before World War I. In 1917, mobilization summoned hundreds of civilian educators to serve. Civilian physical training directors, most notably Dr. Joseph Raycroft, replaced Koehler as dominant cultural producers until 1920. These civilians changed the character of Army physical training, redefined fitness along the lines of functional combat efficiency, and introduced now-familiar concepts such as measurable fitness standards. Tradition waxed and innovation waned after the war. Cultural inertia and the earlier system's bureaucratic entrenchment produced a wholesale reversion to Koehler's original formulation of the Army's physical culture in the interwar years. Debates about masculinized national health and the deployment of martial physical culture, both in practice and in rhetoric, to improve the body politic grew in volume and intensity during this period. New martial "prehabilitation" programs arose, fueled by surprisingly high draftee rejection rates during World War I and the Depression's devastating physical, psychic, and moral toll on US citizens. Two of the most prominent were the Civilian Military Training Camps (CMTC) and Civilian Conservation Corps (CCC). The CMTC linked physical fitness explicitly with citizenship. The CCC sculpted men's bodies and helped remasculinize men's public and self-images, often under the direction of Army leaders.

As in World War I, the Army's physical culture changed significantly during World War II. Because the Army failed to retain lessons learned during its earlier experience, officers and civilians responsible for physical training had to rapidly relearn how to prepare a mass conscript force for war. Primary emphasis in the Army's physical culture returned to functional, combat-oriented training and its producers rediscovered standardized testing. Again, professional physical fitness educators and athletic coaches, such as Theodore Bank and Charles McCloy, pushed changes based on state-of-the-art thought in the physical education community. Their empirical, data-driven approach to crafting a physical training system with performance standards came to be hailed as the "new physical training concept" by later cultural producers. The Army's senior leaders meanwhile developed policies that increasingly recognized different body types and degrees of ability, but they also opted to exclude women from the Army's official physical culture when the Women's Army Auxiliary Corps (WAAC, later WAC) formed in 1942. Women exercised instead within a wholly different set of values, assumptions, and practices, revealing the Army's official physical culture to be a fundamentally gendered construct.

The real and imagined battlefield implications of technological advances converged with cultural anxieties over American masculinity and physical fitness after World War II as they had in the late nineteenth century. On one hand, nuclear weapons and other technologies suggested to some the rise of "push-button" war in which the soldier's physical capacity barely factored. On the other, Korean War experiences and deep-rooted convictions in the Army about the centrality of man in war suggested that physical training remained relevant, and that it might even be more necessary than ever. In 1957, the physical culture's chief producers came down firmly in support of the latter camp and reaffirmed basic tenets of the Army's World War II–era physical culture. This moment represented the maturation of the Army's physical culture, the core of which is not much different from the culture's core today.

Yet fitness was not just a soldier's concern in the 1950s. Mass mobilization in World War II and the Cold War's intense ideological struggle kept attention on civilian bodies and their training. However, the acceptable means by which the state could pursue the prehabilitation of its citizenry had changed considerably since the 1930s. Examining several federal efforts to enhance American fitness between the 1930s and 1950s, including the Victory Corps, proposals for Universal Military Training, and the President's Council on Youth Fitness, highlights many of these changes. Over time, the appeal of martial prehabilitation diminished owing to a combination of American social, cultural, and political posturing against militarism and totalitarianism, and a popular understanding of citizenship in which obligations factored less and less. This combination also increased federal reliance on "advisory state" approaches. Examining the character of implemented programs, along with arguments for and against them, helps illuminate relationships between the Army's physical culture and wider American society.

When Private Kahn took his daily dose of calisthenics in 1941, he was performing a ritual rich with meaning, even if he did not realize it. Two generations earlier, his predecessors began participating in calisthenics, contests of strength and balance, and rifle drill. These activities were supposed to sculpt troops into better men, to chisel body, mind, and spirit into something more upstanding, more resilient, and more capable of meeting modern war's demands. A generation later, Kahn's predecessors took their own doses of calisthenics and mixed them with sports, obstacle courses, and hand-to-hand combat training to become American crusaders suited for victory on World War I's Western Front. Kahn's generation and those that followed participated in similar activities, though they were increasingly informed by empirical research and a more scientific approach to programming. Between 1885 and 1957, US Army soldiers and those potentially liable for service took part in projects of man-, soldier-, and citizen-making that continued elevating physical fitness from being a personal interest to a general, societal interest. Individual bodies became constituent elements of the state's health and military power, and the US Army's approach to physical training became a cultural icon. What follows is an exploration of the people and ideas behind that movement and of the unique physical culture they created.

CHAPTER ONE
BODIES AND BATTLEFIELDS
CONTEXTUALIZING MARTIAL FITNESS FOR MODERN WAR

Images of soldiers running, sweating, squatting, pushing, and pulling their way toward physical readiness are ubiquitous in the media and popular imagination today, so it may be surprising to learn that such activities have only officially and regularly been part of the US soldier's life since 1914.[1] In that year, the US Army published its *Manual of Physical Training*. This manual laid out for the first time in the Army's history a comprehensive, professionally developed, uniform system of exercise designed to occupy a permanent position in the training of America's soldiers. Maj. Gen. Leonard Wood, then Chief of Staff of the Army, penned an introduction to this seminal document in which he asserted that "There is nothing in the education of the soldier of more vital importance than [physical training]."[2] Wood's words were undoubtedly genuine. The Chief of Staff was a famously active man, known especially as a companion of Theodore Roosevelt's in the "strenuous life." Hagiographies published about Wood in the lead-up to his presidential campaign in 1920 invariably extolled his "magnificent health and robust physique" that resulted from making "part of the day's work to keep the body in trim."[3] Yet this riding, rowing, and wrestling general officer was an abnormally avid physical culturist among his cohort of military leaders. Likewise, his ideas on physical training's importance were not universally held, especially among older officers. Thus, Wood's confident assertions in 1914 must also be read as an argument for a relatively new idea that still lacked total acceptance throughout the Army. Formal exercise systems were not native to US Army training practices, and the character of systematic training as we have come to know it was not preordained. As Wood observed in 1914, physical training had to that point been a "negligible quantity," owing in large part to the "absence of any well-defined authorized method of procedure" and the total lack of "system and uniformity."[4]

Movement toward system and uniformity manifested most clearly in the manual from 1914, but it began in the 1880s and 1890s. Understanding the system that emerged in 1914, and the patterns and dynamics in Army physical training philosophy and practice thereafter, requires an understanding of the broader context in which advocates devised that system. In the years between 1880 and 1914, social, intellectual, and cultural anxieties intersected with struggles to prepare for combat on new battlefields rendered more dangerous and demanding by technological developments. Physical training, which was experiencing a popularity explosion in American society, seemed to be a means by which to address all of these problems. Simultaneously, a professionalization movement among physical educators created new philosophies, knowledge, and practices that influenced the systematic training of soldiers in both direct and indirect ways.

Central to the broader context in which the US Army's physical culture originated was a set of social, intellectual, and cultural concerns that gripped Americans in the latter decades of the nineteenth century and the early decades of the twentieth. These interlocking concerns produced a broad anxiety about the nation's human material. Speaking generally, this anxiety manifested in fears of degeneration and a loss of American virility and vitality. In a world often conceived of in terms of social Darwinism, the degeneration of a nation's human material was a critical problem, and perhaps even an existential one. Of America's declining human material, men's bodies composed the most important portion. As historian Kristin Hoganson observes, many Americans believed that the health of the nation and its political system depended on the robustness of its men and their "manly character."[5] Degenerating male bodies therefore posed problems for the nation, but also for the US Army specifically. This anxiety over the nation's human resources is especially interesting because it remains with us today, even if it manifests somewhat differently. Contemporary concerns about high obesity rates, the national security implications of those rates, and the billions of dollars Americans spend annually on diets and exercise all signal the enduring relevance of the body politics' fitness.

American men, and Western men in general, struggled to navigate a gender geography in flux in the late nineteenth century. The crisis was especially acute in white middle-class America. The sources of this crisis were many, but class and economic issues were crucial. To a middle-class Victorian of the mid-nineteenth century, "manliness" had meant self-restraint, character, and a good work ethic. To these qualities, the American Civil War added military service and combat experience. This was the era of the "self-made man."[6] In many ways, industrialization, corporations, management systems, and depressions made the achievement of Victorian manliness very difficult for many men. Fewer men were self-employed, more were trapped in sedentary clerical jobs, opportunities to prove oneself in war grew rare, and hard work and restraint did not insulate men against the effects of market failures beyond their control. Industrialization also changed the nature of some jobs by mechanizing production, seemingly integrating workers as pieces of a larger machine with less need for male physicality. This transition, made especially visible in Frederick Taylor's time-and-motion studies, eroded men's ownership of their own time and labor. Meanwhile, urbanization packed Americans into less healthy environments. Men living in these conditions faced more competition for fewer prizes, along with less opportunity for self-mastery and independence in the workplace.[7] Meanwhile, the western frontier's closure, once a man-making space at the border between primitiveness and civilization, denied men their classic option for regeneration.[8]

Even as middle-class men struggled to make themselves in a changing economy, many perceived threats from women suggested a "feminization" of modern man and of America. Women, it seemed, encroached everywhere in the traditional male sphere. Women increasingly entered the once male-exclusive working world in the late nineteenth century, denying men many workplaces as all-male preserves.[9] More and more, women workers provided new competition for men, and men in most workplaces had to modify standards of behavior to account for women. Woman suffrage movements and other forms of political involvement, contemporaries argued, also denied men exclusive claims in the realm of politics.[10] Even as it seemed that men's purview was shrinking, increasingly fewer men could claim political and social power on the grounds of military service in an era when men lacked a major war in which to "prove" themselves, unlike their Civil War–veteran fathers and grandfathers.[11]

Beyond politics and the workplace, changes in child-rearing and family life fanned fears of feminization. Economic changes relocated most men's place of work from the home to a more distant office or factory, so men spent less time in their roles as fathers and male models. The bonds between mothers and their children grew at the same time.[12] Moreover, fewer male role models were available to American boys because women increasingly dominated the teaching profession. Men feared that women's growing control over the development of male children, and the consequent "regime of sugary benignity," would produce a generation of spoiled, physically weak, and morally suspect men.[13] The period's rising consumer culture and its "ethos of pleasure and frivolity," in the words of historian Gail Bederman, further amplified an obsession widely held by American men with "softening."[14]

Fears shared by many white middle-class men about feminization manifested in another, related concern: "overcivilization." Fast living, feminization, and fewer opportunities for self-making threatened to render men too soft and too refined. In response, white middle-class men in the late nineteenth century increasingly celebrated the primitive. This strategy served a social and cultural purpose by defining distinctly masculine virtues as crucial to the nation's vitality.[15] However, according to Bederman "civilization" also had a racial meaning at the time. In this formulation, civilization was a stage of development beyond savagery or "barbarism." Anglo-Saxons had achieved their advanced status as a civilized people through a long Darwinian struggle.[16] Overcivilization's chief threat in this sense was that soft men made for a soft race, a race unworthy of the evolutionary ladder's top position. Industrialization, urbanization, and the frontier's closure denied men traditional sources of struggle and hardening, demanding that new spaces be found and new methods developed.

By the turn of the century, many white men, especially those of the middle class, began centering definitions of manhood on bodies in response to this complex of anxieties. In this corporeal configuration, an unstable, performative masculinity steadily displaced the earlier, inward-focused self-made-man ideal.[17] More and more, proving one's masculinity demanded constant effort and visible proof. The earlier ideal of a self-made man acquired a physical element by the late 1870s as an outward manifestation of inner strength. However, by the turn-of-the-century, men tended to view physicality as an end to be pursued rather than as a natural byproduct of proper manhood. Men may have doubted the possibility of achieving their forefather's manly virtues, but through gymnasium work they could at least produce the appearance of a virtuous inner life.[18] In the best-case scenario, such work might even strengthen morals as it strengthened muscles.

An irony of the turn toward a more bodily-centered masculinity was that American men simultaneously grew more anxious about their bodies and physical capacities. Men viewed as increasingly effeminate, overcivilized, and living soft lives in mentally overstimulating modern society seemed prone to breaking. Americans quickly invented a medical diagnosis for this culturally based fear: neurasthenia. Though the idea of nervous disease had been discussed since at least the 1830s, it became well defined as an important problem, even a "near epidemic," in the 1880s after the publication of George Beard's book *American Nervousness.*[19] Beard defined nervousness not as a mental illness or an excess of emotion, but simply as "nervelessness—a lack of nerve force." Extreme nervousness led to neurasthenia, or "nervous exhaustion."[20] Beard employed bank account and battery metaphors to explain the condition. Some people were blessed with large accounts or batteries (reserves of nerve energy), and others made due with little. In either case, drawing too much on those accounts or batteries led to bankruptcy or depletion. Nervousness manifested in a wide range of symptoms ranging from dyspepsia and fatigue to premature baldness.[21] Its appearance nearly everywhere in America, according to Beard, was not surprising.

Beard chiefly blamed modern civilization for American's susceptibility to nervous exhaustion in the late nineteenth century.[22] He argued that constant activity brought on by steam power, the telegraph, the periodical press, social institutions, and the "indulgence of appetites and passions" overstimulated men, especially "brain workers."[23] At the same time, men's physical activity decreased due both to economic changes that required less manual labor and to increasing culture and refinement. Confronted with constant overstimulation, these weakening bodies possessed smaller reserves of nerve energy. Beard saw the signs of this pernicious problem everywhere, even in the American man's reduced capacity to hold his liquor, as evidenced by his poor "bottle-power" in comparison to an English man.[24] Neurasthenia was, however, also something of a badge of distinction because only the most civilized peoples (a concept freighted with cultural and racial meaning) were susceptible to its force. Neurasthenia did not seem to afflict more "primitive" peoples, those whose passionate and powerful manhood, according to Beard, both strengthened bodies and disqualified them for civilization.[25] Beard's solution was not to throw out civilization, but rather to leverage its tools to develop new technologies and social customs productive of "strength and vigor."[26]

Embedded in the neurasthenia concept was a potential solution. If bodies could degenerate, then they could also regenerate. Methods designed to encourage regeneration varied widely and came from multiple sources. One of the more famous proposals came from G. Stanley Hall, an American educator and vocal expert on psychology and pedagogy. He argued beginning in the late 1880s that educators could utilize "recapitulation" to help American boys. Hall's recapitulation theory presumed an evolutionary ladder up which human races could progress. Anglo-Saxons had supposedly reached the top rungs, but the modern world denied them the chance to experience the highly physical and passionate earlier stages. Therefore, Anglo-Saxons grew up intelligent, but lacking in passion and power, making them susceptible to neurasthenia. Hall proposed encouraging "primitivism" and "savagery" in young boys by allowing misbehavior, reading bloody stories, and even fighting in controlled environments. This process supposedly molded boys into men while inoculating them against the degenerative forces of modern civilization.[27]

More visible signs of regeneration efforts appeared in America's late-nineteenth- and early-twentieth-century physical culture. This culture, in line with the period's bodily focused masculinity, promoted sport, health remedies, body building, and more. With the right diet and exercise, men could cultivate proportions like Eugen Sandow, the world's "perfect man."[28] Americans could harness science and hard work to engineer their bodies so as to appear strong and vital, and in the process cultivate those same qualities. The idea was not to turn back the clock to an idealized earlier time, but to leverage modernity's tools to fashion new ways of fitting civilized men to a new time.

Biological thought helped translate these broad cultural anxieties spurred by economic, social, geographic, and political change into a national crisis. Although Charles Darwin's book *The Origin of Species*, published in 1859, made no attempt to apply evolution to explain the behavior of people or groups, many Americans and Europeans did just that from the 1870s to the early twentieth century. Social sciences and politics informed by biological concepts framed global politics as a struggle for survival in a world ruled by the iron law of natural selection.[29] National survival in such a world depended simply on strength, the definition of which contained racial and gender components. Therefore, American power depended upon the strength of white American men—the exact population whose masculinity the modern world seemed to threaten most.[30] War thus held a paradoxical significance in late-nineteenth-century American thought. On one hand, war posed a threat to national survival if American manhood was indeed weakening. This was especially true given the likelihood of massive conscription in the imagined wars of the future because a broad swath of the male population needed to be fit to fight. On the other hand, war could also be a vehicle for toughening the latest generation of American men, who were denied both a frontier and their forefathers' crucible of combat. In either case, biological thought heightened the national significance of strong male bodies.

Doubts about the strength, character, toughness, and vigor of American men were of particular concern to many young US Army officers because they coincided with military concerns over combat's evolving character and changing battlefield geometry. These changes derived chiefly from new weapons technology such as smokeless powder, high explosive, rifling, small arms magazine loading systems, and quick-firing systems for artillery. Taken together, these advances increased the range and lethality of artillery pieces and made the ordinary infantryman a much deadlier combatant. Equipped with a small caliber, breech-loading, magazine-fed rifle, the infantryman of the late nineteenth century significantly outmatched his predecessor of just a few decades. The modern infantryman could carry more ammunition, achieve a higher rate of fire with greater accuracy, enhance his chances of survival by operating from the prone or within field fortifications, and remain essentially invisible when using smokeless powder and remaining stationary. The lethal zone in front of defensive positions grew along with the expanding effective ranges of weapons, which increased the time assaulting troops spent exposed to fire and the time over which morale deteriorated. In addition, smaller units on the defense using rapid-firing weaponry generated volumes of firepower superior to that generated by larger units in earlier eras. Because fewer soldiers were needed to generate effective fires and concentrated attacking formations invited heavy casualties, troop densities on typical battlefields plummeted, falling from one man per 257 square meters during the American Civil War to one per 2,457 in World War I.[31] Survival on this ever-more-lethal battlefield depended on dispersion.[32] But while spreading out and seeking cover may have preserved lives, it damaged morale by denying soldiers the support and mutual observation of their comrades. Dispersal also limited leaders' ability to control units and sustain the momentum of an attack. With friend and foe alike invisible, individual soldiers found themselves isolated, vulnerable, and rooted in place. Modern small arms and artillery ushered the earlier age's densely packed ranks of colorfully uniformed troops into a deadly obsolescence.[33] Likewise, combat's evolving character and the new battlefield geometry yielded increased physical, mental, and emotional trauma, placing ever greater demands on the human body.

Military leaders and theoreticians in the latter third of the nineteenth century were keenly aware of the challenges posed by these new weapons technologies and battlefield modifications. Indeed, the limitations on offensive maneuver at the tactical level became the "tactical problem of the day" in the aftermath of the Franco-Prussian War (1870–1871).[34] Even before this, US officers, like their European contemporaries, recognized the need for adaptation. As early as the 1853, US Army-commissioned boards studied the problems posed by new technology and recommended tactical solutions. The American Civil War's massive bloodletting reveals the inadequacy of those early solutions and their inability to resolve tensions between the need for dispersion on one hand and for command and control on the other.[35] Later in the century, some theoreticians in the US and throughout Europe argued that the defense's superiority was so great as to be insurmountable, at least in the near term. Jan Bloch is the best-known representative of this school. In his book *Is War Now Impossible?* and his earlier multivolume study, Bloch argued that the defensive superiority generated by new weapons technologies would yield a bloody stalemate on a vast battlefield. Victory in such a war hinged on exhausting the enemy's economic resources and reserves of will. In Bloch's formulation, the use of force had little utility in national policy.

The argument advanced by Bloch and other like-minded theoreticians never earned a place in the period's mainstream of military thought. Military leaders simply could not accept such a hopeless future. Successful offensive strategies depended upon an army's ability to succeed on the tactical offensive, at least sometimes. So instead of Bloch and company, Napoleonic and Prussian models guided the thoughts of most European and American theoreticians in the late nineteenth century. The Napoleonic and Prussian models demanded aggressive action to achieve conclusive results, with the former placing emphasis on élan and the latter on firepower and initiative.[36] The alternative, theoreticians argued, was passivity and a return to the indecisive wars of the seventeenth and eighteenth centuries.[37] The battlefield may have become deadlier, but to most military thinkers this was just another surmountable obstacle. No complete consensus emerged on the best solution to the new battlefield's tactical problems, but a dominant intellectual position formed between 1870 and 1914. Some historians have labeled this position the "cult of the offensive," though the term is misleading because it characterizes turn-of-the-century military leaders as irrational, self-defeating, and ignorant.[38] Military leaders and theorists were not ignorant or irrational. Rather, they were trying to solve massive problems with the material, intellectual, and cultural resources at hand, and some were unfortunately slow learners.

The solutions these theorists proposed derived generally from two propositions. First, weapons technology benefited the attacker as much as the defender. Colonel G. F. R. Henderson, an influential British military theorist at the turn of the century, advanced ideas typical of this position: "Neither smokeless powder nor the magazine rifle will necessitate any radical change. If the defence has gained, as has been asserted, by these innovations, the plunging fire of rifled howitzers will add a more than proportional strength to the attack."[39] Simply put, the advantages accruing to the offense and defense through technological innovation canceled each other out. The second proposition was that man remained both the constant in war and the dominant factor in combat. Henderson made this argument too. Magazine rifles and other innovations "introduced a new and formidable element into battle," he wrote, but "the moral element still remains the same. Weapons improve, but human nature remains the same."[40]

Moral forces run as *the* key thread in turn-of-the-century military literature.[41] Depending upon context, the concept held two closely related meanings. Moral forces referred to a wide range of intangibles, including morale, the feeling of confidence present in a force, skill, training, resilience, judgment, and the "inherent strength of [an army's] national character."[42] Moral forces were not a new idea in military literature. Clausewitz emphasized them in his writing, for instance, and many authors before him paid moral force close attention, too. Still, these forces assumed a marked prominence in the late nineteenth century following from the technology-imposed tactical stalemate that Bloch predicted and many feared. Victory in battle inclines to the side capable of generating greater combat power at the decisive point. Combat power derives from troop numbers, force capabilities such as firepower and mobility, and intangible moral factors. If theoreticians were correct in asserting that technological innovations offset one another, then moral forces could provide the crucial relative advantage that victory demanded.

The French colonel Charles Ardant du Picq's writings epitomized the turn-of-the-century military thought that awarded moral forces the key role in battlefield victory. Ardant du Picq, whose service as an infantry officer began in 1844, recognized the changes new weapons technology wrought on the battlefield. However, Ardant du Picq rejected technology as the crucial determinant in battle. Instead, he emphasized man. Based upon his study of ancient battle and his modern experience, Ardant du Picq argued that "in battle, two moral forces, even more than two material forces, are in conflict. The stronger conquers."[43] Ardant du Picq did not believe that those moral forces came from destructive power. Instead, moral forces derived from confidence, resolution, and "threatening power" in the form of fresh reserves or forces on the enemy's flank or in his rear.[44] Men needed to be made strong in order to project moral force against the enemy, and to resist the terror and fear inherent in combat. Ardant du Picq advanced several methods to improve an army's moral force, but discipline was his central theme. Ardant du Picq defined discipline as a "state of mind" and a "social institution" built over time that "made men fight in spite of themselves."[45] Nations and armies needed to find new means by which to instill discipline, and thereby attain superior moral force.

A Prussian artillery shell fired near Metz in August 1870 cut short Ardant du Picq's career as a military theorist. His book, *Battle Studies*, was published posthumously and achieved wide readership and influence in the French military with its second edition in 1903.[46] Ardant du Picq's writing resonated with the pre-1914 generation of military officers who were preoccupied with similar tactical problems. *Battle Studies* did not decisively impact military thought before 1903, but Ardant du Picq's work was representative of a broader, transnational trend in military thought at the dawn of the twentieth century. Just as in France, most military theorists in Britain, Germany, the United States, and elsewhere promoted moral forces as essential to victory on the modern battlefield.[47]

Military thinkers drew on more than abstract theory to support their conclusions about tactics and moral forces. Wars fought by European powers between 1870 and 1914 furnished practical experience open to interpretation. The Franco-Prussian War of 1870–1871 that claimed Ardant du Picq's life provided the first major data point. French and Prussian forces employed similar weapons technology and tactics, though the extended order's value remained open to question. Maj. Wilhelm von Sherff, a Prussian officer writing from experience in the Franco-Prussian War, highlighted the debate between "new" and "old" tactics. Sherff and like-minded military men argued that rifling required forces on the offensive to adopt an extended or "individual" order or else suffer catastrophic losses, but that new weapons also enabled loose formations to achieve a sufficiently high rate and volume of fire at a given point to triumph over a more tightly packed opponent. For Sherff and others like him, the offensive was still alive and preferable.[48] Armies needed new tactics to make the offensive work, and those tactics hinged on improving individual soldiers through training in order to offset the psychological penalties of the empty battlefield.[49]

Not everyone agreed with the conclusions Sherff and others drew from the Franco-Prussian War. Advocates of what Sherff termed "old" tactics defended the continued relevance of close order on the basis of moral forces. Only in close order and under the control of leaders, advocates argued, could men face the terror of battle and still advance. However, close order did not mean quite the same thing by the late nineteenth century as it did in the Napoleonic wars or in the American Civil War. Where the old basic unit had been the battalion or even regiment, the basic unit in later close-order systems was the platoon or company. These smaller formations allowed for greater flexibility in employment and would be spaced more widely on the battlefield. In such a system, close order did not mean marching toward the enemy shoulder-to-shoulder, but advancing in longer, thinner lines at a quick walk or run while making use of available cover.[50]

The British experience in the Anglo-Boer War (1899–1902) challenged the close-order orthodoxy, even in its updated form. On the veldt, hidden Boer defenders decimated British formations that advanced in tight formations and relied on cold steel. The British colonel G. F. R. Henderson, who observed part of the campaign and had earlier argued that new technologies benefited the offense and defense equally, responded to continental criticism of the British army by pointing out that "the flat trajectory of the small-bore rifle, together with the invisibility of the man who uses it, has wrought a complete revolution in the art of fighting battles."[51] Henderson insisted that infantry now had to attack in successive lines of skirmishers in an extended order. Henderson observed that troops in close order might achieve a local numerical superiority, but he argued that those formations would take enormous losses that would likely undermine the close-order formation's moral power.[52] As a result of the British experience in South Africa, contemporary military thought swung toward open-order formations as the solution to the old problem of crossing the deadly zone, a zone that continued expanding due to progressive improvements in weapons technology.

Infantry actions in the Russo-Japanese War (1904–1905) stalled and then reversed the Boer War–induced swing toward skirmishing. Western military theorists and leaders could dismiss the Anglo-Boer War as abnormal, or as a brawl between an army geared for colonial warfare and an irregular opponent. In contrast, the Russo-Japanese War pitted two modern militaries equipped with modern weaponry against each other. Even if the Japanese were considered racial inferiors, their German-provided training and largely Westernized military practices made them near-peer competitors in the eyes of most European military thinkers. The ensuing combat closely approximated the future of battle many theorists had earlier envisioned.[53] Military leaders seeking the offense's continued viability found much on Manchuria's and Korea's battlefields to support their theories. For instance, US officers admired the infantry's aggressiveness, the use of the bayonet, the growing impact of field artillery and machine guns on battle, and both armies' tactical adaptability under changing conditions.[54] In particular, the Japanese army furnished examples of successful infantry assaults on entrenched positions. Artillery fire did not eject Russian defenders from their trenches, but close infantry combat did. Commonly, infantrymen sapped their way forward toward enemy defenses over several nights under the cover of darkness. Once in position and receiving supporting fire, Japanese infantry charged forward in mass to overwhelm their opponents at close quarters. In some ways, this experience upset part of Ardant du Picq's theory. Ardant du Picq argued that little *actual* close combat occurred because one side or the other would break purely on the basis of moral force. However, the modern battlefield created an environment in which close combat occurred often because lethal fires kept troops fixed in their entrenchments and rendered them unable or unwilling to flee in the face of an assault.[55] Close combat in entrenchments thus added a new layer to existing theories about the criticality of moral forces. Now soldiers needed not only superior moral force to engage the enemy, but also superior physical force to defeat him in individual combat and eject him from defensive works.

Archibald Becke, a former British Army officer and an author of several histories, captured the most widespread and persuasive pre–World War I interpretation of Russo-Japanese War tactics in his book *An Introduction to the History of Tactics, 1740–1905*, published in 1909.[56] Like many military theorists of his time, Becke concluded that the attack was much preferable to the defense, and that offensive action was still possible on the modern battlefield. Becke argued that artillery and supporting infantry fires were necessary in an attack, but that Japanese success hinged on the Japanese soldier's superior *"fighting power,"* which derived from his high levels of "training, courage, intelligence, self-reliance, and patriotism."[57] Positions and weapons were not decisive in war, he argued, but rather the *men* who occupied those positions and used those weapons. This exhortation had echoed throughout military theory since at least 1870.

The Japanese army suffered heavy casualties even with superior fighting power. Becke and many of his contemporaries accepted these high casualty rates as the price of victory on the modern battlefield. For instance, Col. Frederic Maude, one of Becke's contemporaries, argued that successful assaults depended on soldiers being trained to "know how to die" and not "how to avoid dying."[58] Becke and others extended this need for bloody-mindedness beyond soldiers and their superiors to the whole people of a state. If people wanted victory, and a decisive one especially, then they had to be willing to pay the price.[59] Predictions about a major future war's character reinforced the need to steel not only soldiers but also the whole citizenry. Bloch and others forecast a protracted, attritional struggle. In such a war, conscription would fill the military ranks. Widespread conscription brought the human cost of war home to a society. Conscription also meant that most soldiers would have little time to prepare before finding themselves on a very lethal battlefield.

On the eve of World War I, a half-century of military thought grounded in experiences on the battlefields of Europe, Asia, and Africa suggested a few key lessons. Of these, the most significant was that the offense remained possible and desirable. Despite rifling, smokeless powder, small arms magazines, and other technological developments, even frontal assaults made by infantry against entrenchments could succeed if certain conditions were met. For instance, soldiers might follow the Japanese example and patiently sap their way toward enemy trenches while properly timed and coordinated offensive artillery fires suppressed defenders. However important these preparations were, though, the key determinant of success was man, and specifically the concentration of *moral* forces at a critical point. Superior moral forces derived from the discipline, resilience, and psychology of individuals and units. The new battlefield posed a serious challenge to this formula, though. How could militaries sustain or improve their moral forces, and those of a whole nation, in the face of higher casualty rates and more challenging battlefield conditions without traditional means such as close-order formations and tactics?

Historians have since proposed several ways by which modern militaries sought to improve their human material. For example, some argue that a mystical (and irrational) reverence for the offensive seized military leaders, civilian elites, and publics in the decades leading up to World War I. This reverence allegedly produced a "cult of the offensive" in which European military and civilian elites blindly promoted the offensive on the basis of myth. The cult simultaneously generated security dilemmas while predisposing elites to logics that preferred war in order to address those dilemmas.[60] In this formulation, the self-deception underwriting the cult of the offensive was a means by which militaries and states improved their human material psychologically by teaching soldiers and citizens to accept the offensive's horrors in hopes of securing victory. Other historians, such as Michael Howard and Antulio Echevarria, argue that military leaders followed a "compelling rationale" in emphasizing the offensive spirit.[61] After all, armies needed to attack at the tactical level in order to achieve positive objectives at the operational and strategic levels, and attacking meant crossing the deadly zone. Instead of an irrational cult, Howard found that militaries used doctrine rationally to predispose officers and men toward attacking and to instill the confidence necessary to succeed in spite of heavy losses. Thus, statements such as French Colonel Louis de Grandmaison's in 1911—that the offensive depended upon "cultivating with passion everything that bears the stamp of the offensive spirit. We must take it to excess: perhaps even that will not go far enough"—may have reflected intentional action based on a realistic assessment of probable battlefield conditions.[62] Echevarria points to a more concrete, though narrow, method of improving human material: weapons drills. He argues that fire discipline training, especially for machinegun crews, developed confidence and a union of man and machine that kept soldiers focused on definite tasks under stressful battlefield conditions.[63]

However, Howard, Echevarria, and others have overlooked another tool nearly every modern military force leveraged at the turn of the twentieth century—physical training. This tool was more concrete than doctrine and more widely applicable than weapons drills, but its particular character was not eternal, universal, or predetermined because military theorists and leaders sought solutions within their cultural environments. Those men seeking ways to improve an army's human materiel called upon period ideas about the nature of masculinity and about relationships between the body, mind, and spirit. As US Army leaders in the latter half of the nineteenth century scoured their cultural terrain in search of answers to the "tactical problem of the day," they encountered programs designed to sculpt bodies in specific ways that were growing in popularity. Many of these programs already bore a martial edge. Physical training promised to strengthen the individual soldier's body, discipline individuals and units, and bolster any organization's moral force. Physical training also held wide appeal outside the military, unlike weapons drills. This appeal was important because it implied ways to make whole populations stronger and more resilient, thus preparing them for the demands of a future war in which success probably depended on heavy conscription. Given these points, embedding US Army leaders in their wider cultural milieu must precede the story of how the US Army in particular came to value and practice physical training.

Much of that cultural milieu congregated around another problem akin to the "tactical problem of the day": widespread anxiety about modern man not being as strong, motivated, resilient, or self-sacrificial as his forebears. German military officer and author Wilhelm Balck addressed this issue directly in his treatise on tactics from 1908, in which he argued that units appeared to be growing more brittle. Where units in the Franco-Prussian War could sustain 25 to 33 percent casualties and function, similar-sized units in the Boer War seemed unable to sustain casualties above about 7 percent.[64] Balck explained that the "nerve-racking impressions of the battlefield" had grown over the recent decades owing to extended lines, the suddenness of entering combat, and the decreasing ability of officers to control dispersed formations. However, individual soldiers were also growing more susceptible to the battlefield's impressions. "Steadily improving standards of living," Balck observed, "tend to increase the instinct of self-preservation and to diminish the spirit of self-sacrifice." Also, the simple "physical powers of the human species" were "partly diminishing."[65] Balck's observation lays bare an interaction between the period's "tactical problem of the day" and one of its major cultural phenomena—a crisis of masculinity. The concern Balck elucidated was a trans-Atlantic phenomenon. In the decade preceding World War I, US officers similarly voiced concerns about men's "progressive deterioration," the "over or under indulgence in work or play," the destruction of man's "calmness and deliberation under fire," and the erosion of military virtues such as "courage, mutual confidence, and self-sacrifice."[66]

As did their European contemporaries, US Army officers seeking to improve the military's human material, and perhaps the nation's as well, accessed tools extant in society and culture. There, fears of degeneration had spurred the development of regenerative practices, many of which involved bodily improvement and contained obvious martial potential. Thus, early advocates of "scientific" physical training for the US Army were not thinking, speaking, and writing in a vacuum. Instead, they belonged to and were surrounded by a booming American physical culture consisting of popular and professional elements.

The people and organizations shaping popular physical culture were many and varied. Most were secular, but some key producers of physical culture were religiously motivated. For example, the "Muscular Christianity" movement encouraged bodily improvement as a means of developing character, manliness, and the vigor necessary to work in arduous mission fields at home and abroad. The movement's millennial message held that man was responsible for his own salvation and that he could approach perfection through training of body and soul.[67] For the secularly inclined, the period's plethora of health and fitness magazines made the contours of popular physical culture visible. Featuring increasingly risqué cover art and photos, these magazines promoted a wide variety of exercise programs, diets, daily practices, and more for both men and women that ranged from pure quackery to cutting-edge science. Magazines also provided an advertising vehicle for makers of tonics, "parlor gymnasium" equipment, and books on exercise.[68] Bernarr Macfadden's *Physical Culture* epitomized the genre, though several predecessors predated its rise in the 1890s.[69] Exercise crazes such as bicycling, Indian clubs, wall-climbing, and more regularly gripped the American public in this period. Gymnastic and calisthenic exercise systems also competed for the American public's favor. Most of these systems originated in Europe, two of the most popular being Swedish gymnastics and German Turner gymnastics. Dudley Sargent's American individual strength training machine system entered the competition near the turn of the century as well, though it assumed a distant third place.[70] A construction boom accompanied the boom of interest in physical health. Public gyms, many ornate and elaborate, appeared in American cities and towns alongside ethnically aligned Turnenhallen and *Sokol* facilities.[71] Ultimately, turn-of-the-twentieth-century Americans found themselves surrounded more and more by messages about and the trappings of physical fitness. Popular culture's vectors were various, ranging from the religious to the purely commercial, but they shared a promise of regeneration and a premise of man's perfectibility.

A sports and athletics craze, for both participating and spectating, accompanied the growing American fascination with physical training. Much of the sports craze originated in colleges and universities, and thus among America's middle and upper classes, but deepening obsessions with football, rowing, baseball, and more extended beyond student bodies to seize whole communities. By 1890, it had become fashionable to speak of colleges "as if they were schools for forming ball-players, oarsmen, and athletes," according to Edward Hartwell, a forefather of American physical education.[72] Organizational and business structures soon grew up around athletics that accelerated a transition from pure amateurism to professionalism in sports, though Americans generally clung to an amateur ideal in rhetoric at least.

The sporting craze had many sources, and sport itself served many purposes both outside and inside the US military. For instance, one scholar posited in 1917 that sport provided a safety valve for the American energy and pioneer spirit pent up after the frontier's closure.[73] Turn-of-the-century political and cultural elites certainly promoted sport as a vehicle for renewing society, preparing future leaders, and socializing American youth.[74] Other historians have argued that sports acted like a "social glue" that bonded a diverse nation and helped build a unified national American myth.[75] Whatever its origins and appeal, the athletic side of American physical culture permeated the US military and powerfully influenced the thinking of many US Army leaders.[76] However, sports came heavily laden with cultural assumptions that were occasionally at odds with the values and assumptions motivating advocates of "scientific" physical training in the US Army.

Advocacy of "scientific" physical training in the Army must be understood within the context of a concurrent push for professionalization in the physical education field. Physical educators, many of whom were physicians and physiologists, wanted to separate themselves in the last two decades of the nineteenth century from popular physical culture, antebellum health reform movements, and the competitive athletics craze. The paths toward expert status blazed by physical training advocates in the Army and physical educators in American society were closely related, and they often intersected. Within the Army, physical training began gaining traction after 1885, following the US Military Academy's appointment of Herman Koehler as its Master of the Sword.[77] Physical educators also took a major step toward professional status in 1885 with the founding of the American Association for the Advancement of Physical Education (AAAPE). Pioneers such as William Anderson, Edward Hitchcock, Tait McKenzie, James McCurdy, Dudley Sargent, and others instituted the organization to discuss the "underlying principles of the new profession." The AAAPE's founders believed that most teachers were "individualists" and "missionaries" interested in pressing their own special theories of health and fitness.[78] Such a chaotic discourse needed discipline, especially because no licensing measures existed. The AAAPE's protoprofessionals sought to establish this discipline, earn society's trust and confidence, and distance themselves from a long-associated history of health reform movements. To do so, they asserted an expertise rooted in scientific knowledge that promised benefits to the whole of American society.

The social benefit physical educators touted in the late nineteenth century had two components, which historian Roberta Park labels *hygienic* and *educative*.[79] Presenters at a landmark physical training conference held in Boston in 1899 described both succinctly. Speaking before the assembled body of the region's educators and the nation's physical education authorities, the US commissioner of education, William Harris, defined hygiene as the pursuit of making "the most of the body for human purposes." Harris argued that physical training, which he defined as the "conscious or voluntary training of the muscular side of our system," played a crucial role in hygiene by improving students' wills. Improvement of will occurred through voluntary processes, such as muscle-strengthening exercise, that also "call[ed] into action the higher nervous motor-centres of the body and brain."[80] Improvement and development warrants, referring vaguely to how bodies grew and character formed, undergirded educative arguments for physical training.

Harris's claims reflected the positions of the field's protoprofessionals, who combined antebellum ideas about the nature of the will with new developments in biological science and evolutionary theories.[81] The presentation following Harris's at the conference of 1899, given by the widely respected physical training pioneer Edward Hartwell, reveals both the composite basis of the educative functions and the expansive mission conceived of by early physical educators for their profession. Hartwell, a medical doctor with an interest in history who served as the director of physical training in Boston schools and as Johns Hopkins University's gymnasium director, was a leading authority on the effects of exercise on the human body and mind. Research trips throughout America and Europe, and the influential series of reports that followed beginning in 1885, also gave Hartwell cachet as an expert on pedagogical practices.[82]

Hartwell began his address in 1889 by asserting that physical training deserved stature at least equal to mental and moral training as "an integral and indispensable factor" in education. "Muscular exercise is at once a means and an end of mental, and moral, as well as of physical training," he asserted, because "without bodily actions we have no means of giving expression to mental power, artistic feeling, or spiritual insight. Without muscular tissue we cannot live or move."[83] Hartwell supported his argument with a detailed explanation of the appearance and function of muscle fibers. By 1889, research in biology seemed to have validated the older "blacksmith's arm" analogy, which found that exercise enlarged, hardened, and strengthened muscle fibers while making them more responsive to the nervous system. Conversely, disuse led to "wasting" or atrophy. In his remarks, Hartwell paid particular attention to the connection between muscle fibers and the "nerves and centres" that transmit stimuli, and then continued by way of analogy in asserting that the cells and centers of the nervous system and brain similarly strengthened or atrophied depending upon use. Hartwell reasoned that in order to strengthen the brain, physical trainers needed to identify the muscular activation sequences that triggered actions in particular brain regions.[84] The new scientific findings and theories Hartwell discussed seemed to provide a definitive and direct link between the body and the mind, which had long been regarded as the seat of will. Exercise strengthened muscles as well as the nerves and cells that made the mind work. Muscular training was therefore fundamental to human mental and moral development, and it was up to physical training professionals to unlock the most efficient and effective means of training all three domains at once.

The means available were many and diverse, ranging from sports and dance to free play, but Hartwell and most of his fellow protoprofessionals advocated gymnastics. Trainers struggling to define themselves as experts on the basis of scientific knowledge and unique skills found gymnastics appealing because they were, in Hartwell's words, more "comprehensive in their aims, more formal, elaborate, and systematic in their methods," and more productive of "solid and considerable gains" than any other alternative.[85] Gymnastics systems came in many different forms based on ethnic origins and the use of apparatus, among other factors. Indeed, debate raged in the latter half of the nineteenth century over which of the many possible systems was best, and what in fact constituted an "exercise." Yet these diverse systems shared a few characteristics in common. First, most attended to the needs of a broad population, male or female, and of the whole person. Gymnastics were not generally designed to create elite athletes or train the select few. Second, gymnastics systems were geared to produce symmetrical development of participants along the lines of fixed standards of physical perfection. Finally, all gymnastics systems were formal and subject to strict control by instructors. Experts were supposed to be able to prescribe exercises to correct specific bodily deficiencies, strengthen particular muscle groups, and, in some cases, even cultivate certain mental and moral characteristics. Americans especially embraced the idea of collecting precise bodily measurements and prescribing targeted exercises to generate desired outcomes.[86] This idea manifested in many American systems, including Dudley Sargent's and, in the US Army, Herman Koehler's. The supposed precision in gymnastics gave physical education protoprofessionals a strong claim to unique scientific knowledge and methods.

In contrast, sports and their popularity posed problems for physical educators in the late nineteenth century, both inside and outside of the Army. Many physical educators recognized the potential value of sports, especially their assumed provision of social training in skills such as teamwork. However, school athletic programs and the intercollegiate competition model seemed poised to overshadow physical education in the 1880s and 1890s. Athletic coaches, a body also staking out claims to professional status, competed directly with physical educators for institutional resources, prestige, and power. Intercollegiate competition imperiled faculty control of athletics, thereby putting the educative premise of physical education in jeopardy.[87] Sports also posed some philosophical challenges. For example, sports were inherently spontaneous, and thus a challenge to science-based claims to expert status made using gymnastics' native characteristics of control and precision. Also, competition's dynamics tended to focus attention on the development of the elite few over the ordinary many. Still, trends in physical education thought moved gradually toward an embrace of sport in the early twentieth century, partly in response to growing Progressive-era social and societal concerns, and partly out of recognition of sports' much greater popularity relative to gymnastics.

The Army's first efforts to introduce formal, systematic physical training must be understood within the intellectual and cultural environment to which physical education belonged. Many environmental influences can be understood as indirect. Army physical training advocates wrote and thought in the context of the period's popular physical culture and of physical educators' push for professional status. Other influences were direct. For instance, the US Military Academy's Herman Koehler, a product of a Turner normal school, contributed to constructing the physical education profession through articles, conference participation, and organizational service. Many military advocates and system designers also received formal training at institutions such as Sargent's Springfield College. Additionally, comparable trends in thought on physical training manifested in both the Army and the wider physical education world. Like physical educators, Army physical training advocates combined new scientific findings with older ideas about will, character, regeneration, and mind-body mutualism by way of reasoning through analogy. From the beginning, Army preferences for scientific prescription and highly formal exercise systems also faced challenges from popular pressure for sport. Much like their contemporaries in physical education, Army physical training advocates gradually accommodated athletics to a greater degree over time. Still, differences also existed. For instance, preferences for formal, highly controlled systems of exercise persisted much longer in the Army than outside it.

In summary, the US Army's physical culture rooted in systematic physical training emerged within a larger social, cultural, and intellectual context. Nineteenth-century anxieties over America's health, understood chiefly in terms of the nation's perceived masculine quotient, prompted fears of degeneration. By the turn of the century, Progressive-era social and societal concerns added new anxieties while amplifying and modifying the old. All of these anxieties seemed to jeopardize the nation's survival, or at least its vitality. Could America survive and thrive in a highly competitive world? Were its men capable of enduring the demands of modern war? But where problems existed, so did solutions. Among these was bodily improvement. In a world fixated on social degeneration and efficiency, gymnastics and sport promised regeneration, renewal, discipline, order, character, morality, and more. Faith in modernity suggested a way forward for Americans—not returning to an idealized past, but leveraging science and technology to develop men in new ways for a new world.

Army officers were particularly attuned to the dangers and opportunities in this wider context. Like physical educators and many national leaders, some of these officers turned to physical training and drew on popular physical culture and the professionalizing field of physical education. The direct benefits of physical training seemed obvious. Soldiers could march farther, carry more, and fight harder if in better physical condition. Physical training's less direct benefits were just as desirable, if not more so. Physical training's potential for moral and mental development, and for cultivating discipline, appeared to be a pathway toward improving the Army's human material, which seemed necessary for success on the future battlefield. The Army's central position in the overlapping fields of man-, soldier-, and citizen-making amplified the potential value of human improvement through exercise. The Army depended upon a fit and resilient male population to fight a war using conscription, and the Army could be an agent to help create a more fit and resilient population. Creation of appropriate exercise systems for the Army, which established the basis of the Army's durable physical culture, resulted from the labors of a small set of physical training advocates whose identities and ideas are the subject of the next chapter. However, it is crucial to remember that those advocates worked within and drew on a specific cultural and military context unique to the turn of the twentieth century.

CHAPTER TWO
ORIGINS OF A US ARMY PHYSICAL CULTURE, 1885–1916

Lt. Col. Charles Greenleaf, the Army's assistant surgeon-general, made a shocking claim before a convocation of physical education's early luminaries in the spring of 1891. Greenleaf first iterated the "popular belief" that soldiers exemplified the benefits of physical training. Surely the care taken in a soldier's selection, his need to "endure the hardship of campaigns in every variety of climate" and still triumph in combat, and his discipline, habits, and diet made a soldier the "model of physical perfection." Nonetheless, Greenleaf claimed, the soldier "cannot be regarded either as an athlete or even as a well trained man physically."[1] Greenleaf attributed this failure chiefly to an absence of "systematic gymnastic training."[2] Yet even as Greenleaf made these remarks, a movement was afoot within the US Army to rectify the problem. That movement's nucleus resided at the US Military Academy, but its voices bubbled up from across the force in professional journals and popular periodicals. The movement crested with the publication of the Army's first physical training manual twenty-three years after Greenleaf sounded his warning. In 1914, the US Army established an official physical culture for the first time, and it was based on systematic training.

A small clique of men was responsible for producing this physical culture. Analyzing their publications between 1885 and 1914 along with their relationships in light of their immediate professional contexts reveals four key features of the culture they fashioned. First, Army physical training advocates valued expert knowledge. They strove to ensure that actual training conformed to that expertise instead of happenstance and folk wisdom. Second, a soldier's psychologic development was valued at least as much as his physical development within this new physical culture. Third, their culture prioritized unit fitness over individual soldier optimization. Finally, their culture worked from an assumption that the human material to be sculpted would be of relatively high quality because the small US Army could enlist men selectively. In most ways, this culture reflected contemporary assumptions, beliefs, and practices in the professionalizing field of physical education. However, the Army's physical culture and American physical education had begun diverging by 1906 for institutional and cultural reasons. Ultimately, the physical culture represented by the Army's manual of 1914 responded to the beliefs of its producers about the value of fitness in modern war—and that notion of fitness extended well beyond bigger biceps and stronger lungs. But why did members of the US Army become interested in physical training in the first place?

Much of that interest had European roots. In the wake of the Franco-Prussian War, commentators advanced theories to explain the Prussian victory. One theory held that superior Prussian education accounted for the outcome. A representative example of this argument appeared in a letter written to the editors of the *Army and Navy Journal* in 1872. Its author, known to history as T. Gentz, argued that only one component of the superior Prussian education mattered—physical education, both in and out of the army. Integrating Prussia's victory into a longer history of conquests by hale northern nations, Gentz insisted that even in modern warfare "muscular power and a hardy constitution" remained relevant. Human bodies put machines into action, and gymnastics imparted "firm nerves and a manly spirit" to its practitioners. The stronger arm could "take the steadier aim and deal the more forcible blow," the "stout shoulder" bore more weight, the stronger legs leapt ditches and charged uphill better, and superior constitutions saw soldiers through the "brunt of the dusty battle."[3] Gentz went on to argue that the United States would also benefit from gymnastics, especially as a part of military training. With the frontier's closing, Gentz argued, "it is time that gymnastics should raise us a new generation of men."[4] Positive impressions about the desirability and utility of gymnastics persisted in parts of the US Army through the following decades. Writing twenty years later, systematic training advocate Capt. James Pilcher made an argument similar to Gentz's. "When the superior physical training of one of the parties to so great a contest as the Franco-Prussian War is known to have been the force that turned the tide of victory in its favor," Pilcher wrote, "the United States cannot afford to reject it."[5]

Even before 1871, US Army officers were aware that European militaries used gymnastic training to improve their soldiery. For instance, the Delafield Commission's Capt. George McClellan, who traveled Europe as a military observer between 1855 and 1856 before gaining his "Young Napoleon" sobriquet, had praised the French army's physical training manual from 1847 and its gymnastic school near Vincennes.[6] Maj. Richard Delafield, the commission's leader and subsequently the US Military Academy's superintendent, acted on these findings. In 1858, he directed Lt. J. C. Kelton to develop a "systematic course" of training for West Point's cadets based on systems in use at military schools in Paris and Vienna.[7] Praise for systematic gymnastic training came to Army officers through civilian sources as well. For instance, physical education pioneer Edward Hartwell commended Prussian practices in his influential report on the state of physical education from 1886. "In the interval between Jena and Sedan," Hartwell declared, Prussia had "demonstrated most clearly and strikingly the power and worth of comprehensive and scientific 'training.'"[8]

Some American officers viewed systematic training as a way to prepare soldiers for the new empty battlefield's demands that were created by the need for troop dispersal in the face of increased firepower. Assistant Surgeon-General Greenleaf insisted that soldiers themselves, lacking the "elbow touch" of linear warfare, had begun by 1891 to "feel the necessity for physical activity and endurance in attacking an enemy or in defending himself."[9] Pilcher, also a medical officer, similarly argued that the "soldier's physique" had more than ever "become indispensable."[10] Fortunately, Pilcher insisted, modern knowledge and science made it more possible than ever to precisely and efficiently condition bodies for combat. This way of thinking fit perfectly with the contemporary turn in American high and popular culture toward activity, dynamism, and masculinity. Similarly, these ideas harmonized with a movement in American higher education toward physical education and sport. If colleges and universities took interest in fitness, should the US Army do so too?[11]

However, not everyone in the Army agreed with the premise of systematic physical training or the means of implementation. Nor did most officers possess the expert knowledge needed to employ systematic training. Many senior Army officers had long acknowledged the connection between physical fitness and soldiering, but they rarely made methodical efforts to improve soldier fitness. Instead, they assumed that soldiers' bodies best adapted to the rigors of soldiering by soldiering. Lt. John Kulp captured this idea of incidental training when he complained that the older generation of officers believed "the shovel to be the best gymnastic apparatus for soldiers."[12] Some members of this older generation also considered systematic physical training to be a fad, possibly a dangerous one, and therefore not a necessity.[13] Thus, dedicating precious training time to exercise outside of traditional drill made little sense.

Others saw utility in physical training but did not know how to structure programs or lead exercises. Such shortcomings typically inclined officers toward either extreme emphasis on popular sports and field days or dull repetition of the drill manual's limited setting-up and rifle exercises. Maj. Gen. Leonard Wood, the Army's outgoing chief of staff in 1914, stressed the consequences of these conditions in his preface to the physical training manual of 1914. He wrote that despite the well-intentioned efforts of many commands, physical training's benefits would "remain a negligible quantity" without a "well-defined authorized method of procedure" that imposed "system and uniformity."[14]

Desire for system and uniformity in training informed by expert knowledge also existed at the Army's lowest levels. For instance, Lt. Frank Besson warned just prior to the publication of the manual of 1914 that Army officers were aware of physical training, but that they needed more specific guidance. Besson counted five manuals in publication dedicated to military exercise, yet none resided in the headquarters library of the Hawaiian Department where he served, and he knew of no officers who owned copies. Besson had seen copies of then-Maj. Edmund Butts's *Manual of Physical Drill* occasionally in company libraries. However, he believed that officers were only familiar with the fifteen pages that described rifle drill and contained accompanying sheet music. Even these exercises were rarely employed, Besson observed.[15] According to Besson, units usually resorted to using the seven setting-up exercises in the drill regulations, but these tended to "do more harm than good" owing to a lack of knowledge and enthusiasm. Too often, Besson remarked, physical training amounted to little more than a squad of men, "blouses unbuttoned and hats jammed down on their heads, going through these, the same monotonous exercises day after day, each man with a funereal cadence all his own."[16]

Wood and Besson both proposed similar solutions. First, the Army should compile the best of what had been written on military physical training since the 1880s into a single, comprehensive manual. Next, the Army should require all commanders to make that manual's system a universal part of every soldier's regular education. Publication of the Army's physical training manual of 1914 was an attempt to do just this. Its pages, steeped in a rich broth of ideas and practices concocted by physical training advocates, crystallized and institutionalized a physical culture more than thirty years in the making. Taken together, the manual's methods, guidelines, definition of fitness, and underlying assumptions compose a physical culture. This culture was the product of a long history and a particular moment. A small group of men, mostly associated with the infantry branch and the US Military Academy, produced that culture over three decades. Examining their backgrounds, relationships, ideas, and contributions to actual physical training practices in the Army yields insights into the nature of the culture that materialized in 1914.

None of these cultural producers exercised a greater or more enduring influence than Herman Koehler, who served as the US Military Academy's Master of the Sword from 1885 to 1923. His impact on the Army's systematic-training-based physical culture in its nascent years was both deep and wide. For instance, Koehler's manuals and his articles in professional military and physical education journals largely determined official training practices and decisively shaped the thinking of most Army officers on the subject of exercise. Although he was not the first to claim that the Army needed systematic, standardized training, Koehler's prominence in martial physical training discourse waxed over the years the Army edged closer to sanctioning an official physical culture. The Army's seminal *Manual of Physical Training* of 1914, in which the Army formalized a physical culture, was essentially an amalgamation of his two earlier books from 1892 and 1904. Perhaps this was not surprising, given that Koehler was a member of the three-officer board that authored the document.[17] Beyond his publications, Koehler's influence also derived from his Academy position and the men he instructed. West Point was particularly significant to the early history of the Army's physical culture because for decades it was the Army's sole center of expertise in physical training. Also, its graduates greatly influenced the Army's policies and day-to-day life in its various units from the bottom to the top of the institution. As Master of the Sword, a position responsible prior to 1885 only for teaching swordsmanship and other physical skills, Koehler became the school's father of physical education and, in many ways, the Army's as well.[18] Koehler was the Army's only dedicated expert in and practitioner of physical training, and he personally instructed more than thirty-five classes of West Point graduates, who went on to fill leadership roles ranging from platoon leader to chief of staff of the Army. Through his publications, institutional influence, and personal instruction, Koehler came to dominate the accreting body of philosophy and practices that was coalescing into a well-defined physical culture at the turn of the century.

Prior to Koehler's arrival in 1885, West Point's administration had taken tentative steps toward incorporating systematic physical training into its curriculum. These steps helped position West Point as the Army's center of expertise on the subject, but they left ample room for improvement. Kelton's European-inspired program of 1860 had cadets of all four classes performing calisthenics and gymnastics, though the Academy discontinued it in 1861 with the Civil War's onset. After 1861, cadets did not follow a systematic program of training, but they were required to spend time in the gym pursuing whatever caught their interest. Gymnastics languished at West Point until 1877 when the superintendent, Gen. John Schofield, recommended its resumption.[19] The recommendation idled until a Board of Visitors report in 1881 criticized gymnasium conditions at the Academy. "There was no exhibition of exercises in the gymnasium," the board noted, and "the whole furnishing is unsatisfactory." The board's members declared that the "value of this class of exercise for whose profession requires good physical development cannot be doubted." They then proposed the construction of a new gym and creation of a department that would make gymnastics training a "positive requirement" for every cadet.[20]

The report jolted the Academy's administration into action. The superintendent directed Lt. Edward Farrow, an instructor in the Department of Tactics, to draw up a training program. Farrow's system, which included gymnastics and swimming, became a part of cadet development in 1882.[21] Farrow directed training until he departed for a new assignment in 1884 and was replaced by Lt. Henry Kirby. Koehler later criticized Farrow's program because there "was but little system" in the course and because it "lacked many of the fundamentals of a rational training system." However, as Koehler also observed, Farrow and Kirby deserved credit for "breaking up the pernicious practice of permitting Cadets to use the gymnasium as they saw fit," and for raising the Academy's appreciation of physical training as a necessary component of cadet development.[22]

In 1884, the death of Master of the Sword Antone Lorentz created an opportunity to put West Point on equal footing with other institutions of higher education, many of which were rapidly incorporating physical education into their curricula. Lorentz had done little to advance systematic training in his twenty-seven-year tenure and must have left much to be desired, seeing as how he was replaced in practice if not in title by Farrow in 1881.[23] The search for a professional educator to replace Lorentz led to George Brosius, the Milwaukee Normal School's director and coach of the Milwaukee Turnverein's award-winning 1880 team.[24] Brosius declined the offer, citing his work in Milwaukee, but recommended his nephew, protégé, normal school graduate, and "best man of the Frankfurt class"—Herman Koehler.[25] Academy officials offered Koehler the position. He accepted and began instructing in 1885.

Koehler, only twenty-five years old, was an impressive candidate by dint of his physical prowess alone (he boasted flexed biceps nineteen-and-a-half inches around), not to mention his education and credentials.[26] A talented gymnast, Koehler placed second overall at the 1880 international Turner Festival in Frankfurt. While observing another meet a year later, Koehler learned that the man who beat him in 1880 was competing. Despite not having trained, Koehler entered the competition and won first place in a field of more than three hundred contestants.[27] Koehler also bore an educational pedigree that qualified him as a professional physical educator, unlike any of his predecessors at West Point. Moreover, he possessed practical experience, having worked since 1882 as a school gymnastics director in Oshkosh, Wisconsin.

Koehler immediately set about constructing a system of physical training for West Point's cadets. He expressed the philosophy behind this program and his broader concept of fitness in an article written for the Academy's centennial in 1902. Koehler's aim was to counteract the pressure placed on cadets by their program of study, which he deemed a "mental strain" that was "fraught with danger to the physical welfare of the cadet." Koehler planned to do this by building up the weak so that they might "have an even chance with the naturally strong," sculpting sound bodies that might yield sound minds, and nurturing energy and strength reserves upon which cadets could call in times of stress. The first objective of Koehler's system was general health, though he sought simultaneous cultivation of "strength, agility, precision, self-reliance, courage and endurance."[28] Because physical training had a fundamentally educative purpose at West Point, Koehler intended his system to raise the general standard among the Corps of Cadets. Endeavoring to "turn out record-breaking strong men, or skilled acrobats" was "wrong in every particular" in Koehler's opinion because focus on elites did the majority harm through neglect. To this end, he laid down a principle that recurred through his later work as well: "The greatest good to the greatest number, and only at the expense of those who can afford it."[29]

Physical training's share of the Academy's curriculum grew throughout Koehler's tenure. Beginning in 1885, fourth-class cadets received three weeks of daily drill upon arrival at the Academy, and then three drills of forty-five minutes a piece and three periods of fencing instruction per week from October through June. The upper three classes were not required to attend drill, but they were encouraged to do so in the winter months.[30] The benefits accruing to cadets were obvious. For instance, the 1889 Board of Visitors gushed in their report that it was "exceedingly difficult to believe that the gymnastic exercises performed by the fourth class could be the result of only one year of practice under instruction by Professor Koehler. The feats of agility were simply wonderful; they are valuable chiefly as evidence of sound, muscular, trained bodies."[31] Most of the exercise system under which cadets toiled appeared in Koehler's *Manual of Calisthenic Exercises*, published in 1892, which later formed the basis for the Army's manual of 1914.[32] Koehler pushed continuously to make physical training mandatory for all classes so that gains made in the first year would not be lost in the latter three. He finally realized this objective in 1905 and simultaneously had boxing and wrestling added to the curriculum.[33] In recognition of his contributions and the value of his work, West Point's superintendents and Board of Visitors requested repeatedly beginning in 1889 that Koehler be granted a commission. Congress agreed in 1899, commissioning Koehler as a first lieutenant. In 1901, Congress also made Koehler's post permanent by law. Furthermore, the law required that the Master of the Sword to henceforth act as "instructor of military gymnastics and physical culture," and that Koehler's successors be officers of the line specially selected for the post. Koehler received subsequent promotions to captain, major, and lieutenant colonel in 1905, 1917, and 1920, respectively.[34]

Koehler's system reflected its creator's background in Friedrich Jahn's Turnen, which was a German system of gymnastics that Jahn created in the early nineteenth century after witnessing the Prussian army's disastrous defeat at Jena in 1806. Jahn subsequently participated in Prussian educational reforms as a leading physical trainer.[35] Major aims of those reforms included instilling national pride and preparing Prussian men for a future war to throw off French dominance. Thus, whole body improvement for a broad population, not the creation of elite athletes, was at Turnen's core. Turnen also harnessed exercise as a means of promoting well-trained citizens that were faithful to the nation and prepared for war.[36] Two waves of German emigres fleeing government crackdowns in Prussia and elsewhere brought Turnen to the United States, first in the mid-1820s and later following the revolutions of 1848. In the United States, Turnen clubs became centers of ethnic German communities, but they also strove to Americanize their message. Turners earned national recognition for their service in the Union Army during the Civil War, helping propel their system of gymnastics to prominence.[37] Later, Turners attempted to integrate their system into American schools, placing them in the midst of a late-nineteenth-century nationwide debate about the best means of training American youth. This "Battle of the Systems" pitted Turnen against many other competitors, including Ling's Swedish Gymnastics and a homegrown system of machine exercises developed by Dudley Sargent. Turnen ultimately lost this battle in the first decade of the twentieth century, owing in part to its ethnic associations but primarily to its strong emphasis on apparatus work, which was impractical for many schools.[38]

Although the Turners eventually lost in the Battle of the Systems, Turnen was alive and well at the US Military Academy after 1885 and the US Army baked it into its official physical culture in 1914. Understanding the core elements of Turnen is therefore helpful for understanding the core elements of the Army's physical culture. A typical Turnen syllabus for male students included six classes of exercises: marching; calisthenics; "heavy work" with dumbbells, rings, and other implements; apparatus work; gymnastic games; and some popular physical activities such as track-and-field competitions, swimming, fencing, boxing, and more.[39] This typical syllabus emphasized general body development and prescribed progressively more difficult, complex, and active exercises. Formality also characterized a Turnen session. One instructor normally led large groups through structured and rhythmical sequences, often using commands.[40] Turnen clearly inspired Koehler's emphasis on general health and his principle of doing the greatest good to the greatest number. The material in the manual of 1914 could have also been pulled directly out of a Turnen syllabus, as it matched the six typical categories of exercise.[41] Turnen's high degree of formality, emphasis on discipline and broad populations, and overt military focus must have appealed to Academy officials and Army officers congenial to physical training alike.

In a time when most of the Regular Army's officers earned their commissions from West Point, Koehler's long tenure as Master of the Sword gave him a unique ability to promulgate his Turnen-derived system throughout the Army. Between 1885 and 1900, Koehler instructed every West Point cadet personally.[42] As the Academy's physical program expanded, especially after 1905, Koehler acquired several assistants, but he retained control over the program's structure and continued delivering instruction personally. By 1919, only two hundred West Point graduates on active duty had not received personal instruction from Koehler, and all of those entered the Academy prior to Koehler's arrival in 1885.[43] If officers were leading physical training or writing about it after 1889, then their only likely frame of reference was Koehler's example and system. Dissemination through discipleship was an intentional strategy. In the absence of a secondary education program for physical instructors, Koehler believed that West Point graduates needed to enter the Army prepared to lead training as local experts.[44] The Army refused to establish an official physical culture from the top down before 1914, so Koehler tried to spread one from the bottom up.

Koehler's disciples, joined by like-minded advocates of systematic training, propagated a consistent physical culture through praxis and print. A gymnasium construction boom on Army posts in the 1890s provided proponents of systematic training opportunities for practice. Initially funded by profits from post canteen sales, gymnasia enabled all-weather, year-round physical training.[45] With few exceptions, gymnasia built specifically for systematic training first appeared at the Army's three recruiting depots: Columbus Barracks, Davids Island, and Jefferson Barracks.[46] These buildings came equipped with all the tools necessary for strengthening the bodies and minds of American soldiers at the turn of the century. Tools ranged from "light work" implements such as dumbbells, barbells, rowing machines, and Indian clubs (wooden bowling pin–shaped instruments of varying weight) to technical gymnastic apparatus such as parallel and horizontal bars. A lieutenant or captain at each post was detailed to direct training in these gyms, usually with the assistance of a few noncommissioned officers.[47]

Koehler believed that such "splendidly equipped gymnasiums" removed the "chief obstacle" to systematic physical training. However, there remained the question of how to put these resources to best use.[48] Junior officers detailed as instructors enjoyed no training apart from what they received as cadets at West Point or as college students elsewhere. Several publications offered some guidance. Koehler's manual from 1892 was popular, for instance, as was British author Archibald Maclaren's book *Physical Education*. Koehler attempted to fill this gap in 1904 with his *Manual of Gymnastic Exercises*, but ultimately the Army did not mandate any specific practices or a consistent system before 1914. Young officers in control of gymnasium instruction thus enjoyed wide latitude in determining the nature of training at their posts. This was a major responsibility. Koehler charged these young officers with remembering the importance of their duty to lead critical training, on which the "success or failure is dependent entirely upon themselves."[49] Many rose to the challenge. Gymnasia created spaces for officers to encounter, experiment with, and lead physical training. Several innovators, most with experience as gym directors, published their systems in print. By 1913, at least four of these were available as full manuals: Constantine Chase's *Physical Drill for Foot Troops* (1897), Edmund Butts's *Manual of Physical Drill* (1897), Enoch Garey's *Manual of Physical Drill* (1911), and Merch Stewart's *The Physical Development of the Infantry Soldier* (1913). Each system differed in some specifics, but the culture each manifested and promulgated was remarkably consistent with Koehler's, including key elements such as the pursuit of the greatest good for the greatest number using progressive, systematic, formal training.

The most influential of these gymnasium instructor-innovators was Edmund "Billy" Butts. An 1890 West Point graduate who had enjoyed Koehler's tutelage, Butts was given charge of gymnastics training at the Columbus Barracks recruiting depot in 1893. He found that physical training occurred at the depot, but that there was no "systematic drill." Instead, soldiers were "'turned loose' in the gymnasium" under the lax supervision of noncommissioned officers. Under these conditions, Butts felt that the "results could not but be more harmful than beneficial."[50] Butts quickly set about constructing a regular training program. He also improved the gymnasium while filling it with new equipment purchased using funds from the Post Exchange and elsewhere. Soon, each of the depot's four companies was sweating through thirty-five-minute drills five days a week under Butts's direction. These drills included a variety of activities ranging from calisthenics to dumbbell exercises. In designing his drills, Butts sought to "avoid that constant repetition" that made work "mechanical and tiresome," while also aiming to engage every soldier's whole body to promote symmetrical development.[51]

Butts's performance earned him recognition among peers and superiors alike. After he spent fifteen months at the Columbus Barracks, the Headquarters Department of the East, encouraged by its adjutant general, Col. Samuel Breck, detailed Butts in 1894 to travel to various posts and establish training programs. Butts spent a few months each at posts throughout the East, Southeast, and Middle West departments doing so.[52] This experience challenged Butts to craft a standardized system that could be applied in a wide range of conditions. By 1895, Butts had also become something of an expert for his peers. Earlier that year, the Department of the East required each post to place an officer in charge of physical training. Several of these newly appointed officers wrote to Butts seeking advice and guidance.[53]

Butts applied his knowledge and experience to respond to these requests in two ways. First, he published an article in 1895 in the *Journal of the Military Service Institution of the United States* offering his peers some generic advice. Butts directed physical training instructors to secure and improve gym facilities initially, and then prepare themselves as athletes and disciplinarian drill instructors, develop a cadre of assistants, and read a good reference manual such as Koehler's *Manual of Calisthenic Exercises*.[54] Butts also began work on a practical manual that would enable "any officer to give regular and beneficial instruction to his command."[55]

Just three years after being detailed to tour posts and establish training programs, Butts published the first edition of his *Manual of Physical Drill*. The manual was a practical guide designed by Butts to "systematize physical training in the army."[56] The system's foundation was a "simple and progressive" five-exercise-set arrangement without rest between exercises. Butts applied this structure to a wide variety of exercises, though the core drills consisted of calisthenic, rifle, dumbbell, and gymnastic apparatus work. Wall-scaling, rope-climbing, and other activities with obvious practical military value were also included as "essential to the athletic training." While "athletic games and contests" occupied about 20 percent of the manual's pages, they were relegated to the back of the book, confined to track-and-field events, and given only as "matters of general interest and information."[57] As in Koehler's scheme, officers led the drills in Butts's system using commands. Butts recommended that officers drilled their units in thirty-minute sessions at least four times per week. Ideally, whole companies would go through the drill together, though Butts allowed for battalions or even regiments to exercise together if the lead instructor had several officer assistants.[58] Butts furnished two ten-day example programs, one for units without much gymnastic apparatus available and one for units with fully equipped gymnasia.[59] However, as in Koehler's manuals and the later manual of 1914, Butts left the specific content of each "thirty minutes' drill" up to instructors.

From its organization and purpose to its recommendations on dress and hygiene, Butts's manual reflected Koehler's unmistakable influence. Not only did Koehler instruct Butts during the latter's cadet years, Butts also sought Koehler's advice when detailed to Columbus Barracks in 1893 and praised Koehler as "one of the best authorities on physical culture in this country and certainly one of the most successful instructors."[60] Butts's system differed from Koehler's in only a few regards. For instance, Butts placed more emphasis on rifle drill than did Koehler, and he was more open to athletic contests held during field days. However, Butts's definition and valuation of fitness, along with the means he thought best to achieve it, generally matched Koehler's. The differences were more a matter of nuance than substance. Prior to 1914, Butts's *Manual of Physical Drill* achieved a level of influence in the Army equal to or greater than any of Koehler's manuals, but the physical culture it advanced was chiefly Koehler's creation.

Koehler, Butts, and others developed and spread a coherent physical culture that yielded similar systems of exercise, but these cultural producers struggled to get the Army to put that culture into practice. Wholly systematized training throughout the Army proved difficult to realize. Gyms may have appeared on posts and recruiting depots may have instituted physical training in the 1890s, but articles in professional journals at the time indicate that commanders often resisted incorporating systematic and formal physical training, or simply knew too little about it to do much besides permit competitive sports. For instance, Lt. Robert Smart, an assistant surgeon, complained about this situation in 1901 when he bemoaned the lack of a "compulsory system of physical exercise" in the Army. Speaking about the drill required at recruiting depots by that time, Smart remarked that what physical drill did exist was "wrong because [it was] unsystematic."[61] Exercise was encouraged, but it was left up to local commanders and was neither structured nor ordered. Smart recommended that authorities superior to post commanders make daily exercise compulsory, and then turn that training over to men "instructed specially in this branch of military science" at proposed training centers run by military medical officers.[62]

Three years later, Koehler issued similar complaints in the *Infantry Journal*'s inaugural issue, writing that the "proper physical training of the enlisted man" had been "written about, discussed and talked over for a long time, but as yet, except in a few instances, little of lasting value has been accomplished."[63] Koehler rejected reliance on competitive athletics, and advocated instead using the "splendidly equipped gymnasiums" at most posts to execute systematic, supervised physical training.[64] In 1905, Fort Snelling's superintendent of athletics, Maj. Robert L. Bullard, observed that there was excitement over sport in the Army, but few commanders arranged training to rationally build better bodies. "The present state of athletics or physical training in the army," Bullard alleged, was "unsystematic, irregular, and uncertain in the extreme."[65] By 1907, little had changed. Koehler again wrote to the *Infantry Journal* complaining that commanders did not treat physical training with the "degree of seriousness commensurate with its importance."[66] According to Koehler, company commanders did not integrate physical training into daily schedules and did not compel most of their men to participate in what little training commanders did schedule. Furthermore, senior commanders "considered their duty ended with the issuance of orders pertaining to the subject."[67]

The challenge confronting the Army was not one of resources, but one of will and organization. By the end of the first decade of the twentieth century, the Army had well-equipped gymnasiums on most posts and was building more. Several manuals were in print that laid out exercise systems specifically for Army use. The Army also had a body of officers able to put those systems into practice, whether they were medical officers or West Point graduates with rudimentary training as instructors. Yet the Army lacked a central authority to control and direct training. Koehler and others pointed to contemporary European practices as a possible model. One example was British Army's Gymnastic Staff at Aldershot, which was established in 1860 as a central school with a permanent staff to train instructors for every regiment in the British Army.[68] Establishing such a center for the US Army was problematic, so much so that Lieutenant Colonel Greenleaf argued in 1891 that the creation of a permanent organization required an act of Congress. Without a legal basis, he predicted, a permanent organization's future would be forever in jeopardy, subject to the whims of each new senior Army authority.[69]

Assuming that such a law could be passed, Greenleaf suggested the US Military Academy (USMA) as a prospective location for such a center. This argument made sense in 1891 purely from an organizational and bureaucratic perspective. An Academy chair would require few new resources to stand up, and the organization would be well positioned to transmit training practices into the Army through each year's graduating class. Pointing to the US Naval Academy as an example, Greenleaf argued that the leader of such an organization should be a medical officer well versed in anatomy, and capable of precisely, efficiently, and safely honing the human body.[70] Yet West Point did not have a department of physiology and hygiene like Annapolis. Instead, it had a Master of the Sword. Despite this, the argument for West Point as the seat of a permanent physical training center made more sense every year. As Koehler's reputation and influence grew, and as his tenure lengthened into seeming permanency, there seemed no better choice. Additionally, Koehler enjoyed the patronage of West Point's superintendents, who advocated for Koehler in the Army's highest echelons. Koehler's manual from 1892 was the product of such lobbying, as was the USMA-dominated board that produced the manual of 1914.[71] Still, congressional action or, more realistically, firm commitment and orders from a senior Army leader was necessary to make systematic training a fixture across the Army.

Movement toward such a top-down directive began in the mid-1890s thanks to a trio of senior leader sponsors: Gens. Nelson Miles and Franklin Bell, and President Theodore Roosevelt. The directives these three leaders issued did not resolve all existing problems, but they moved the organization toward a standardized training model. Miles took the initial steps, first as the commander of the Department of the East between 1894 and 1895, and later as commanding general of the United States Army from 1895 to 1903. In the former position, Miles had a hand in assigning Butts to his educative tour of army posts, requiring athletics officers at each post, directing units within his department to conduct regular physical training, and publishing several pamphlets and circulars on training.[72] As commanding general, Miles continued promoting the benefits of physical training as something of a celebrity fitness role model and enthusiast. Perhaps his most notable stunt in this role was his surprise eight-hour, ninety-mile horseback ride in July 1903, just a month before his mandatory retirement at age sixty-four. Miles supposedly rode the first thirty-five miles in record time in temperatures as high as one hundred degrees. He arrived in Fort Reno "fresh as the 34-year-old officer who had been his companion," having definitively proven his fitness by doubling President Theodore Roosevelt's recent forty-five-mile Laramie-to-Cheyenne ride, which had been considered "quite a physical feat."[73]

More meaningful orders came down from one of Miles's successors as Army chief of staff, Maj. Gen. Franklin Bell. An 1878 West Point graduate, Bell is notable for being perhaps the most educated of senior officers in the early twentieth century on physical education. Although he graduated from West Point before Koehler arrived, Bell experimented with the use of gymnastics apparatus to train his troops as a cavalry lieutenant in the 1880s. He later spent a summer studying physical culture and training under Harvard's Dr. Dudley Sargent, one of the fathers of American physical education.[74] Bell's experiences in the Indian Wars and Spanish-American War motivated his continued interest in physical training.[75]

Convinced of the need for improving the American soldier's physical fitness, Bell, as the incoming chief of staff, was the driving force behind General Order 44's issuance in March 1906.[76] This order required cavalry, infantry, and field artillery units in the Regular Army to conduct physical training in garrison and in the field. Gymnastics, athletics, bayonet, and "kindred exercises" were required in garrison, while practice marches were required in the field. Furthermore, all company-level units had to conduct one practice march per week at a minimum of at least twelve miles, plus a monthly march of three consecutive days when in an active field training period.[77]

Bell also partnered with President Roosevelt, himself a famed proponent of the strenuous life, in performing fitness "stunts" to promote the value of exercise. For instance, the two competed in the fifteen-mile "Muldoon Challenge" in February 1908, which Bell won.[78] In November of that year, Roosevelt and Bell appeared together at the War College. Both men delivered messages about the "desirability of officers keeping in fit condition at all times," and then Roosevelt invited the General Staff officers and War College students present to join him on a "stroll" that afternoon. Unable to refuse, the fifty-eight officers present followed the president on a "bully tramp" through thick woods, up and down rocky cliffs, and across a chin-deep stream.[79] A month later, Roosevelt issued Executive Order 989, which required an annual physical exam for Marine officers that consisted of a fifty-mile march.[80] One year earlier, Roosevelt had also directed Army officers to take physical fitness tests. This was partly in response to a report from the Philippine Department's inspector general that found only two of nine colonels fully fit for duty. The War Department's answer was to require all field-grade officers annually to ride thirty miles a day for three consecutive days, though coastal artillery officers and some staff officers were permitted to walk fifty miles over three days instead. The riding requirement remained on the books until 1917.[81]

Miles, Bell, and Roosevelt made physical training more visible in the Army, and they also made it mandatory in limited ways. But what they did not do was specify *how* commanders should conduct physical training. Thus, Koehler and others continued complaining even after General Order 44's issuance that commanders did not take physical training seriously, and that the Army needed to systematize its practices. Pressure mounted, as did interest among senior leaders. Bell's successor as chief of staff, Maj. Gen. Leonard Wood, took the next step by directing the publication in 1914 of the Army's *Manual of Physical Training*. Seeking authors for this manual, the Army turned to its internal expert at the US Military Academy, just as Lieutenant Colonel Greenleaf had recommended in 1891.

The resulting manual, officially authored by a small board but chiefly Koehler's product, equipped officers responsible for training in philosophical and practical ways. Philosophically, the manual described fitness and ascribed it value. Practically, the manual posed advice on hygiene issues, gave guidance on structuring training programs, and dictated exercise methods. Several manuals may have come before, but none equaled the manual of 1914 in breadth, depth, specificity, distribution, and official endorsement. Appropriately for an expression of and foundation for a physical culture, the manual of 1914 began with a definition of fitness. The authors conceptualized the elements of this definition as a pyramid capped by the supreme component of discipline. The pyramid's foundational layers were fourfold: general health and bodily vigor; muscular strength and endurance; self-reliance; and "smartness, activity, and precision." The latter qualities were described as "physical expressions of mental activity."[82] The first two elements, both hygienic and physical, formed a base for the second set of elements, which were psychological. Once the soldier obtained "robust health" and an awareness of his increased strength and endurance, then he needed to be "taught how to value the former and how to use the latter to best advantage."[83] This knowledge translated into self-reliance and self-consciousness. The manual's authors intended for soldiers to exercise not just their muscles but their minds as well. Instructors exercised minds chiefly by insisting on "precision and exactitude." Doing so supposedly cultivated "essential soldierly qualities" such as self-respect, neatness, and grace, which "combined spell discipline."[84] Fit soldiers were mentally and physically healthy, strong, and resilient. Fit soldiers were confident in their abilities, in complete control of their bodies and minds, and willing to submit themselves to a unit's needs.

The manual provided instructors with more practical advice regarding hygiene and programming, which was typical of training guidance found in period professional physical education and the popular press.[85] For example, the manual counseled that exercise should occur in open air, preferably "pure, dry air," whenever possible.[86] Other advice equipped instructors to teach their charges proper breathing techniques and to recognize the onset of exhaustion. In the interest of completeness, the manual's authors recommended the best time of day to exercise (never after a meal), the best clothing to wear while exercising (flannel), and the healthiest way to recover after drill (sponging the body with tepid water) too.[87] In terms of programming, the manual's authors offered general direction but stopped short of dictating a schedule beyond providing a sample five-day program. Instead, they gave those responsible for training leeway to build programs that took into account their soldiers' aptitude and condition, and the facilities and time available. This was an enormous responsibility. Officers needed to take their work seriously and "not for an instant lose sight of the fact that to them has been intrusted [*sic*] a part of the soldier's training which is of great importance."[88] The manual did include some guidance to help structure programs. For instance, instructors should work extensor and flexor muscles in paired exercises, seek harmonious and symmetrical total-body development, and ensure that every day's work "dovetail into the next and be progressive."[89] The "setting-up exercises," a series of calisthenic drills, formed the core of every session. Instructors could add various types of apparatus and skill work to this core. Grouping and sequencing exercises fell to the instructor's discretion. This latitude might seem odd for a document that purported to standardize physical training practices across the Army. However, the manual's authors wanted to account for the variety of conditions in which units might train.[90] Too prescriptive a program might allow officers to make excuses for not doing physical training at all if local conditions did not match those assumed in prescription. Flexibility in programming therefore enabled standardization of physical training itself across the force.

In contrast with the hygienic and programming sections, which were essentially compilations of suggestions, the manual dictated how to perform exercises and drills. Of the manual's 335 pages, 319 contained exercise instructions, guidance on issuing commands, and photos and drawings illustrating movements and positions. The instructions were comprehensive. For instance, the broad jump alone required four pages and three images to explain.[91] Specificity enabled focus on precision and exactitude—supposedly vital to building discipline—and allowed amateurs to employ expert-developed movements properly. According to the manual's authors, every exercise had a "function peculiarly its own" that had a "certain effect upon a certain part of the body."[92] While officers could arrange those exercises according to general guidelines, they lacked the expert knowledge to design movements capable of producing such precise results. Maj. Gen. Leonard Wood, writing in the manual's preface, therefore discouraged any "departures" from the manual that were "at variance with its methods generally."[93]

The resulting institutionalized physical culture embodied in the manual of 1914 expressed a body of ideas that had accreted over nearly three decades, and that were chiefly birthed and shepherded by Herman Koehler. Four salient elements characterized that culture. First, the culture valued psychological qualities at least as much as physical qualities in defining fitness. Second, the culture prioritized a unit's average capabilities over optimizing any individual's physical capacity. Third, the culture built on an assumption that experts possessing specialized knowledge and training were essential to fitness. Finally, the culture's producers assumed that the Army's recruits were of generally high quality, though in need of refinement. These characteristics mostly reflected the culture's heritage from the second generation of American physical education. This second generation had emerged after the American Civil War, but transition to a third generation that embraced sport and play to a greater degree was underway by 1906. As a result, a divide emerged between physical training practices prevalent in the Army and those in higher education and wider American society.

Additional cultural analysis turns on investigating the qualities valued in the culture and each quality's relative value. To begin with, the Army's first institutionalized physical culture valued a soldier's psychological qualities at least as much as his physical qualities, and it assumed that physical training could address both. As reflected in the manual of 1914, Koehler and others presented the benefits of physical training as a pyramid. Physical qualities formed the pyramid's foundation. None of these qualities was surprising or new: strength, endurance, improved posture and appearance, agility, gracefulness, general health, resilience to disease and injury, and muscular efficiency. However, advocates of systematic training claimed to be able to produce bigger gains faster by leveraging the latest advances in the professionalizing fields of physical education and training for the sole purpose of improving bodies. The application of new methods also addressed the pyramid's second level: confidence, courage, self-reliance, and willpower. Koehler labeled these "psychologic" qualities. For him, intentional development of specific psychologic qualities was the "essential difference" between military and civilian physical training, and a key goal for military training.[94] The Army's manual of 1914 summarized these qualities using one of Koehler's well-worn sayings: they induced "men to dare because of the consciousness to do."[95]

At the top of the pyramid perched the culture's ultimate psychologic quality: discipline. The definition of discipline in this physical culture reflected an understanding of what the future battlefield might demand of the soldier, and of how physical training could prepare soldiers for that battlefield. Contemporary theorists of warfare worried over the corrosive effects on command and control created by the need to disperse due to the deadliness of modern weapons. If not in close order, how could units sustain the momentum of an attack? How could soldiers overcome the psychological trauma of combat? Systematic physical training advocates responded with a type of discipline that combined individualist and corporate aspects. Reading Butts's and Koehler's definitions together sheds light on how this combination worked. Butts stressed individuality. "With all the discipline that is instilled [in military training]," Butts cautioned in 1904, "we do not want the American soldier to lose his individuality—that individuality which makes him the greatest soldier in the world."[96] In contrast, Koehler stressed subordination, as evident in his description of a disciplined soldier as an "interdependent and dependable effective unit, with a direct and definite responsibility to the state."[97]

With its veneer of drill, systematic physical training seemed to foster Koehler's subordination more than Butts's individuality. The ideal training sessions imagined and depicted in these works always had men in ranks responding in unison to commands issued by forceful, disciplinarian paragons of physical fitness. Yet Koehler's and Butt's positions were closer than they at first appear. Koehler did not seek blind or unthinking obedience, but the "intelligent, voluntary subordination of the individual in an equal degree with every other individual."[98] Subordination was an individual decision, compatible with American ideals of individuality. Physical training taught men to control their bodies and to respond to commands. Self-control helped men willingly submit themselves to authority and the unit's needs while retaining their individuality, and thus the confidence to act on their own initiative if necessary. Physical training conditioned bodies and minds alike, the combination of which was supposed to enable a bottom-up discipline productive of aggressive team-based action on the battlefield.

The logic behind promises of improving psychologic qualities also underwrote promises about making soldiers more moral. Period beliefs closely linked strong bodies and strong minds. Much as training muscles to submit to the will was thought to develop discipline, exercise was thought to strengthen both muscular and moral fibers. Noted psychologist G. Stanley Hall expressed the muscles-morals connection clearly in a paper he delivered in 1894: "You cannot have a firm will without firm muscles; and there is nothing so dangerous for morals as to have the gap between knowing what is right and proper and health and the doing of it, yawn; and it always yawns if the muscles get weak."[99] Koehler made similar comments in a draft of the manual of 1914, writing that "it is the physical that determines the destiny of the intellectual."[100] Thus, physical trainers also saw themselves as cultivators of vigorous, moral, and active masculinity.

Moral development helped commend the idea of systematic exercise to otherwise skeptical senior officers. Not only did exercise improve discipline and behavior, but it provided a healthy alternative to vice.[101] Many of the authors urging the Army's adoption of systematic physical training made this argument, though sometimes in overly simplistic ways. For example, Lt. A. B. Donworth, one of the young officers assigned as a gym superintendent, related his own college experiences in an article from 1897. Donworth wrote that maintenance fees for damaged school property had been on the rise at his college, but the opening of a "fine gymnasium" on campus curtailed vandalism. The reason, according to Donworth, was that the students were so tired by evening from exercise that the "property remained unmolested."[102] Most advocates, like their counterparts in civilian education, made more sophisticated arguments that linked muscle fiber and moral fiber. One of their most commonly invoked analogies was the "blacksmith's arm." This analogy drew on the observation that the more a blacksmith used his arm muscles, the stronger they became. Physical education advocates reasoned that exercising man's will by the disciplined and mutual action of mind and matter could similarly strengthen that will.[103] Connections between exercise and moral behavior would only grow more influential as a justification for physical training in the years to come.

A second key feature of the new culture's definition of fitness was an emphasis on organizations over individuals. In an article published in 1904, Koehler asserted that other armies had adopted physical training in the interest of improving whole-army efficiency. Koehler argued that the US Army, like others, was "most invariably dependent upon the average man," so the "standard of physical excellence which may be attained is dependent directly upon the efforts made to develop the average man and the man who is below average."[104] The point of physical training was to raise the average level of fitness across an organization, not to maximize individual physical performance. As Capt. L. S. Upton observed a year later in reflecting on his Spanish-American War experiences, systematic training could ensure "that each man will be developed and made an efficient physical unit in the army machine." The whole idea of physical training, Upton argued, was to "give all soldiers a proper physical development and sufficient stamina to make them equal to a required military task with the least number of ineffectives."[105] To make his point, Upton compared two theoretical battalions, one containing the Army's best sprinters, and the other focused on training its average men. If both ran a mile, the battalion focused on its specialist sprinters would lose a larger percentage as fall-outs than the other, making it militarily inferior. Even Butts's bragging about his trainees' muscle growth revealed his stress on organizations—his statistics only highlighted average gains across units.[106]

Valuation of an organization's average level of fitness above the individual's capacity also manifested in an injury- and exhaustion-avoidance mindset. "Underdoing is rectifiable; overdoing is often not," cautioned the authors of the Army's manual of 1914, echoing one of Koehler's maxims.[107] Systematic training advocates viewed injury and exhaustion as a double threat. First, because improved unit efficiency was the ultimate goal of training, injuries were counterproductive. Injuries kept men from training and degraded a unit's combat effectiveness. Second, injuries and exhaustion could make soldiers dread physical training. Monotony posed a similar threat. Training advocates regarded enthusiasm and focus as key to developing psychologic qualities. If soldiers dreaded training, then they would not participate enthusiastically or focus their efforts.[108] Moreover, dread and dissatisfaction worked against the creation of a team mentality conducive to discipline.

A third key feature of the Army's first official physical culture concerned physical trainers' qualifications. Systematic physical training was premised on claims of scientific, expert knowledge. Only by precisely applying specified methods could trainers help soldiers achieve promised psychologic, physical, and organizational benefits. Such precision was beyond the reach of people unversed in the nuances of a human body's composition, arrangement, and operations. Some training advocates, almost exclusively medical officers, argued before 1914 that only physicians possessed such knowledge. Pilcher, one of the medical officers who first promoted systematized training, made this case in his seminal article of 1892 by noting that many of the day's "best teachers of physical training" held medical degrees, and that regulations in the British Army and elsewhere required medical officer supervision of gymnastics. Pilcher argued that medical officers were uniquely equipped to obviate the "danger of injury from the abuse of exercise" and to diagnose "defective parts" of soldiers' bodies.[109] However, while many of the period's famed physical educators held medical degrees, not all did. Similarly, not all medical officers had mastered the latest methods of physical training. Finally, given the imbalance between the number of men to be trained and the number of medical officers available, a requirement for all training to be led by medical officers was impractical. Other experts needed to be found or made.

The most efficient and effective system most advocates proposed resembled European establishments, especially the British Army's program at Aldershot. This program, created and directed by experts assigned to the British Gymnastic Staff, certified trainers who then returned to their regiments and served as physical training specialists. As noted earlier, ideas for a similar program in the US Army invariably identified West Point as the obvious proponent and Koehler as its director. Though not a physician, Koehler could claim the necessary expert knowledge thanks to the professionalization of physical education. Yet hopes for a similar "postgraduate" course in the US Army had died out by late 1904.[110] Instead, Koehler and his compatriots settled for relying on West Point graduates as local specialists. Educated by Koehler and his staff as cadets, Academy graduates were theoretically equipped to apply a centrally constructed system of training.[111] This stopgap solution to the expertise problem worked so long as cadets and commanders alike took physical training seriously, and so long as commanders only assigned those men most interested in the work as training officers. However, this solution also had drawbacks. For example, it produced a limited pool of potential trainers that was not easily expansible. Also, potential instructors equipped with the latest knowledge were invariably the youngest officers in a unit, and thus they lacked influence over unit training.

Finally, producers of the Army's first official physical culture assumed that the Army's recruits were of a generally high quality, even if they harbored doubts about wider American society. The period's cultural producers tended not to explicitly reinforce the popular perception of the enlisted ranks being peopled by society's dregs. However, the culture's nearly complete focus on improving the rank-and-file's physical fitness and the absence of disciplinary training for officers imply some paternalist assumptions about the qualitative differences between the two populations. As an example, Butts, ever the American fighting man's promoter, observed in 1895 that the Army's human material was "of the highest order." New recruits entered with sufficient foundations of strength and endurance, each "well developed in his uncouth way." Butts therefore charged physical trainers with making the most of this raw material, sculpting each soldier into a "magnificent specimen of physical manhood."[112] A decade later, Capt. Guy Palmer delivered a similar assessment of the American soldier. New recruits possessed solid foundations, though they lacked "grace, agility, and a knowledge of how to use their strength" and displayed unevenly developed bodies. "Latent qualities exist in these men," Palmer observed, but they needed a "course of systematic and wise instruction to bring them out."[113] Systematic training advocates generally converged on the idea that to be ready for modern war, the American fighting man, but not his officers, needed honing and to be made more efficient.

For all their confidence about the quality of the average recruit, systematic training advocates regularly hinted at their doubts about the quality of men in wider American society. Sometimes these doubts reflected anxieties springing from the period's dominant Darwinian racial theories. Maj. Henry Kilbourne, an army surgeon, sounded such an alarm in a paper for a panel on military physical training during the 1897 Association of Military Surgeons conference. Alongside presenters proposing systems of training and debating the place of athletics in the Army, Kilbourne warned that the average quality of the American population was decreasing due to racial mixing. The "swarthy, low-browed and stunted people now swarming to our shores" were problematic, he cautioned, because physical training could only enhance what was already naturally available. Perhaps Butts's superior American recruit would become a thing of the past.[114] Other anxieties sprang from the neurasthenia crisis seemingly gripping American and Western European societies. Koehler himself gave voice to these concerns in a draft of the Army's manual of 1914, writing that the "primitive and simple methods of life" that had cultivated a "physical and moral hardihood" in American men were under threat from modern conveniences on one hand, and urbanization on the other. Koehler estimated that as a result, less than 50 percent of men aged eighteen to forty-five were physically healthy enough to serve.[115]

Those men most responsible for constructing a physical culture around systematic training assumed they would sculpt generally high-quality raw material, even as they echoed the era's concerns about the suitability of most men for modern war. Rarely did these cultural producers give any written consideration to mass mobilization's implications for their physical training systems. The closest most came was a vague hope that men introduced to physical training in the service would take their fitness knowledge, skills, and enthusiasm out into American society, thereby "preconditioning" the next generation of soldiers for service. One of the clearest expressions of this hope is found in then-Capt. Merch Stewart's *Physical Development of the Infantry Soldier* (1913). A prolific author, veteran of the Spanish-American War, and future West Point superintendent, Stewart argued that all able-bodied male citizens between the ages of eighteen and forty-five were liable for military service, so all were obligated to improve their fitness.[116] Yet exhortation could not replace planning for an influx of lower-quality recruits, especially given that the Army included few expert trainers and had only a limited, fixed pipeline for producing new trainers. Thus, differing perceptions of human material in and out of uniform suggest that this physical culture was geared chiefly toward a small standing army's needs.

Apart from training manuals, nothing more clearly illuminated the outlines and elements of the Army's first official physical culture than did debate over sport's place in the military at the turn of the twentieth century. This debate's influence on the Army's physical culture and physical training practices also persisted through subsequent decades, as later chapters demonstrate. Enthusiasm for sport and systematic physical training grew up together in the decades following the American Civil War. The sporting movement in the US Army chiefly resulted from grassroots interest and organization. Soldiers' interest in athletics coincided with a sporting craze in late-nineteenth-century America. Soldiers' interest also coincided with military reform movements, especially after the Spanish-American War, and with social reform movements that painted sport as an alternative to vice.[117] More specifically, the military's sporting germ arguably originated at the academies before spreading throughout the larger force, a key inflection point being the inaugural Army-Navy football game in 1890. In the 1890s, officer attitudes toward sport shifted from toleration to a willingness to experiment and athletics became part of the duty day for some soldiers. By the 1900s, sport enjoyed "unqualified acceptance" as one of the "essential elements of soldier training," according to historian Steven Pope.[118]

Linked by one historian as synergistic trends, sport and systematic physical training also represented two different, though related, physical cultures.[119] Systematic physical training sought to organize and rationalize training practices from the top down, and it emphasized average unit performance. Sports arose from a bottom-up popular movement and typically celebrated the elite individual athlete's performance. Systematic physical training activists such as Koehler and Butts saw both opportunity and peril in sports. On one hand, field days and athletic competitions built esprit de corps, celebrated physical activity, and encouraged interest in training among many soldiers. On the other, competition inclined leaders to focus on their star athletes and pushed soldiers to specialize instead of seeking harmonious, balanced development. A few critics went further, arguing that sports were "mere play" as opposed to the "serious nature" of a soldier's calling, so the "kindergarten methods" of sport could not advance training.[120] Ultimately, negotiation of the sports issue by producers of the Army's physical culture clarifies many outlines and contours of their own physical culture.

Paired articles under the title "Athletics in the Army" in a 1905 edition of the *Journal of the Military Service Institution of the United States* captured the potential and problems nearly all systematic training advocates perceived in sports. In one article, Capt. H. Hawkins expressed deep concern about the proliferation of field days and their pernicious effects on soldiers' bodies and command climates alike. Field days, common features of Army life by 1905, set aside a day or more from regular training so that entire units could participate in and observe athletic competitions. Hawkins described this application of athletics as submission to a sporting craze or fad, and he argued that commanders were wrong to think of these days as physical training. Only men who could already run well or play a sport participated, while the rest of the unit's men "merely clap their hands at the performances of their representatives."[121] The elite competitors benefited little from participation in terms of exercise, though they risked injury, and the rest did not benefit at all. In the other article, Maj. Robert Bullard claimed that enthusiasm for sport reflected a deeper concern about physical training and development present in American society at the time. On the whole, Bullard found athletics to be a potentially positive tool for shaping fit bodies appropriate for soldiering. However, Bullard took issue with the Army's unsystematic use of athletics, which was neither entirely recreational nor entirely for training. Athletics, he argued, must be "subordinated—better—completely swallowed up in the idea of training" and turned from "sport, play and trifling, to training and the serious business of preparation for war."[122] Both Hawkins and Bullard recognized the need for physical training and the potential role athletics could play in it. Yet both also expressed concern about how enthusiasm for sports could derail more serious and constructive means to build better bodies.

Bullard's and Hawkins's efforts to find appropriate ways to apply sport were typical of systematic training advocates at the turn of the century. For instance, Koehler and Butts also wrestled with the role of athletics in physical training. Their thoughts on the subject are worth exploring, given the influence both men wielded in the production of the Army's physical culture. Over more than a decade of writing, Butts consistently argued in favor of athletic competitions. While inaugurating physical training at Columbus Barracks in 1893, Butts also inaugurated regular post field days. As late as 1905, Butts still hoped for a time when these post field days might culminate in department or all-Army championships equal in import to the annual Army Rifle Competition.[123] Butts valued all kinds of field day competitions. However, he advised that the bulk of the events be military in nature, such as wall-scaling or tent-pitching, and involve as many members of a unit as possible.[124] Every officer, and especially young graduates of West Point, had a duty to encourage all kinds of athletic activities, according to Butts.

Still, "national sports" such as baseball and football also found favor with Butts. The benefits he perceived in "national sports" were many: building esprit de corps, inspiring emulation of fit athletes, and providing alternatives to vice, among others. Butts also saw sport as a way to simultaneously build discipline and individuality. Comparing ball players and skirmishers, Butts contended that both must be "subservient to and united with" the team's efforts, and yet able to take "quick and prompt individual action" on which success often depends. "An able player on the ball field will not forget his tactics on a field of battle," Butts wrote, "and an able captain of a ball team will make an abler captain in the deadlier game of war."[125] Given his cadet reputation as a remarkable athlete, his enthusiasm is not surprising. Yet for all of the eloquence Butts invested in celebrating sport, it never figured as more than a complement to the core of his system—methodical, disciplinary gymnastic training. For instance, consider the composition of his manual. Track-and-field training information earned a chapter, and intercollegiate and amateur track-and-field records earned a page, but both were appended to the end of the manual and added simply "as matters of general interest and information."[126]

Tension also existed in Koehler's opinion of sport. Intercollegiate athletics blossomed at West Point during his tenure as the Academy's Master of the Sword, led by an interest in football, as was the case in so many other institutions of higher education at the time. In fact, Koehler served as head coach of the Army football team from 1897 to 1900 and remained involved with the team in later years.[127] Koehler also oversaw the institution of mandatory intramural athletics for all cadets in 1920, a practice that continues to the present day. Yet Koehler also argued against athletics in the wider army. For instance, in an article published in 1904 Koehler urged the Army to adopt a system of training that would raise the physical standard of all its members, but remarked that "it is needless to add that competitive athletics do not and can not do this."[128] Though a fan of the sort of field days Butts advocated, which Koehler labeled "organization competition," Koehler also argued against the proliferation of field days on units' training calendars.[129] Similarly, Koehler worked to advance sport at West Point, but ignored the topic in his manuals of 1892 and 1904, and only briefly covered track-and-field events in the Army's manual of 1914.

How does one explain the disapproval of sport in the Army voiced by one of the most influential figures in the history of West Point athletics? Features of the systematic physical training culture Koehler fathered are key to solving this puzzle. Physical training in the Army was supposed to improve a unit's average fitness and symmetrically develop all soldiers, while simultaneously promoting discipline and other psychologic qualities. Koehler believed that competitive athletics, in contrast, targeted small populations of men for specialized development who were usually already fit. Competition also inclined participants to focus on victory over training, which posed increased risks of injury. Competition's seductiveness also threatened to take time and attention away from the serious business of physical training.

West Point was uniquely capable of avoiding these hazards of sport according to a manifesto Koehler wrote in 1909 on the "theory and practice of athletics" at the Academy for its nascent Athletic Council. In this paper, Koehler argued that West Point's physical training goal had always been to develop the "very highest possible standard of general excellence of the mass of its students."[130] Competitive athletics could support that objective, he asserted, because West Point already had a mandatory systematic training program for all cadets and the Academy's supervisory organizations were dedicated to keeping sport aligned with the developmental mission. In short, *all* cadets developed a foundation of fitness in systematic training, and then those that desired additional challenges could try out for competitive sports teams. This aligned with his consistent position that competitive athletics, while potentially valuable, should "never be more than an *incident* in the system of training of soldiers."[131]

Conditions in the Army did not match conditions at West Point, so Koehler doubted that competitive athletics could remain incidental. If all commanders were not dedicated first and foremost to systematic training, and the Army's highest authorities did not make such training mandatory, then competitive athletics would spin out of control. Koehler's experiences at the Academy likely reinforced his beliefs. After all, his manifesto of 1909 responded directly to competitive athletics having spun out of control at the Academy a few years prior. While the Academy's superintendent, Col. Hugh Scott, had been away on an extended absence in 1908, members of the Army Athletic Association had threatened to cancel the annual Army-Navy football game over a player eligibility dispute with the Naval Academy. For Scott, this was the last straw. The Army Athletic Association, founded in 1892 as a private booster organization that funded competitive athletics and scheduled competitions, had grown too independent and lacked a stake in the Academy's core educational and developmental mission.[132] Scott responded by establishing his own Athletic Council comprising the commandant, the Master of the Sword, and various officers from the superintendent's staff.[133] This council directed the activities of the newly rechartered Army Athletic Association, bringing competitive athletics under the tight supervisory control Koehler extolled as one of two key reasons why competitive sport could be part of a cadet's daily life, but not necessarily a soldier's.

Producers of the Army's first official physical culture reflected American physical education's second generation in their views on sport, emphasis on psychological qualities and group fitness, and logical linkages between mental, physical, and moral qualities. Capitalizing on the American public's fascination with health, strength, and fitness in the decades following the Civil War, this generation claimed expert knowledge based on physiology, evolutionary theories, and traditional practices associated with ethnic groups. Scientific training and knowledge set this generation apart from its forebears, though much of the earlier millenarianism of antebellum health reformers endured. The leading thinkers of physical education's second generation included physicians as well as self-styled physical educators or trainers, much like the population of principals behind the Army's physical culture. Historian Roberta Park has shown that second-generation physical education claimed two functions: a hygienic function and an educative function. Physical education goals were broad and comprehensive, including physical, mental, and moral development. These ideas match language Koehler and his peers consistently used. Second-generation physical educators also stressed the need to direct exercise toward specific goals, and to confine exercise within tight limits set by experts who prioritized physical, mental, and moral development over victory in competition.[134] Like Koehler, Butts, and other Army training advocates, second-generation physical educators endorsed sport, but only as a complement to gymnastics and other types of disciplinary training.[135] Similarly, physical educators also struggled against the constant threat of sport's popularity overwhelming their serious goals in physical training.

Identifying these common roots is important in light of the eventual divergence between the Army's physical culture and American physical education. Where the Army's institutionalized physical culture remained stable, American physical education moved into a third generation around 1906 that embraced sport to a much greater degree. Many factors propelled this move, such as the increasing influence of social science and psychology over physiology, the pressure of popular culture, the growth of professional and college sports, and the rise of the play movement and child development theory.[136] The Army's official physical culture proved more resistant to change. Resistance stemmed partly from the decisive influence Koehler and his disciples exercised on policy, and partly from the overlap between military values and practices and the gymnastics and psychologic outcomes touted by second-generation physical education. More and more, fitness in American physical education and wider American society meant "normal" social development and a healthy body. In the Army, antebellum and even earlier values endured. Fitness in the Army meant health, strength, resilience, confidence, and discipline. Psychologic qualities were just as important as physical qualities in this model. Fitness also continued to include logic that transcended the individual: fitness was an obligation owed to the unit and nation; improving the unit's weakest link remained the top priority; and a fit body was in part one placed in willing submission to the group's needs.

Ultimately, the physical training manual of 1914 makes clear that the Army had come a long way in addressing Greenleaf's warning in 1891 that the American soldier was something less than a model of physical perfection. Though Koehler and his compatriots still complained about the implementation of systematic physical training and the dangers of the field day, the Army as an institution had decisively embraced their mode of physical training. Such training seemed well suited to the perceived demands of the modern battlefield. There, mass mattered more than quality by 1914, but a higher-quality mass trumped a lower-quality mass. While the scale of war grew, loss of the "elbow touch" in combat demanded more of the individual soldier. Discipline seemed critical, given the corrosive effects of battle's enhanced physical and psychological challenges. Yet discipline taken too far and made too strict could also squelch the individual initiative that also seemed necessary when every soldier had essentially become a skirmisher.

Producers of the Army's physical culture promised to give American soldiers a competitive edge in this environment. By using expert knowledge of the body and mind to construct systems of training, these cultural producers planned to sculpt stronger bodies and minds than had been possible using older, incidental modes of physical training. Though not intended to make individual supermen, the new physical training augured an improved average level of fitness for whole units. Men accustomed to subordinating their bodies to their will, and their will to the unit's needs, could enter modern battle confident of success, if not survival. Disciplined and enhanced bodies, minds, and morals—such were the assurances of this physical culture. But given the limited capacity to produce certified trainers, the growing divergence from thought and practice in American physical education, and the assumption of building from relatively high-quality human material, how truly ready was this culture for the demands of mass mobilization and modern war?

CHAPTER THREE
THE US ARMY'S BATTLE OF THE SYSTEMS, 1914–1920

World War I is commonly remembered as a machine war or an industrial war, but it was a war of flesh and blood as well. Many strands of technological change converged during the Great War that rendered battlefield conditions vastly different from those of a century prior. Machine guns, rifles, huge artillery concentrations lobbing high explosives, and more drove soldiers underground and created strangely empty battlefields. In the generation before 1914, most of Europe's leading military thinkers had posited an aggressive offensive mindset as the best way of overcoming the advantages new weapons technologies gave to the defense. According to this body of thought, the strategic offensive was necessary to win a war, and this depended upon offensive success at the tactical level. If opposing forces possessed similar technology, then triumph would go to the side whose men were stronger, faster, more resilient, and more motivated.[1] Consequently, firepower could enable offensive action, but the margin of victory lay with man. European militaries had looked to physical training systems for decades as a way to gain that critical, qualitative edge in manpower.

Most European militaries expanded their physical training systems during World War I and the US Army followed suit. Physical training was a major element of every US soldier's preparation for war. Koehler's physical culture guided it, at least initially. For instance, both Koehler and his system were fixtures at preparedness camps in the summers of 1915 and 1916; also, his *Special Regulations No. 23: Field Physical Training of the Soldier* became a staple training aid for many junior officers in 1917. Experience in combat only reinforced the value leaders inside and outside the military affixed to physical training. When noted physical educator Luther Gulick returned from a visit to the American Expeditionary Forces in Europe in 1918, he brought a message for his fellow physical educators: physical fitness in war had become more important than ever. Gulick dismissed certain prewar theories that suggested modern war would be one of machines and that the improved ability to kill from a distance devalued physical strength, speed, and endurance. Nothing, he argued, could be further from the truth. The willingness to do or die counted, but "plain physical capacity" was equally vital. Victory went to the man who could endure longer, march farther, and fight harder. Gulick declared that even in the land of the machine gun and artillery shell, man's physical fitness remained the "foundation of all success in war."[2] Even as leaders continued to emphasize physical fitness, the ways of building up that foundation changed drastically between 1917 and 1918. In that narrow window, an insurgent corps of civilians entered the scene and challenged the physical culture the Army had so recently sanctioned as official after thirty years of development.

Ultimately, mobilized civilians displaced Koehler and his compatriots as the Army's primary producers of physical culture between 1917 and 1920. The relative decline of Koehler's institutional power began in 1917 when the newly created Commission on Training Camp Activities (CTCA) took charge of recreational athletics and physical training in the Army. Unfettered by the Army's conventions and existing physical culture, and bearing fresh ideas from the world of physical education about what physical training could be, the CTCA's civilian cadre crafted a new physical culture. This new culture was more inclusive of varied activities, more focused on combat-oriented functional fitness, and more concerned with efficiently sculpting the individual soldier into an effective fighting machine. Such efficiency seemed critical within the context of a perceived manpower crisis engendered by surprisingly high rates of draft rejections for physical and mental inadequacy. As the war drew to a close and in its immediate aftermath, the CTCA's leaders attempted to cement their physical culture as the Army's own. Yet supplanting Koehler's physical culture proved more difficult than expected.

As conscription began swelling the US Army's ranks in the late summer of 1917, the Army struggled to deliver sufficient physical training to its new recruits. At the beginning of 1917, the Army counted approximately three hundred thousand men in uniform in either the Regular Army or the National Guard. By November 1918, that population exploded to nearly 3.9 million.[3] The bodies and minds of those recruits needed strengthening, toughening, and sculpting, but the Army lacked an expansible corps of physical trainers able to meet the demand. Despite the Army's embrace of the physical culture developed by Koehler and his compatriots, it had not invested in a training pipeline to create and certify trainers. Calls for a central school on the British Aldershot model had come to naught and

Koehler's alternative proposal for a "postgraduate" course at West Point had withered by 1904.[4]

Instead of a central school, the Army had opted to rely on West Point for the production of its physical trainers. Young West Point graduates, all beneficiaries of Koehler's instruction, assumed various duties at their new units as athletic officers and gymnasium directors. Though this system worked reasonably well in the prewar Army, it proved wholly inadequate to the challenge of mass mobilization.[5] West Point's accelerated program turned out hundreds of new officers during the war years, but their physical training education was curtailed, other duties quickly consumed their time, and they were simply too few in number. Without a central school for physical trainers, the Army could not equip newly enlisted and commissioned citizen-soldiers with the knowledge and skills to lead training. Thus, the Army was incapable of expanding its corps of physical trainers to meet the demands of mobilization.

Similar shortfalls in other areas ranging from logistics management to psychological evaluations challenged the Army's ability to mobilize on such a vast scale. To make up for these shortfalls, the Army, and President Woodrow Wilson's administration more broadly, turned to civilian elites staffing new, ad hoc organizations.[6] The CTCA was one such organization, and it rapidly assumed responsibility for the care of soldiers' bodies, minds, and morals. Wilson established the CTCA on April 17, 1917, just eleven days after the United States entered World War I, and charged it with preventing the spread of venereal disease among soldiers. Simultaneously, the Department of the Navy established a nearly identical commission to provide healthy recreational outlets for its sailors.[7] According to the Army's CTCA, victory would come through "man-power and manhood," so the commission dedicated its efforts to cultivating both.[8]

In part, the CTCA's existence revealed the obligation the Wilson administration felt toward young men it drafted into service. America's youth were called in unprecedented numbers for a cause portrayed in highly moralistic terms. Accordingly, those men should be moral warriors and return home bearing only those scars "won in honorable conflict."[9] The CTCA's campaign against venereal disease and the immoral influences traditionally associated with military encampments by Americans helped assuage the public's concerns about entrusting its young men to the military.[10]

The CTCA's mission also revealed two other impulses in the Wilson administration's management of the war effort. Efficiency was the first of these. Rumors at the time held that venereal disease ravaged the armies fighting in Europe—supposedly, the Austrian army alone had lost upward of sixty-seven divisions worth of men to it.[11] Reduction in venereal disease rates therefore seemed an excellent way to minimize wastage. Fewer soldiers put out of action by preventable disease meant more bodies available for military operations. Additionally, the soldiers themselves would be more efficient if content and engaged instead of bored and left to their own devices. The second impulse was toward social engineering on a massive scale. Progressives in the Wilson administration perceived an opportunity to reshape American society using soldiers and their training camps as a vector. Instead of introducing men to vice, military service could teach men healthy alternatives. Soldiers could return home with their bodies "strengthened and more virile," their minds "deepened and enriched by participation in a great, heroic enterprise," and their spirits enhanced by values "which come from a full life lived well and wholesomely."[12] After the crusade in Europe, American soldiers could bring the crusade home as the vanguard in a campaign of national uplift.

Both impulses were evident in the ideas and actions of the CTCA's director, Raymond Fosdick, and the man to whom the CTCA answered, Secretary of War Newton Baker. Both were Progressives keen on improving American morals and leveraging social engineering for reform.[13] Fosdick, a New York city official who had made his name investigating European and American police systems, first encountered the problem of morality in military training camps in August 1916. That summer, US soldiers deployed to the Mexican border found themselves bored in a hot and desolate land. Alcohol and prostitutes helped fill the dull hours. Alarmed by reports of vice, the War Department dispatched Fosdick as a special agent to study conditions.[14] Fosdick's report earned him the chairmanship of the Army's CTCA and of the Navy's parallel commission in 1917. Fosdick waged his subsequent campaign against venereal disease and immorality on many fronts. For instance, the CTCA established in-camp alternatives to vice such as libraries, clubs, and hostess houses. The organization also used repression, as in their agents' heavy-handed dealings with communities near training camps when rooting out illegal liquor sales and prostitution. Simultaneously, the CTCA worked at the development of soldiers as moral men through educational programs, singing, sport, and more. Such diverse lines of effort demonstrate that Baker, Fosdick, and their chief subordinates conceived of their mission in broad terms and were willing to pursue their objectives aggressively by many means.

Athletics instantly emerged as a key tool in the CTCA's grand campaign to combat venereal disease, improve efficiency, and remake American society. Sports and exercise fulfilled the CTCA's immediate mission of providing healthy alternatives to vice. Soldiers could spend their energy in exercise and their spare time playing in or spectating at sporting events. Such arguments had long been among the justifications for recreational athletics, gym construction, and systematic physical training in the military. Additionally, sporting events could tie training camps and their local communities together more tightly through wholesome competition, which advanced the CTCA's vision of reshaping society. Athletics also enabled the CTCA's Progressive leadership to pursue what historian Nancy Bristow has identified as one of their prime objectives: cultivation of an active middle-class masculinity to counter the feminization wrought by industrialization and urbanization.[15] Ideally, soldiers would take their new knowledge of and zest for physical activity back to their communities after discharge. Veterans could be vectors for revitalizing, and remasculinizing, an enervated American society. Finally, athletics seemed to have obvious and direct military relevance. At least three decades of cultural, intellectual, and institutional momentum ensured that many of the Army's leaders were receptive to athletics, even if the Army's official physical culture separated athletics and training. The CTCA, dedicated to "educat[ing] the men to be better fighting organisms," capitalized on this moment and on easy analogies in claiming that athletics could make men fit to fight and keep them that way.[16]

Responsibility for athletics fell to the CTCA's Athletic Division, headed by Princeton's Joseph Raycroft.[17] This division, and Raycroft specifically, displaced Koehler between 1917 and 1920 as chief producer of official Army physical culture. The CTCA's authority and reach made the displacement possible. Part of that authority derived from the professional credentials Raycroft and others like him brought to bear. A member of the University of Chicago's first graduating class in 1896, Raycroft earned his doctoral degree in medicine from Rush Medical College in 1899. He later returned to Chicago as a full professor and served for twelve years as the university's medical director. In 1911, Raycroft became Princeton's second chairman of health and physical education, a position he retained until retirement in 1936. Among many other accomplishments at Princeton, Raycroft championed expanding the school's intramural athletics. He based his Princeton program partly on arguments that unhealthy students lowered the efficiency of the institution as a whole and that healthy bodies were essential for "clear thinking, clean living and efficient citizenship."[18] He also called on physical educators to design outcome-oriented curricula instead of prescribing general programs. For Raycroft, physical education's ultimate purpose was training the person to "get normal control of himself and to adapt himself to his environment."[19] At Princeton and in the Army, Raycroft championed a holistic, educational approach to physical training intended to produce positive mental, moral, and physical effects in its subjects.[20] Raycroft's belief in holistic education belonged to physical education's third generation, which had diverged from the thought and practice informing the Army's physical culture around 1906.

The Athletic Division differed from benevolent organizations such as the Young Men's Christian Association (YMCA) and Knights of Columbus, which facilitated recreational athletics in camps and overseas, by aggressively interceding in military training.[21] In May 1917, less than a month after the CTCA's creation, Raycroft laid out his understanding of the problems facing physical training and his proposed solutions in a memorandum for the Army's General Staff. This memorandum reveals Raycroft's desire to fundamentally change Army physical training practices. In it, Raycroft asserted that the US Army had to rapidly mold the "raw, untrained material from civil life" into men ready for "technical military training." In brief, the problem was to bring men up to "a condition of maximum physical and mental efficiency in the shortest space of time." Raycroft urged a "simple, intensive, uniform" training program to develop the "body control, physical reserve and endurance demanded by modern warfare."[22] According to Raycroft, doing so necessitated an increase in scale, more central control, further standardization, and the use of "more varied types of physical activities" beyond the disciplinary exercises Koehler's culture promoted.[23] The Athletic Division's leaders prided themselves on their open-mindedness to any methods, whatever their source, that would help them achieve their goals.[24] Crucially, Raycroft and his community of newly empowered civilians were unfettered by Army traditions and many of the assumptions that underwrote the Army's existing physical culture.

To fulfill this vision, Raycroft initially recommended using the Army's internal resources to build up a cadre of physical trainers in the British mold through a central Physical and Bayonet School. He envisioned this central school training and certifying instructors in courses ranging from one to four weeks in length. As in Britain and Canada, such a school could grow and shrink its capacity based on demand, thereby creating an expansible training pipeline.[25] From the beginning, Raycroft attached a great deal of importance to training trainers. He stressed that success in physical training depended upon the spirit and expertise shown by instructors. Expecting Koehler and his limited cadre of young West Point graduates to teach all the new conscripts and recruits would be inefficient, not to mention physically impossible. Instead, Raycroft wanted experts such as Koehler in a school where they could "teach other men to teach."[26] Raycroft also proposed the establishment of a physical training control board in Washington to develop the thought, practice, and systems to be taught at the central training school.[27] Though this board never formed, the CTCA's Athletic Division filled the role, temporarily replacing West Point as the de facto agency for development and promulgation of physical training systems.

Much of Raycroft's vision for the Army's future physical training infrastructure reflected his study of programs in use by Allied forces. In drafting his memorandum of May 1917, Raycroft had focused his studies on the British and Canadian systems, and even briefly visited a Canadian training camp.[28] This was not a new or novel approach. Aldershot had served as a model for physical training advocates within the Army for decades. Civilian physical educators newly interested in military physical training repeatedly pointed to Aldershot as a model too. After all, it demonstrated the feasibility of an expansible central school for trainers, and its curriculum was informed by lessons learned on the battlefields of World War I.[29]

Prompted by Raycroft's memorandum, the War Department dispatched Koehler to Toronto in June 1917 to study the feasibility of implementing a system like the Canadian Army School of Physical and Bayonet Training in the US Army.[30] The curriculum Koehler encountered differed from his own in many respects, even if both built from a foundation of disciplinary physical exercise. For instance, the Canadian system reflected its British roots by incorporating both formal and recreational athletics. Bayonet and hand-to-hand fighting figured prominently as well.[31] Koehler issued a negative report upon his return that convinced the War Department that it was "not considered possible to establish a course . . . on the scale suggested."[32] What exactly Koehler found unfeasible or undesirable is not known. However, Koehler had expressed hostility in the past to turning over any part of Army physical training to civilians, so he may have found it impractical to build such a school just using the military's limited pool of uniformed experts, given the urgency of mobilization.

Subsequently, the War Department dispatched Koehler to officers' training camps instead of putting him in a school as Raycroft urged. Koehler spent two to four weeks at these camps, giving special instruction to selected candidates.[33] Graduates of Koehler's crash course could, in theory, lead exercise sessions in accordance with *Special Regulations No. 23*, published in May 1917.[34] This practice essentially perpetuated the Army's existing instructor training program, but where Koehler spent four years preparing West Point graduates to lead physical training, he now spent at most four weeks with candidates. Several factors compromised the effectiveness of this arrangement. First, Koehler simply could not train enough officers himself. Training at most a few hundred men during each two-to-four-week iteration did not produce a corps sufficient to meet the needs of the Army's rapidly swelling ranks. Second, other duties tended to consume these officers once they arrived at their units, making them unavailable for service as physical training instructors.[35]

Because the War Department did not initially follow through on Raycroft's recommendations, the Athletic Division's head shifted his efforts to promoting a second scheme. Perceiving that Koehler's assignments to the camps signaled the way forward, Raycroft moved to place his own men in training camps. The Athletic Division would recruit leaders of college athletics and insert them into camps as athletic officers responsible for organizing training and sports. This plan followed the model set by Koehler while capitalizing on a feature common to most Regular Army camps, especially those overseas: athletic councils.[36] By 1917, athletic councils had been in operation for about two decades. Army officers on those councils were charged with organizing and supervising recreational athletic competitions. Raycroft's proposal would put civilians at the head of similar councils that simultaneously organized training and athletic competitions while educating officers on how to do the same in their regiments, battalions, and companies.

Preparing and positioning new athletic directors posed some challenges. For example, the CTCA could not force commanders to accept these men. To get around this, the CTCA, with Secretary Baker's authorization, wrote to camp commanders offering "the right, if they so desired," to "invite the services of trained athletic coaches" in order to "stimulate and promote the development of a knowledge of the organization and conduct of athletic sports."[37] However, the Athletic Division reserved responsibility for recruiting and managing civilian athletic directors. Rolled out first at officers' training camps, the program proved popular and rapidly expanded to cover all training camps. By November 1917, the CTCA's athletic directors operated in sixteen Army and sixteen National Guard cantonments.[38] This training cadre reinforced the Athletic Division's institutional control over physical culture production. Over the following two years, they extended Raycroft's influence down to the division level and below, built a school system from the ground up, and used their laboratory of human material to develop a comprehensive system of military physical training.

This influential group initially included physical educators, coaches, and athletic trainers pulled mostly from institutions of American higher education at the outset of the war. The War Department designated these experts as "civilian aides" to camp and division commanders. For the most part, camp commanders enthusiastically welcomed them, and most received the title of "athletic director."[39] Their duties involved building and leading athletic councils, as well as coordinating the work of YMCA and Knights of Columbus physical directors who were already organizing recreational activities. In August, the CTCA expanded this program by adding boxing experts to serve under the athletic directors as special instructors.[40] Raycroft prided himself on recruiting men as athletic directors, special instructors, and advisors based purely upon their qualifications in the subject matter. This led to the recruitment of some unorthodox trainers, including professional prizefighters, a "Scotchman who had lived in Japan" and there earned a fifth-degree black belt, and a "couple of noted knife fighters" from a lumber camp in Mississippi who were "very tough guys," according to Raycroft.[41] Merit-based recruitment reflected Raycroft's commitment to efficiency. Yet it occasionally cut against the Progressive morality project, such as when rough-and-tumble instructors failed to model the honorable masculine ideal the CTCA sought to cultivate.[42] However, the use of these instructors demonstrated Raycroft's functional, combat-oriented definition of fitness that characterized the physical culture he helped craft.

Inserting civilians into military organizations triggered a running debate about whether the athletic directors should remain civilians or receive a commission, and if they should deploy with their divisions. In part, this debate reflected negotiations over the athletic director's role. The CTCA's initial pitch to camp commanders emphasized the athletic director's responsibility for organizing and promoting *sport*. Yet clearly Raycroft and others in the CTCA imagined a larger role for their directors. In this regard, the title "athletic director" was somewhat misleading; one Athletic

Division inspector observed in 1918 that most of a director's work, and the "most important part" of that work, was in physical training.[43] Were these civilians really just supposed to promote sports, or did their duties blend recreation and training?

Preserving the athletic directors' civilian status offered several advantages. For instance, a civilian aide could sometimes get the ear of a general more easily than could a captain or major on staff because they retained a unique expert status in their area of proficiency instead of appearing as just one more junior officer among numerous others.[44] Many of the CTCA's senior leaders therefore believed that civilians could potentially push the Athletic Division's agenda more effectively by generating more traction with decision-makers at the division level and below. After the war, Raycroft's former executive officer, John Griffith, recalled that Raycroft's civilian status opened generals' doors, which helped him convince key leaders of the value of physical training.[45] Secretary Baker also viewed civilian status as an asset, at least at first. As he observed in June 1917, civilians not only enjoyed potentially better access to senior officers, but they could also build closer relationships with soldiers than could officers.[46] Close relationships helped athletic directors advance the Athletic Division's agenda and spread its emerging physical culture.

Civilian status also imposed liabilities, though. Some of these were trivial or merely annoying. For instance, Fort Gordon's athletic director, Thomas Browne, complained about receiving extra scrutiny from sentries, being unable to purchase clothing from the quartermaster, and difficulties in securing memberships at a nearby country club. Other liabilities posed a greater threat to the Athletic Division's mission: Browne also reported that some officers resented being instructed by a civilian, and many objected to him inspecting their physical training programs.[47] Commissioned athletic directors could, in theory, more effectively institutionalize and police their systems of exercise and athletics by their own authority.

Despite the advantages that Raycroft apparently enjoyed as a civilian, he argued for commissions for his athletic directors as early as May 1917. Raycroft believed that his directors deserved the pay, privileges, and respect that came with a commission. He also believed that commissions increased the likelihood of keeping his directors in the Army on a permanent basis, thereby enhancing their long-term influence on physical training practices and policies after the war.[48] Finally, Raycroft believed that his division's responsibilities extended beyond recreational athletics, and that commissioned physical trainers could make claiming a stake in basic military training easier. Raycroft's and Fosdick's exertions convinced Baker to reverse his position and authorize some commissions in December 1917.[49] In January 1918, fourteen athletic directors received commissions as captains and were assigned duties as "physical training officers."[50] More followed in 1918, and a few of these physical training officers even deployed to Europe with their divisions.

Beyond winning physical training officers some new power in military units, commissions also helped resolve occasionally fractious relationships between the YMCA's agents and the CTCA's representatives. In camps, directors from both organizations found that they shared overlapping areas of responsibility and that their relationships were not well defined. This sometimes led to conflict, as when one YMCA regional secretary suggested to a camp physical director that he organize athletics at his camp so as to impede the CTCA's newly arrived athletic director's participation.[51] Conflicts led to a series of letters and meetings between the top leaders of both organizations in late 1917. These exchanges produced an agreement that required directors in the various camps to develop harmonious working relationships. The agreement implied a superior position for the CTCA's athletic directors, who were responsible for coordinating athletics for commanding officers. Yet the agreement forbade the athletic directors from issuing orders to their YMCA counterparts.[52] Relationships between directors became more vertical and formal as the CTCA's representatives gained commissions. The debates between these organizations are further evidence of the role the CTCA perceived for itself in military training. Unlike the YMCA, which worked chiefly to improve soldier morale, the CTCA viewed itself as a part of the War Department responsible for the "military efficiency of the soldiers."[53] In following this logic, the CTCA's Athletic Division positioned itself as the preeminent authority on physical training and athletics by early 1918.

CTCA athletic directors and physical training officers, along with their YMCA physical director compatriots, entered service with many shared ideas shaped by civilian education and experience. Over time, these ideas gelled into a coherent physical culture. For the most part, this was a bottom-up process that resembled, in Raycroft's words, a "great laboratory experiment in the development of human material."[54] Physical educators and athletic coaches initially applied their knowledge and experience to improve soldiers within the unique conditions that each camp presented. As these volunteers and their military counterparts hashed out practices at the local level, they shared their experiences through organs such as the US Army War College and the *American Physical Education Review* journal.[55] The CTCA's Athletic Division also served as a central clearing house for information. Camp athletic directors remained in regular communication with the Athletic Division's office in Washington, DC, and the Athletic Division issued weekly bulletins to their men in the field that included policy guidance and highlighted best practices.[56] In the spring of 1918, the CTCA also began holding regional conferences for their camp athletic directors and boxing instructors. These conferences were intended to give directors opportunities to discuss common problems and develop solutions.[57]

Raycroft standardized these practices as they cohered into a training system over time. This was among his top priorities from the moment he assumed leadership of the Athletic Division.[58] Initially, Raycroft envisioned a central school fulfilling this role. Although the War Department initially declined to build such a school, Raycroft never gave up on the concept. In April 1918, the Athletic Division once again proposed an Aldershot-like central bayonet and physical trainer school along the British model, plus expanded duties for physical training officers. Raycroft grounded his argument in a review of the Athletic Division's accomplishments to date, and in an awareness that the military would eventually assume responsibility for the services civilians had until then provided. Baker approved the recommendations. In July, he directed the Athletic Division to coordinate with the General Staff's Instruction Branch to develop the plans further.[59] Coordination bore fruit that September in the form of *Training Circular No. 19: Organization of Physical and Bayonet Training.* Among other items, the circular advised that units form Physical Training Boards under commanding officers to supervise and coordinate athletic and physical training activities. The boards included a chairman, who was a staff officer directly responsible to the commander for physical training, the physical training officer, and selected physical and bayonet training officers, advisers, and instructors.[60] These were precisely the organizations Raycroft had advocated in his April arguments. Functionally, they combined recreational and physical training activities under one body. The boards also consolidated the power of the Athletic Division's officers and directors within camps and units.

Another pathway to standardization emerged organically by the summer of 1918. Since late 1917, many camps and divisions had formed schools under their athletic directors to create physical and bayonet trainers.[61] In the summer of 1918, Raycroft capitalized on these small schools to take concrete steps toward building a central school for the entire Army. In June, Raycroft received authorization to put a test school at Rich Field, Texas, into operation, formally charged with improving air crews' physical capabilities. Every aviation field and ground school dispatched three men to attend. Officers and civilians detailed by the Athletic Division conducted the training under the advisement of the War College's Training Committee.[62] In August, the General Staff's War Plans Division's Training and Instruction Branch authorized a wider "coordination course of physical training."[63] Raycroft selected Camp Gordon's school, run by Cap. Thomas Brown, as the host. Camp Gordon's school had become a robust operation since late 1917. With a staff of more than thirty, the school educated physical training officers for Camp Gordon units as well as classes of noncommissioned officers. Graduates of these latter classes numbered at least fifteen hundred and were supposed to pass on the Athletic Division's nascent system to the recruits under their charge.[64]

Fifteen months of effort culminated in the Athletic Division gaining a central school, though it was ostensibly temporary. The Athletic Division's physical directors, hand-to-hand fighting specialists, and boxing instructors were the first to attend. Raycroft later recalled that this temporary school represented a major step toward standardizing Army physical training along the lines of the Athletic Division's emerging system.[65] Not only did it increase the likelihood of the Army opening a permanent central school, but its graduates received a special certification and returned to duty with recommendations for commissions in the Reserve Corps, further institutionalizing the Athletic Division's system and its associated physical culture.

Movement toward centralization and standardization of physical training under Raycroft's model continued even as the war drew to a close and the CTCA demobilized. As part of that demobilization in 1919, the CTCA recommended establishing a permanent course in physical instruction. The General Staff's War Plans Division concurred and directed that the emergency course at Camp Gordon transfer to Camp Benning.[66] Raycroft believed that the Benning school marked a "great step upward" in promoting a "comprehensive standardized physical . . . athletic and bayonet training" throughout the Army on a "permanent basis."[67] Veterans of Raycroft's Athletic Division staffed the new school, including senior instructor Maj. John Griffith, who was Raycroft's former executive officer.[68] Five officers each from the Infantry, Cavalry, Field Artillery, Coast Artillery, and

Engineers attended the Benning school's first class between September 8 and 30, 1919. The purpose of this class was twofold. First, it was a testbed for Raycroft's forthcoming manual, which many anticipated would replace the *Manual of Physical Training* of 1914.[69] Indeed, the course's content matched Raycroft's later manual exactly. Second, its officer graduates were supposed to establish similar courses at their service schools to propagate the physical culture nurtured at Benning's central school.

Between 1917 and 1919, Raycroft and his civilian compatriots displaced Koehler as the Army's primary producers of physical culture. Beginning with a broad charter to improve the minds, morals, and muscles of America's soldiers, the CTCA's Athletic Division leveraged its influence and access at the War Department's highest levels to reshape physical training in the Army. Koehler stayed active throughout this period and his ideas and practices remained relevant. For instance, elements of Koehler's earlier manuals were reprinted for use in 1917, and Koehler himself moved from camp to camp conducting training with all the vitality and energy he had always displayed. Yet Koehler could not be everywhere. In place of the old Turner and his West Point disciples, civilian educators and coaches wielding fitness philosophies from the physical education community flooded in. Over time, their ideas coalesced through an institutional framework of conferences and schools, built from the ground up, that came to fulfill Raycroft's original vision of a central proponent. Civilian ascendency had major consequences for the Army's physical culture, but what ideas informed the work of those civilians, what sort of physical culture did they sculpt, and how did that culture differ from Koehler's?

As before, context is key to understanding this new physical culture, hereafter referred to as Raycroft's culture in acknowledgment of his central role in conceiving, shaping, packaging, and promoting it. Four elements of that context were especially relevant to the formation of Raycroft's culture. First, the men who created it entered the Army in a time of acute emergency with orders to address that emergency. Second, those men revered efficiency—maximum gain toward a specific outcome in minimum time with minimum waste. Third, the producers of Raycroft's culture approached their duties from the perspective of *educators*, not merely trainers. Finally, Raycroft and his partners understood their mission to be part of a broader enterprise concerned with the morality and masculinity of young American men.

Concerning the conditions under which Raycroft and his team entered service, the War Department called upon these men soon after the United States entered World War I and charged them with preparing for combat an army growing more massive by the day. The CTCA's civilians believed that they belonged to a world where "everything is necessarily subordinated to the need of creating an efficient fighting force."[70] That force was preparing to embark on a difficult and dangerous task. Shortly, its troops would enter the war in Europe alongside and against veteran forces with years of experience. Raycroft held that physical training was a way to compensate for inexperience. He and his colleagues hoped that an effectively leveraged, comprehensive system of exercise could put American recruits near the level of German veterans in terms of mental readiness, physical preparedness, and "fighting spirit."[71] Thus the men of the CTCA were not much concerned with the need for instilling iron discipline or controlling regulars. Their understanding, or perhaps imagination, of the modern battlefield and combat differed from the way prewar regular officers understood battle. Officers such as Edmund Butts who promoted physical fitness prior to 1917 emphasized unit fitness. In contrast, CTCA leaders focused on the individual fighting man. This was reflected in *Training Circular No. 19*'s stated purpose: the "development of the greatest possible individual efficiency and power in offensive combat."[72] A battalion's average marching speed was less important in this construct than the soldier's grit, aggressiveness, and close-combat skills.

Reverence for efficiency appeared frequently in texts and practices produced by the CTCA's physical training experts. In a presentation delivered to the Athletic Research Society shortly after the war, Raycroft named three elements of efficiency that guided his approach to developing a military physical training system: a clear conception of the work's purpose, suitability of the means and methods of administering work to achieve that purpose, and standards of measurement to mark progress toward the ultimate purpose. In that same speech, Raycroft rejected as too general the promotion of overall strength, vigor, and discipline that he understood to be the purpose of prewar Army physical training. Raycroft believed that more focus was necessary, specifically on advancing a soldier's basic military training and his physical education.[73] Physical training could do more than strengthen muscles and minds; it could make soldiers ready for combat.[74] This was the basis of Raycroft's repeated assertion that one differentiate between *exercise* and *training* when developing a military physical training system. Exercise for the sake of exercise was inefficient. Instead, everything needed to contribute to building a competent, lethal soldier.

However, Raycroft and his compatriots do not appear to have made any significant efforts to compile data on actual physical requirements for combat or to determine what specifically soldiers needed to be able to do. In reflecting later on their process of creating a training system, Raycroft laid out broad objectives, but never mentioned specific requirements such as being able to move a given load over a given distance.[75]

Raycroft defined soldier physical fitness in his manual of 1920 using four categories that aligned with his training system's broad objectives. First, fit soldiers demonstrated excellent bearing. They were poised, neat, alert, well disciplined, and precise in their movements. Second, fit soldiers possessed physical and mental control. They were coordinated and could respond to commands and changing situations rapidly. Control of body and mind granted soldiers "initiative, persistence, shiftiness, resourcefulness, willingness to give and take punishment, nerve, strength, and endurance." Third, fit soldiers could fight unarmed and with a bayonet. Raycroft specifically defined fitness here as a soldier's ability to "acquit himself creditably in a three-round bout with a skilled boxer of his own weight." Finally, fit soldiers could demonstrate achievement of minimum standards in a test that involved running, jumping, climbing, throwing, and negotiating obstacles.[76] Mental health also appeared occasionally in Raycroft's definition of fitness. He believed that sports and training toughened minds, provided outlets for competition and entertainment, and prevented soldiers from "getting stale" or giving in to the anxiety of combat, which was a route to shell shock.[77]

Raycroft's rejection of exercise for its own sake and his desire to align the means of physical training with desired outcomes reflected his background as a physical educator. He shared this background and its attendant perspectives with the Athletic Division's other experts. Raycroft believed that the purposes of civilian and military physical education were very similar, except in some of their specific outcomes. Likewise, he believed that the problems both military and educational institutions faced were "fundamentally the same." That problem was, in short, how to leverage physical activities to prepare a person for success by developing crucial qualities, whether physical or not.[78] Koehler and other early advocates of physical training in the Army had voiced similar ideas, but the qualities sought by these two generations differed. Koehler's generation focused more on the group and the individual's role in that group, while Raycroft's focused more on the individual himself. Physical educators of Raycroft's generation were also willing to use a much wider range of physical activity in pursuit of their outcomes. For instance, the Athletic Division promoted activities once appreciated purely for their recreational worth, such as sports, as valuable augmentations to the soldier's "formal training."[79] This willingness reflected the heritage of the playground movement and physical education's embrace of sport, both trends that had manifested after the paths of civilian physical education and military physical training diverged around the turn of the century.

Raycroft and his compatriots also demonstrated an awareness of their role in a larger social engineering enterprise when crafting their system. The CTCA was dedicated to cultivating an active middle-class masculinity in the men of the American Expeditionary Forces (AEF). In turn, the AEF represented America in the world. An article published in the *Independent* in 1917 captured this prevailing perspective: the AEF was a model for the world of "a composite, human standard of our national ideals."[80] Soldiers needed to be masculine, morally wholesome, and physically fit to meet this standard. Yet those responsible for getting soldiers up to such a standard shared a considerably dimmer view of the quality of American men entering the service than had Koehler and Butts. Based on high draft rejection rates and personal observations in camps, Raycroft found that many recruits were "awkward" for not having had a chance to play and undergo athletic training as children.[81] Social, moral, and physical consequences followed. Such a perspective contrasted with Butts's late-nineteenth-century assertions that recruits were high-quality raw material merely needing refinement and sculpting. The Athletic Division, on the other hand, perceived a gap to be bridged using physical activity. Their charge was to turn "narrow-chested clerks," "lean-visaged philosophers," and the "book-keeper and the street-car motorman" into soldiers ready for the modern battlefield. Their tools were exercise, sports, and teaching men how to "get bumped, and not to mind it."[82] The drive to cultivate a more physical and active masculinity in new recruits influenced the structure of Raycroft's system and pervaded the physical culture his system exemplified.

The clearest expression of Raycroft's system is in his book published in 1920, *Mass Physical Training*, and in the operations of the Camp Benning Physical and Bayonet Training Course in September 1919. In writing his book, Raycroft surveyed the programs of instruction fashioned by the various divisional and camp schools that had grown up under the Athletic Division's supervision since 1917. Regular communication with the Athletic Division headquarters and cross-talk in various channels between athletic directors and physical training officers had introduced a good deal of consistency to these programs. Raycroft combined the programs into a single system and tested it during the Benning school's first class. He regarded the result as the "first detailed and comprehensive scheme of Physical Training to be adopted by the army."[83] The War Department originally intended to publish Raycroft's book as an official document. However, postwar budget cuts and downsizing forced the manual into private publication.[84] Despite its private publication, the General Staff's War Plans Division under Maj. Gen. William Haan approved the book and directed that its "contents form the basis for the training and instruction of the military service of the United States in the subjects included."[85]

Mass Physical Training's body of subjects was much broader than that of its predecessor from 1914, the *Manual of Physical Training*. Raycroft's system covered six general categories of activity: physical drill, group games, drills in personal contact, individual efficiency tests, mass athletics and competitive games, and bayonet training. In contrast, the manual of 1914 ostensibly embraced ten subjects, but five of those fit within the rubric of Raycroft's "physical drill." Three other subjects received minimal coverage: running, athletics, and boxing and wrestling. Whereas setting-up exercises and gymnastic exercises formed the basis of Koehler's program, functional training for individual combat readiness characterized Raycroft's, as evidenced by exploration of each subject in detail.

Physical drill was the first subject Raycroft addressed. This comprised Koehler's setting-up drills and other routines from Koehler's earlier system. In fact, Raycroft simply adapted his drill from Koehler's manuals.[86] Adaptation was not direct, though. At least one CTCA athletic director had found Koehler's physical drill to be a mixed bag. "He has a mass of material both good and bad," this director observed, but instructors tended to pick the bad more often than the good and failed to redeem the drill with expertise as could Koehler.[87] Raycroft and his partners therefore had to simplify and modify Koehler's drill to meet their goal, which was to enable someone besides the system's creator to conduct effective training. One of Raycroft's greatest deviations from the preexisting system was the lesser emphasis he placed on physical drill. In Koehler's system, the setting-up drills were central to the entire physical culture. In contrast, Raycroft considered physical drill useful only for disciplinary training and education in bodily control, not for exercise.[88] Recruits might benefit from improved posture and responsiveness to commands, but ultimately physical drill was merely "kindergarten work."[89]

Mass Physical Training's second subject encompassed a wide variety of group games. All games were selected for simplicity of organization and their popularity in addition to their educational value. Raycroft intended ten of the simplest for use in regular drill periods. Examples of these include relay races, tug-of-war, and a mass participation version of red-rover called "Over the Top." *Mass Physical Training* covered another eighty-three games in its later chapters, many of which instructors could also adapt to drill periods, though most filled supervised athletic periods and leisure time. Additionally, group games included a series of skirmishing and quickening exercises. Many of these were taken directly from French and British practices: bear crawls, goose steps, standing long jumps, and more. Moving on the modern battlefield required soldiers to crawl, dash, dive, and run while stooped forward. Skirmishing drills strengthened the muscles needed for such unusual activities. Quickening exercises also prepared men to react rapidly to commands. For instance, an instructor might yell, "out of my sight," in the eponymous game to prompt his men to drop whatever they carried and scurry for the nearest tree or hole. Raycroft advised that any men remaining visible be singled out and made to "feel conspicuous."[90]

Raycroft gave two explanations for including group games in their many forms. First, he considered them useful for making soldiers combat-ready in a physical sense, but even more useful for developing mental qualities. Games, skirmishing drills, and quickening exercises presented soldiers with rapidly changing conditions, whether due to competition or the instructor's commands. Soldiers had to perceive change, make decisions, adapt, and respond rapidly. Physical exercise thus achieved mental effects by training "concentration of attention, quick thinking and instant execution."[91] Morale building and mental health also justified group games. Raycroft asserted that in the Athletic Division's wartime experience, its directors found that such games were more effective than anything else in "preventing discontent and homesickness" during training or after returning from the front lines.[92]

After the setting-up drill and group games sections, *Mass Physical Training* diverged sharply from its predecessor of 1914 with more than fifty pages on personal contact drills. Many activities fell under the personal contact rubric, including wrestling, hand-to-hand fighting, and boxing. Again, this training was intended to develop mental as well as physical qualities: aggressiveness, personal grit, mental and physical alertness, confidence, and the "ability and willingness to carry on in spite of punishment."[93] Treatment of hand-to-hand combat training in the Raycroft and

Koehler manuals highlights differences between their physical cultures. In the manual of 1914, boxing and wrestling made a brief appearance, but were "not recommended as an obligatory part of the enlisted man's training."[94] Koehler encouraged boxing and wrestling for their value in strengthening muscles and self-confidence, but he did not consider them a key element of physical training. In contrast, Raycroft dedicated nearly half his manual to physical contact and combat training, emphasizing a gritty, individual warrior paradigm. The "spirit of hand-to-hand fighting," Raycroft wrote, "is that of grim, watchful determination." Raycroft advised that aggressiveness and determination were keys to success, and that "principles of sportsmanship and consideration" for the opponent had "no place in the practical application of this work."[95] Like Koehler, Raycroft valued the physical and mental benefits of combat training. However, he also appreciated the functional benefits of the skills themselves. This physical culture valued an individual soldier's ability to control a prisoner and strike, strangle, or trip an enemy combatant. Each manual's imagery made the differences between Koehler's and Raycroft's systems obvious: Koehler's depicted gymnastic contests between opponents in gym clothes, while Raycroft's featured combatants locked in mortal combat.

Later in the manual, Raycroft continued his emphasis on aggressiveness and the realities of combat with a chapter on bayonet training. Raycroft considered this "invaluable in the basic training" of all soldiers, regardless of branch or duty, chiefly because it developed confidence, determination, and a "fighting spirit."[96] The Army had trained its soldiers in bayonet fighting for years. However, Raycroft's manual was the first instance of bayonet training featuring as a component of physical training. This fact highlights the functional fitness focus in Raycroft's physical culture. Discipline and obedience were not enough—soldiers must be ready to kill. *Mass Physical Training* drove this point home repeatedly. "In a bayonet assault," Raycroft wrote, "all ranks go forward to kill or be killed, and only those who have developed skill and strength by constant training will be able to kill."[97] Even if few soldiers ever found themselves in true bayonet combat, the spirit of the bayonet held value culturally, much like General Pershing's emphasis on rifle marksmanship and open warfare.[98]

Differing emphasis on activities within any given training session also illustrates variances between Raycroft's and Koehler's physical cultures. In his manual, Raycroft left the construction of daily and weekly programs up to individual instructors, much as Koehler had done. This freedom allowed instructors to meet the specific needs of the groups being trained and to adapt that training to local conditions. Simplicity and enabling physical training anywhere under any circumstances were central design principles, after all. However, Raycroft did give some guidance on the apportionment of time within a daily drill based on wartime best practices. In this guidance, he advised spending well over half of any given hour-long session in combat-oriented activities: boxing, hand-to-hand fighting, physical efficiency tests, bayonet fighting, and skirmishing exercises. In contrast, the setting-up drill occupied as little as ten minutes.[99] Again, this highlighted the differences between Koehler's and Raycroft's physical cultures. The former revered disciplinary drill, while the latter valued combat-centric functional fitness.

Three other elements of Raycroft's system especially characterized the physical culture produced by the CTCA's Athletic Division and distinguished it from Koehler's: boxing, athletics integration, and individual efficiency testing. Raycroft and his compatriots attached great significance to these elements, each of which were vital components of the larger system. Accordingly, the definitions and valuations of fitness in Raycroft's physical culture are exceptionally visible in these elements when examined closely. Of the three, boxing was perhaps the Athletic Division's signature initiative. Following the British example, pugilism figured prominently in Raycroft's system and in the CTCA's publicity campaigns because Raycroft and others regarded it as having an "intimate connection with bayonet fighting."[100] Parts of this connection were very direct: the "long point" bayonet attack corresponded with a "left lead" in boxing, as did a rifle butt strike with a "right-hand counter." Bayonet fighting was merely "boxing with a gun in your hands," according to the Athletic Division's boxing training film.[101] Other connections were less direct, but still key to Raycroft's definition of martial physical fitness, such as developing the quality of aggression.[102] More than most sports, boxing cultivated quickness, self-confidence, self-control, and toughness in participants. The CTCA's rules even specifically promoted aggressive offense and penalized defensive strategies.[103]

The Athletic Division recruited boxing experts as special instructors, partly to capitalize on star power to popularize their work. Between the instructor corps and the special subcommittee to study boxing formed in 1917, the Athletic Division collected many of the biggest names in the sport at the time, including James Corbett, Norman Selby (Kid McCoy), Robert Edgren, Richard Melligan, and Michael Donovan.[104] Raycroft later wondered at the "galaxy of world's champions" that his corps of instructors represented.[105] In keeping with his dedication to efficiency and his combat-centric, functional definition of fitness, Raycroft repeatedly focused this corps on their primary mission of making "'head up and eyes open' two-fisted fighting men."[106] Mass instruction was key, not the creation of individual ring stars. Instructors were to stress aggressiveness, simplicity, effectiveness, and a willingness to give and take punishment. Soldiers did not need anything fancy, just the six standard blows and the appropriate attitude. "A straight left," advised an Athletic Division memo, "well delivered and backed up by aggressive American determination, is a Boche eliminant in nine cases out of ten."[107]

Incorporating boxing into the Athletic Division's physical training program posed some challenges, though. One was a concern about high injury rates, which could cut against the CTCA's emphasis on efficiency. The Athletic Division took several steps to reduce this risk. Centrally developed standards dictated instruction, and only trained personnel were authorized to deliver and supervise boxing instruction. The CTCA's special boxing instructors were assigned to each camp under the athletic directors, who supervised training. Through intensive small group sessions, camp instructors trained and certified enlisted assistant instructors selected from the ranks. These assistant instructors in turn trained their fellow soldiers. Most soldiers would have experienced mass training, where whole companies or battalions at a time learned the fundamentals of stance, movement, and punching.[108] Bouts were encouraged to give men a real fighting experience and to increase the training's popularity, but matches were only allowed under strict supervision. Furthermore, the Athletic Division created a film to communicate the importance of boxing and to further standardize training. Linkage between bayonet fighting and boxing was the film's central thrust, but it also demonstrated basic boxing techniques.[109]

Boxing posed another potential problem for the CTCA in light of the form of masculinity the commission promoted. The CTCA promised to make men tougher, but also more wholesome. In contrast, boxing was illegal in most states and the prizefighter experts brought on as instructors were rarely paragons of moral righteousness.[110] The commission's public messaging revealed sensitivity to this tension. For instance, its book *Keeping Our Fighters Fit for War and After*, published in 1918, featured an enthusiastic clergyman who declared it "worth a ten-dollar bill to see a man who can take a blow in the face without getting mad" after watching a bout.[111] The book included a similar vignette directed at soldiers' mothers and wives who feared brutalization of their men through boxing. "If you feel that jabbing six inches of cold steel into Germans will make brutes" of your men, the author asked, "what would you think about him if he refused to do it?" The author assured female readers that the bravery, tenderness, loyalty, and other qualities they taught and inspired in their men were still present, but that those men had to kill their foes to protect the innocent. Army training did not make men brutes with a "lust for blood," but rather equipped honorable men with the skills and moral fiber they needed to fight for the "righteousness of the cause."[112] This rhetoric, combined with the focus on efficiency in making fighting soldiers, justified boxing in the commission's broader effort to form better men in the Progressive mold. The CTCA's boxing program fashioned manly warriors—crusaders—who could and would kill in battle, but who possessed the character to control and precisely direct violence.

Boxing underscored core elements of Raycroft's physical culture. Within this culture, fitness was defined functionally in light of World War I's combat and European battlefields. Like Koehler's culture, Raycroft's conceived of fitness more broadly than simply as a measure of physical capacity. Both attached mental and moral elements to fitness, though each culture valued variations of those elements differently. Discipline and obedience were important in both cultures, as evidenced by Raycroft's inclusion of Koehler's disciplinary drill. However, Raycroft and his compatriots prioritized qualities such as toughness and aggression that did not feature in Koehler's definition of fitness.

As with boxing, Raycroft's integration of athletics into his system highlighted core elements of his physical culture. The inclusion of athletics also reflected civilian physical education's zeitgeist. Initially, the CTCA intended its athletic program to encourage the "*largest possible* number of soldiers" to participate regularly in "some form of athletics" during leisure hours, though the program favored those "hard competitive sports that develop the fighting instinct."[113] Athletic directors and military commanders both perceived such great utility in games that they soon pushed athletics into formal training periods too. Sports were certainly not new to the Army in 1920, but Raycroft incorporated them into a formal physical training program in a way Koehler had not. Through the latter half of the nineteenth century, Army leaders had tolerated sports as a diversion for troops. Changing attitudes followed sport's exploding popularity both inside and outside the military in the 1890s, leading officers to argue that competitions helped men become physically fit for war while molding character.[114] However, the Army's official, pre-Raycroft physical training barely addressed sport. Training and athletics had thus proceeded on related but separate tracks, whereas Raycroft integrated them.

Comparing the manuals of 1914 and 1920 illustrates this difference. In the manual of 1914, athletics appeared in a single, slim chapter that mostly warned about the potential evils of athletics. That chapter led with a word of advice: "in order to meet the requirements of the service," military athletics should "have nothing in common with competitive athletics."[115] Koehler was not opposed to sports, but he thought their presence tended to undermine or challenge the physical training mission. Thus, Koehler advised eliminating any events that "have nothing to commend them from a military point of view."[116] The only events that met his criteria were distance running and various jumps. Other activities might have a place in field days, which he counseled holding annually at most, or as pure recreation, but they had no place in physical training.[117] In contrast, Raycroft dedicated nearly half of his manual to athletics. This included chapters on conducting meets and contests, as well as a chapter on the "strategy and tactics" of football, baseball, basketball, and other games. The Camp Benning school's curriculum also reflected the emphasis on athletics. Just under thirteen of its 145 instructional hours were spent on disciplinary gymnastics, while twenty-five and a half were committed to mass athletics and "highly organized games" such as football and baseball.[118]

Moreover, Raycroft and his compatriots frequently cited the perceived merits of athletics in regard to improving soldiers. Raycroft believed that play and games were "immensely important in the making of an efficient man" because they developed valuable mental, moral, social, and physical qualities.[119] Whether used in training or as a leisure activity, Raycroft sensed sport's social function in developing group loyalty, teamwork, and leadership. Additionally, sports were thought to cultivate group loyalty and esprit de corps.[120] Linkages between combat and sports skills also regularly appeared in justifications and statements. Raycroft and his fellows often cited soccer, baseball, and football in this regard. For instance, they asserted that soccer taught balance and a short gait useful for negotiating no-man's land, and that throwing a baseball obviously correlated with grenade throwing.[121] In short, the Athletic Division's members held that nothing "coordinated the personal faculties needed in warfare" like organized athletics.[122]

Integrating athletics reflected the broad educational mission Raycroft and his partners pursued. While Koehler had also described physical training as primarily educational, he put more emphasis on the term "training" than "education." Also, Koehler believed that his disciplinary gymnastics approach was the best way of strengthening bodies and minds, improving unit capabilities, and instilling discipline and obedience.[123] Raycroft and his partners conceived of their educational ends, ways, and means differently. They grounded their ends in an individual's functional combat fitness and agreed that there was more than one way to achieve those ends. Raycroft distilled many of his ideas in critiquing the Army's existing approach to training during a talk given in 1918 to college administrators and physical educators. The core of his critique concerned an old false dichotomy in the Army's physical culture between recreation and training, the latter being defined as disciplinary or hygienic exercise. In his opinion, recreation and training could be combined in an educational mission. For instance, combining sports with basic soldier training could prepare men to react to changing situations and respond effectively under fire. Simultaneously, sports could develop crucial battlefield qualities such as strength, endurance, leadership, and confidence.[124] Several of these qualities differed from those that the Army's earlier physical culture sought to develop. Furthermore, Raycroft argued that the Army's greatest mistake was its tendency to commit to a single form of activity, such as disciplinary drill or gymnasium work, as the basis of its system. Raycroft held that a comprehensive, inclusive system was superior. By combining the educational strengths of various activities, a more efficient and effective system became possible. Raycroft kept faith that sports would not displace physical training as Koehler had feared, but that they could supplement and augment formal military training.[125]

One final element of Raycroft's system that characterized his physical culture and differentiated it from Koehler's deserves attention: individual efficiency testing. The presence of individual efficiency tests reflected the backgrounds of the Athletic Division's personnel. In civilian physical education, such tests had become increasingly popular in the two decades preceding 1917. Testing benefited both individuals and units according to Raycroft. By setting standards, testing inspired soldiers to meet or exceed those standards. Testing also gave officers a snapshot of unit fitness levels and singled out those "inefficient men" in need of "special attention and work."[126] *Mass Physical Training* proposed a modest five-event test done monthly that measured attainment of baseline standards in combat-focused physical activity. Soldiers sprinted one hundred yards, executed a running broad jump, climbed an eight-foot smooth fence, threw a hand grenade thirty yards into a ten-foot-square box, and negotiated a simple obstacle course involving hurdles, barbed-wire entanglements, plank bridges, and smooth walls in less than thirty seconds.[127] Testing progressed through three grades. Each grade used an identical course, but soldiers in the third grade performed without equipment while those in the second and first grades performed with a rifle and with a rifle and light equipment, respectively. Achieving first-grade status also required soldiers to prove their abilities with the bayonet, in hand-to-hand combat, and in boxing. No specific standards defined a passing score in these latter three events, but Raycroft advised weighting most heavily the display of "fighting spirit, determination, and willingness and ability to give and take punishment." The combatives events functioned not only as motivational and confidence-building tools, but also as filters to identify and possibly eliminate those unwilling to apply violence or endure it. According to Raycroft, testing in general identified men requiring remedial training, gave commanders an objective appreciation of unit fitness, and built esprit de corps through interunit competition over pass rates.[128]

Unlike earlier Army physical tests like those designed by Koehler for West Point's cadets, Raycroft and his compatriots specifically designed theirs to align with their perception of real battlefield demands.[129] Raycroft's test measured the effectiveness of the object he and his partners sought in physical training, namely, the fitting of a soldier to combat through the use of physical activity. Raycroft's team identified key soldier qualities, in this case "strength, speed, skill, endurance," and the ability to "creditably" acquit oneself in close combat.[130] Through experimentation and study at various camps, the Athletic Division's members crafted a test to measure those qualities directly. Ultimately, testing implied that fitness was measurable and defined it in terms of individual combat efficiency.

Boxing, integrated athletics, and individual efficiency tests, together with the structural dissimilarities between Raycroft's and Koehler's systems, illuminate a new wartime physical culture that differed in many ways from its predecessor. This culture bubbled up as a collaboration between like-minded civilian physical educators and athletic coaches with guidance and coordination provided by the CTCA's Athletic Division, and Raycroft specifically. During the war years, this culture displaced Koehler's in the Army. It defined fitness in more functional, combat-oriented terms than had Koehler's and evinced a willingness to leverage a wider variety of activities in pursuit of fitness. In a key departure from its predecessor, Raycroft's culture also emphasized maximizing individual combat efficiency over general unit capability. In 1914, the fit soldier was disciplined, obedient, self-confident, and capable of above-average feats of strength and endurance. In 1918, the fit soldier exhibited additional characteristics. He could also give and take punishment, fight barehanded and with the bayonet, react to rapidly changing conditions, and play a number of all-American sports. This culture reflected the conditions in which it developed. Its creators sought to efficiently prepare conscripts for combat with hardened veterans, often without the lavish gymnasiums and apparatus collections that Regular Army posts had accrued since the last decade of the nineteenth century. Furthermore, its creators also pursued a project of social engineering of greater ambition and scope than Koehler and his compatriots had imagined.

Though Raycroft's physical culture displaced Koehler's during the war years, its continued dominance was not a foregone conclusion. The suddenness of its success posed one challenge to the durability of Raycroft's culture. In contrast with Koehler's slow and steady rise to almost complete control of Army physical culture, Raycroft's was sudden, temporary, and occasioned by an emergency. Raycroft's culture did become dominant, and it did determine Army policy from late 1917 through late 1919 at least. Two pieces of War Department guidance, *Special Regulations No. 23* (1917) and *Training Circular No. 19* (1918), show this clearly. Where the former advanced Koehler's system wholesale, the latter decisively broke with the Army's older physical culture, which was organized around unit fitness, in asserting that the purpose of physical training was to develop "in each individual soldier the highest attainable physical efficiency, confidence and power in offensive combat and in military activities related thereto."[131] Despite its dominant position, Raycroft's physical culture did not fully penetrate the Army's institutions and its larger culture because it was mostly developed and implemented by outsiders.

Following the Armistice, the CTCA's leadership had to work quickly and aggressively to sustain the programs it developed during the war.[132] Raycroft began demobilization work in earnest in June 1918, having spent the months since November in France with Fosdick at the secretary of war's direction. As part of this demobilization work, Raycroft tried to transfer parts of the Athletic Division's program to permanent organizations within the War Department. For example, Raycroft collaborated in the creation of the General Staff's Education and Recreation branch. He also urged the establishment of a central instructor school, which he realized in September at Camp Benning, and the transfer of control for *all* athletic and physical training activities at camps to the physical training officers educated at that school.[133]

Raycroft's strategy for earning the official adoption of his physical culture within the Army and making it permanent had three main components: a certified instructor corps, a central school, and his manual. The instructor corps' members would serve as physical training officers in camps, divisions, and service schools. Physical training officers would ensure adherence to centrally developed physical training policy, educate others on the conduct of physical training, and control leisure-time athletics and competitions.[134] In short, they were to continue the work that the Athletic Division's athletic directors had performed between 1917 and 1919, but as commissioned officers. A central school was necessary to create and certify this instructor corps. Raycroft intended for the school at Camp Benning to become a permanent fixture beyond its first iteration in September 1919. The school would give the Army an expansible training pipeline and a means to rapidly propagate new policies through the force. Raycroft's *Mass Physical Training* manual would be the school's cornerstone document. The Army already had a standardized training program in the form of its *Manual of Physical Training* of 1914, but Raycroft wanted to replace it with his own. The old methods were outdated, he believed. His system combined the latest in physical education thought with lessons learned in the crucible of combat. A corps of school-trained instructors could make this a reality over time.

Raycroft's strategy had to overcome several obstacles. First, all of this had to be achieved within the context of shrinking budgets. The CTCA had capitalized on massive government expenditures to build out its physical training and athletic programs beyond the scope of anything achieved by its predecessors. Against this backdrop, the Camp Benning school's continued existence was never a given. Also, most of Raycroft's men left the service after 1919. A cadre of trainers, mostly those certified at the Camp Gordon school and given commissions, remained at Benning and in some units. Yet most of Raycroft's athletic directors were civilians or reserve officers. Their service was no longer needed after the war emergency, so they returned to civilian life. Creation of a new training cadre of commissioned officers through the Camp Benning school was consequently a vital necessity. Additionally, shrinking budgets pushed Raycroft's manual into private publication. As a result, it was not issued widely by the War

Department and, despite the General Staff's full endorsement, it did not appear as official as had *Manual of Physical Training* in 1914.

Finally, and perhaps most importantly, Raycroft had to decisively overcome the Army's existing physical culture. Despite Raycroft's culture having displaced Koehler's in policy and in training camp practices, Koehler's culture persisted during the war. Koehler himself provided instruction in camps and in Europe. His manual remained in publication, and the Army directed its use in the form of *Special Regulations No. 23* in 1917 before the Athletic Division fully took charge. Regular Army officers, most of them West Point graduates, were more likely than any other officer to remain in the service after the war. Nearly all of these had been Koehler's pupils at one time or another, and they had grown up in an Army that equated physical training with Koehler's disciplinary drill. A book published in 1919 on physical training authored by one of those officers, Col. William Waldron, illustrated the persistence of Koehler's culture. Waldron, who simply copied the disciplinary drill chapter from the manual of 1914 and marketed it for civilian use, claimed that the setting-up drill was the "basis upon which the entire system of physical training in the United States Army is founded—the system employed in the physical training of the vast army of over two million men who went to France in 1918 and fought the Nation's battles."[135] Ignoring the Athletic Division's system, Waldron credited Koehler's setting-up drill for all of the physical improvements civilians observed in their returning soldiers.

The permanence of Raycroft's physical culture in the Army was clearly not a foregone conclusion in 1920. That culture was the product of a particular time and of the men who fashioned it. The wartime emergency opened a window of opportunity for new cultural producers to reimagine Army physical training. Combining the latest thought from the worlds of physical education and college athletics with the practices of seasoned Allied militaries, civilian leaders such as Joseph Raycroft and his athletic directors crafted a new training system. Their system responded to the needs of a newly mobilized army of citizen-soldiers rapidly preparing to face veteran opponents. Pursuit of efficiency, a hallmark of Progressivism, informed their efforts. Efficiency demanded matching means to ends while maximizing gains and minimizing waste. In this new physical culture, the individual soldier's fighting ability displaced general unit condition as the chief aim sought.

As a consequence, the system they crafted and the physical culture it reflected emphasized the individual in combat conditions. Where discipline and obedience characterized Koehler's culture, Raycroft's stressed grit, aggressiveness, and a functional definition of fitness. This new culture also embraced a wider spectrum of physical activities as means by which to achieve those qualities. Sports and bayonet training became core components of physical training, both intended to augment and supplement disciplinary drill instead of existing in separate spheres of work. Such inclusiveness echoed both the drive for efficiency and the influence of college athletics and the playground movement on civilian physical education. Whether such a culture developed in wartime for an army mobilizing on an unprecedented scale would be valued after the war remained an open question in the era of downsizing and normalization that followed demobilization.

CHAPTER FOUR
REVERSION, DISAGGREGATION, AND "PREHABILITATION," 1919–1940

Standing before the National Convention of the American Physical Education Association (APEA) in Chicago on April 11, 1919, Col. F. J. Morrow claimed that the recent war had made "evident that one of the leading considerations in military preparedness is the matter of physical power and vigor."[1] Advancing a linkage between service and citizenship, Morrow also asserted that any effort to improve such qualities had to begin by targeting American boys, but that no plan for military training of civilians could succeed unless it "incidentally produces results which are of solid benefit to the individual and to the community under peace conditions as well as under war conditions."[2] Earlier that year, Dr. A. D. Browne made a similar appeal to adjust civilian physical education to meet the needs of military preparedness. Modern warfare demanded much of the soldiers fighting it. "Men are now required to drag themselves over many yards of rough ground without raising the body," Browne observed, and men who had "never had occasion to raise their own weight off the ground" found it necessary to "climb out of trenches, over seven-foot walls, vault, leap and jump over obstacles."[3] Morrow's and Browne's pieces were representative of many articles produced by commentators on physical fitness and combat in the decade following World War I. Nearly all shared a few consistent themes: fitness was a necessity in war; American men were less physically suited for service than once thought; military training proved more successful than civilian training in sculpting men; and national preparedness required a fit citizenry.

The Army's wartime experiences and interpretations of those experiences advanced by military officers, physical educators, and political leaders stimulated change in the Army's physical culture during and after World War I. First, systematic training came to be accepted within the military as a crucial element of basic soldier and unit training. By 1918, the value of such training was unquestionable. Second, civilian educators, who dominated physical training theory and practice during the wartime emergency, had reoriented military physical training on producing capable individual warriors using a wide range of activities. Most observers hailed this system as a smashing success, but its survival was not guaranteed. When civilians departed the service, Army officers content in success and facing budget restrictions returned to the physical culture they knew best—Koehler's. Raycroft's culture faded away in all but a few parts of the US Army. By the 1930s, the Army's official physical culture, propelled by institutional and cultural inertia, and the physical education profession's dominant body of philosophy and practice parted ways once more. Third, the physical training discourse within the Army shifted to the question of *whose* bodies should be built up for battle. The answer, in an age of mass mobilization and industrial warfare, was both the soldier *and* the citizen. Military and political leaders alike perceived a need to deploy the Army's physical culture and its attendant systems elsewhere in citizen-shaping projects designed to prehabilitate potential soldiers. The resulting programs, such as the Citizens' Military Training Camps and the Civilian Conservation Corps, aimed to improve the nation's manpower and embodied lessons learned from the Great War about the need for and demands of total mobilization.

In the late summer of 1919, a cadre of Raycroft's physical training veterans assembled in Camp Benning. Among them were many of Raycroft's top instructors who had earned commissions during the war, including his former executive officer and the Big Ten's future first athletics commissioner, Maj. John Griffiths, and Herman Koehler's cousin, Capt. Carl Brosius.[4] These men gathered at the behest of the General Staff's Training and Instruction Branch to open a special school for physical and bayonet training. Raycroft's advocacy during the CTCA's demobilization over the previous year persuaded the Training and Instruction Branch that making the wartime physical training system permanent would improve the physical condition of the Army's enlisted population and morale throughout the force.[5]

The resulting Physical and Bayonet Training Course pursued a twofold purpose. First, the course was supposed to propagate and perpetuate Raycroft's system within the Army. Consequently, three or four officers from each of the Army's five service schools composed the student body.[6] These newly minted physical instructors would, ideally, return to their service schools and train the next generation of young officers.[7] Second, it helped Raycroft validate his comprehensive training system, which he had spent the summer assembling into a treatise that became his book *Mass Physical Training*, published in 1920.[8] The Benning course's program of instruction followed the outline of Raycroft's later book precisely, furnished many of the photographs used as illustrations, and reflected the functional training approach underlying Raycroft's system. Maj. J. C. Drain, the course director, defined functional development as physical and mental improvement, or the "development of initiative and spirit," through participation in "carefully prepared games and athletic exercises."[9] According to Drain, this approach contrasted with earlier Army practices that pursued corrective, physical enhancement, and recreational goals, but that did not combine practices synergistically. Raycroft's solution, adopted by the Benning school, was to pull together disparate exercise systems and recreational activities under the control of experts who could achieve better, quicker results than had previously been possible.

The variety of activities under an athletic director's purview during the war and the range of subjects covered in the Benning course illustrate Raycroft's concept of functional training. Between 1917 and 1918, CTCA athletic directors assumed wide responsibilities in the divisions and camps to which they were assigned. They advised commanders on issues related to physical training, developed local training programs, led exercise sessions, trained uniformed instructors, supervised boxing programs, and participated in planning and executing bayonet training. Along with partners from the YMCA and other organizations, athletic directors also coordinated recreational athletic leagues and events, and even planned large competitions that often drew spectators from local communities. The Benning course prepared uniformed officer instructors to perform a similarly wide range of functions. Of the 145 hours of instruction students received over three-and-a-half weeks, more than twenty-eight were dedicated to bayonet training. The remaining hours were spread evenly between subjects such as quickening and skirmishing exercises, boxing and wrestling, hand-to-hand fighting, setting-up exercises, mass athletics, physical efficiency tests, and "highly organized games" that included football and baseball.[10] This distribution of time and emphasis highlights the impetus, foundational to Raycroft's culture, to incorporate athletics and combat training into physical training. This approach differed from Koehler's, which had largely separated physical training, combat skills training, and athletics into related but distinct activities. Had the highest hopes of the Benning course been realized, Raycroft's instructors would have been better prepared than their predecessors to direct and integrate a wide variety of activities. Drain promised that the US Army could look forward to beginning the next war with the "splendid physical opportunities" of the German army, along with the benefits of "complete physical and mental training" from uniquely American games and exercises.[11] Indeed, the school's instructors and others anticipated the course and its associated manual becoming official Army practice. The *Infantry Journal*'s editor, for instance, commended a report from the school as indicative of the future of physical training.[12]

Those high hopes were soon dashed. Graduates of the course's first class returned to their service schools but made only a limited impact. A second iteration in March 1920 pulled five officers from each department. The War Plans Division of the General Staff anticipated that graduates of this special course would establish similar schools in their own departments, but such schools do not appear to have become regular fixtures.[13] Raycroft's system did not spread. Postwar consolidations and budget cuts soon shuttered the new physical and bayonet training school, well before it could produce a critical mass of certified trainers.[14] Dreams for a comprehensive trainings system did not survive the era of normalization.[15] Shutting off the inflow of new instructors proved fatal for the consolidation of Raycroft's system in Army practice. Furthermore, most of the instructors trained at Camp Gordon and elsewhere during the war were reservists or emergency officers who departed the shrinking interwar army. Without new, uniformed officers trained to replace them, physical training policy largely fell to regular officers brought up under Koehler at West Point and untutored in Raycroft's system.

Camp Benning's Infantry School was one exception to the gradual passing of Raycroft's system. There, Maj. Gen. Charles Farnsworth, the school's first commandant and a physical training enthusiast, was a vocal proponent for the Physical and Bayonet Training School.[16] When the scheme for training officers of other branches withered, Farnsworth turned his attention to the infantry officers over which he had control. Farnsworth kept Drain and his instructors from the Department of Physical and Bayonet Training employed over the following year teaching courses for Infantry School students. These courses mirrored the program of instruction that had been applied in September 1919 in Raycroft's school. Farnsworth envisioned this program expanding to offer four six-week courses annually at Camp Benning between October and June. In the summer months, Farnsworth intended to disperse his instructors throughout the northern military districts to assist in instruction and to inspect their physical training programs. Instructors were to make similar trips throughout the southern districts between each course iteration in the winter and spring.[17]

Farnsworth struggled to realize this dream in the face of fiscal constraints. In letters between Farnsworth and Raycroft, the former identified several problems. For instance, the War Department frequently turned down, without comment, requests for funds to dispatch instructors on assistance and inspection trips to regional departments. Camp Benning's physical plant seemed to be the most critical problem. Forecasted rainfall during the planned primary instruction period between October and June was of special concern, so Farnsworth had sought a large indoor assembly building where training could proceed regardless of weather conditions. Costs proved prohibitive. Given the small appropriations Congress directed to the Infantry School in 1920 and the likelihood of continued economization, Farnsworth believed the funds required for construction would not be available for several years. On Raycroft's suggestion, Farnsworth instead secured several steel and canvas hangars that partly addressed the indoor training space issue. Filling those buildings with exercise and sporting equipment was another matter entirely, and one still unresolved by mid-1922. However, Raycroft proved instrumental through the mid-1920s in helping furnish the Infantry School's gymnasium by securing funds from those raised during World War I.[18] Thanks to both Farnsworth's and Raycroft's efforts, the Department of Physical and Bayonet Training managed to obtain sufficient manpower and facilities to propagate Raycroft's system in the infantry branch through the 1920s.

The survival of Raycroft's system at the Infantry School made sense. The infantry branch had taken an intense interest in physical training issues since the 1880s. Discussion about these issues appeared far more frequently in the branch's professional publications, such as the *Infantry Journal*, than in those of other branches. Furthermore, many infantry officers took seriously the assertion in *Training Regulations 10–5* of 1922, the basic training regulation for all arms, that athletics and physical training were key elements in every military training program.[19] The Infantry School's leadership saw itself filling a void in physical instruction left by Koehler's retirement from USMA in 1923, but physical training at the school adhered to a gradually diminishing version of Raycroft's model that included competitive sports, calisthenics, and apparatus work. Even if time constraints reduced the hours devoted to topics such as wrestling and baseball, the training philosophy remained true to Raycroft's comprehensive concept: exercise was not for strength alone, but for its "military value, its hygienic or health value, its educational value, mental and physical, for its recreational value, for its moral value, and for its social value."[20] However, the persistence of Raycroft's philosophy and system in the Infantry School's curriculum through the 1920s ultimately proved insufficient for sustaining Raycroft's ideas and practices in the wider Army physical culture.

Wider trends in Army physical training during the interwar years, abetted by organizational forgetting and complacency, bent toward disaggregation. Raycroft's system was notable for its comprehensiveness and integration of calisthenic drills, athletics, close-combat work, and more. In contrast, all of these activities existed on most prewar Army training calendars, but they stood alone as complementary but separate. Thus, Koehler's manuals had paid little attention to athletics, military sport developed haphazardly in a quasi-official status without a central proponent, and bayonet training appeared in separate manuals and occurred in hours outside those designated for physical training.[21] These same features, characterized here as a disaggregation of efforts, reemerged in Army physical training and physical culture during the interwar years.

The first visible manifestation of these trends appeared in *Training Regulations 115-5*, published in 1928, which was the first official Army physical training guide published since Koehler's *Manual of Physical Training* of 1914. Raycroft's book *Mass Physical Training* of 1920 predated *Training Regulations 115-5*, but it exerted very little influence on subsequent manuals. Maj. Gen. William Haan, chief of the General Staff's War Plans Division, had endorsed Raycroft's work, recommended its use in institutions providing physical training, and anticipated that it would "form the basis for the training and instruction" of the Army "in the subjects included."[22] However, in an effort to save both time and money, the War Department published Raycroft's book privately. The manual never gained official status within the Army or full organizational backing as a result. Mentions of *Mass Physical Training* disappeared from military professional journals by the mid-1920s and the authors of *Training Regulations 115-5* made no reference to its privately published predecessor. Indeed, someone reading only the Army's official physical training manuals might never have an inkling of the Army physical culture's wartime interregnum.

Training Regulations 115-5 might have ignored *Mass Physical Training*, but it exhibited a strong historical continuity with Koehler's culture. Published on September 10, 1928, upon the authority of Chief of Staff Charles Summerall, *Training Regulations 115-5* explicitly superseded the *Manual of Physical Training* of 1914. Its preparation occurred under the direction of West Point's superintendent, Brig. Gen. Merch Stewart.[23] Both the place and the leadership under which *Training Regulations 115-5* gestated were significant because Koehler strongly influenced both, even though the famous Master of the Sword had retired in 1923 and passed away in 1927. Koehler had directed all aspects of physical training at the Academy for nearly four decades. He molded the institution's physical culture and those men who took up his work after 1923. Institutional memories and culture virtually guaranteed that the Academy would look to its own heritage and practices, both inseparable from Koehler, when updating the Army's physical training regulations.

Koehler also strongly influenced key individuals, such as Stewart, who were responsible for the creation of *Training Regulations 115-5*. Merch Stewart, an 1896 Academy graduate and former student of Koehler's, made his outlook on physical training clear in his book *The Physical Development of the Infantry Soldier*, published in 1913. In it, Stewart championed the importance of systematic exercise for the infantry soldier. "War," he noted, "is truly a struggle between life and death and, in war, death is caused equally as frequently by sickness and incapacity as by the bullets of the enemy."[24] Because the infantryman was an "independent fighting element" that bore a heavy "burden of combat and march," he had to be fitted to carry on "when every muscle in his body cries out for rest."[25] Much like Koehler, Stewart connected physical fitness with qualities such as will and discipline, and then declared that exercise could develop all of them. Stewart's concept of discipline aligned with Koehler's; it was both the subordination of the body to man's control and the subordination of the man to the team's needs.[26] Development of physical fitness, discipline, and other qualities occurred in three stages according to Stewart: strength and endurance first, then ease and grace, and finally self-confidence, "which comes of a knowledge of his strength and capacity."[27] This progression paralleled Koehler's pyramidal structure. Although Stewart did not advance a system of physical training, he directed readers to other manuals then in publication, all of which Koehler either authored or influenced. Stewart also quoted the Master of the Sword and proposed categories of exercise that matched those found in Koehler's manuals of 1896 and 1904.[28] While Stewart also addressed functional fitness activities such as rushing, crawling, and aiming exercises, these were included for the general physical development of infantry soldiers as activities complementary to but distinct from systematic training. Responsibility for restating the Army's official physical culture thus fell to a disciple of Koehler's leading an organization that remained a posthumous bastion of the old Turner's thought and practice.

Comparing *Training Regulations 115-5* of 1928 and the *Manual of Physical Training* of 1914 also reveals a direct lineage. Little differentiates the two works in terms of format, organization, objectives sought, areas of emphasis, and recommended activities. Many of the demonstration photographs even appear to be unchanged. Like Koehler and Stewart before them, *Training Regulations 115-5*'s authors posited a multilevel hierarchy of objectives pursued through physical training. Physical fitness, according to these authors, was a recruit's baseline requirement that enabled him to execute all of his other duties. Through systematic exercise, recruits developed health, strength, and vigor. Learning to employ those physical qualities "to the best advantages for himself and for the mass for which he is a member" also developed "self-reliance, confidence, self-control, the courage to dare," alertness, precision, and enthusiasm.[29] These intangibles translated into the Koehler culture's ultimate quality of discipline. Physical training in this mode therefore possessed a "disciplinary value" that was "at least the equal to its physiological or military value."[30]

Further examples of continuities with the pre-Raycroft physical culture appear in the methods employed to achieve physical fitness. The authors of *Training Regulations 115-5* briefly addressed activities ranging from gymnastics, jumping, and climbing to rifle exercises, group games, and dumbbell routines. They also advocated including boxing, wrestling, and bayonet drills in training programs.[31] However, the importance of all these activities paled in comparison to the value accorded to traditional setting-up exercises. Unlike Raycroft's dismissal of the setting-up exercises as kindergarten work, *Training Regulations 115-5*'s authors asserted that the drills formed the "foundation upon which the entire course of physical training in the service is based" and that "their importance hardly can be overestimated."[32] The new regulation recommended that setting-up drills comprise a full third of every morning's physical training period, and its authors dedicated nearly two-thirds of the manual's contents to the precise explication of each movement and its associated commands. As had their forebears, the soldiers of the 1930s were to flex, bend, thrust, hop, swing, and squat their way to fitness in mass formation and in response to commands.

A single addition to these "disciplinary physical training exercises," known as mass commands, set the model from 1928 apart from its predecessor from 1914. Pioneered in an officer's training camp in early 1917, mass commands involved men in formation collectively giving preparatory commands and the exercise cadence in response to prompts issued by an instructor. The authors of *Training Regulations 115-5* contended that this practice had "practically revolutionized the old method of recruit instruction, both as to the time required and the efficiency obtained."[33] With mass commands, the "volume and smash" of the combined voices "literally impel[led] every man to extend himself to the limit in performing the movements snappily and precisely."[34] The value attached to these mass commands helps illustrate key features of the physical culture that the authors of *Training Regulations 115-5* promoted. Mass commands did not make the exercises themselves more strenuous. Instead, their value derived from enhancing the disciplinary quality of the drill and boosting self-confidence. Soldiers felt a part of the whole organization, practiced precision in the issuance of clear commands, and learned self-reliance and "assertiveness."[35]

Other elements of continuity between the Army's official physical culture and its prewar predecessor included an emphasis on average unit fitness over maximal individual capacity, and a general wariness about the value of athletics as a part of the formal training program. The former is visible in the methods advocated, the disciplinary objectives sought, and the repeated goal of subordinating the individual to the unit. For instance, the authors of *Training Regulations 115-5* summoned the spirits of Koehler and Butts in asserting that athletics should have "an applicable value" and be "educational" instead of "spectacular" because it was the "ability of the average of the mass that determines the efficiency of a fighting machine."[36] Concerning athletics, *Training Regulations 115-5* staked out a position more friendly to athletics than had its predecessor of 1914, which included in its athletics chapter as many warnings about the potential evils of sport as it did instructions. The authors of *Training Regulations 115-5* contended that use of mass athletics in the Army was "most desirable" on the grounds of both fitness and morale. This aligned with the Army's World War I experience and the contemporaneous flourishing of sport at the US Military Academy.[37] However, the manual downplayed games such as football and baseball as a component of formal physical training. Instead, it stressed mass games and individual contests such as relay races, cane wrestling, and other schoolyard competitions that had also featured in the manual of 1914. This was a far cry from the prominent place sport occupied in Raycroft's manual, even if they shared an emphasis on the educational value of athletics.[38]

Although *Training Regulations 115-5* exhibited strong continuities with an earlier physical culture, it did not replicate earlier manuals entirely. Several matters, though minor, differentiated the manuals of 1928 and 1914 and deserve mention. First, running (or double-timing) made its debut in Army physical training as a beneficial activity. *Training Regulations 115-5*'s characterization of running as being "invaluable in the development of endurance and organic vigor" diverged from the *Manual of Physical Training*'s claim about the extreme risk of injury associated with running and its concomitant warning that instructors "exercise the utmost care in its application."[39] The inclusion of running probably does not reflect much influence from Raycroft's culture. Running was not a major component of Raycroft's *Mass Physical Training*. Also, Koehler had come around to the practice after 1914, claiming in 1919 that no exercise could "develop condition, vigor and endurance, lung and leg power in general" as rapidly as running, so long as care was taken with "green" men.[40] In another contrast, *Training Regulations 115-5* suggested two hour-long training sessions per day, the latter consisting of bayonet or other combatives training and mass athletics, instead of the *Manual of Physical Training*'s single forty-five-minute drill. However, such differences did not represent a significant variance between the physical cultures each manual embodied and promoted. Their definitions of physical fitness remained largely the same, as did the vast majority of the methods recommended to attain fitness.

The trend toward disaggregation in the Army's official physical training system and the general reemergence of Koehler's physical culture, both embodied in *Training Regulations 115-5*, continued up until the eve of World War II. Although the regulations were formally superseded by the fourth chapter of the *Basic Field Manual*'s (*BFM*) first volume, published in 1936, the latter manual did little more than reprint a portion of *Training Regulations 115-5*.[41] Somewhat more change arrived in 1941 with the publication of *Field Manual (FM) 21-20*. The new manual slightly modified the Army's definition of fitness, but only in replacing the discipline capstone with a generic quality of "physical efficiency for military effectiveness."[42] *FM 21-20* continued the disaggregation of physical activities. Sports and combative training did not qualify for coverage, and disciplinary drills in mass formation continued to dominate training periods. The only notable change between 1928 and 1941 was that *FM 21-20* exhibited a turn toward a more functional fitness-based physical culture with the inclusion of obstacle courses and survival swimming. This turn echoed a similar cultural shift around 1917 when the Army began seriously preparing for war. Yet at root, the new manual still reflected the culture Koehler fashioned nearly six decades earlier.

One consequence of disaggregation in the Army's physical culture was that systematic training and sport diverged. The former leveraged the latter less and less. Sport remained enormously popular and a fixture in Army life, but soldiers increasingly played for the sake of playing instead of as a supplement to rational training objectives. Sport became a site only for building morale and for incidental training of soldierly qualities. Still, Americans attached an enormous amount of importance to sport in the military after World War I. Perhaps the most dramatic representation of this valuation was the Inter-Allied Games of 1919. Held in Paris, the games pulled together nearly fifteen hundred athletes from eighteen Allied nations and more than thirty thousand spectators, cementing the place of sport in the US military and helping spread the cause of the "sporting life" to other nations recovering from the trauma of World War I.[43] To reaffirm the place of sport on a scale smaller than an Olympiad, many Army posts also built new athletic complexes. For instance, Fort Benning completed construction of its Doughboy Memorial Stadium in 1925. During a speech dedicating this latest American living memorial, Maj. Gen. R. H. Allen declared that physical training and athletics had been recognized as "vital parts of all military training" and that neglect of either represented a "vital blow" struck at an army's "efficiency as a fighting machine."[44] Summoning long-standing assumptions about the inherent developmental potential of sport, Allen declared that the playing field cultivated qualities key to past and future success: action, teamwork, fighting spirit, the will to win, tenacity, and steadfastness.[45]

The Army's official physical culture increasingly ignored or minimized sport, but athletic competitions remained a regular feature of US Army life between 1918 and 1941. An unofficial, parallel physical culture emerged as a result. Historian Wanda Wakefield's survey of the accounts of retirees who served as junior officers prior to World War II confirms this. Many recalled the great personal and professional importance they attached to sports. One, Lt. Gen. Hobart Gay, even chose to remain in the army after World War I solely because he earned a spot on the Army's prestigious polo team.[46] Another, Gen. Robert Porter, found that young officers *had* to involve themselves in sports if they wanted to establish control and discipline in their units. "If he [the young lieutenant] was nothing but a bookworm," Porter recalled, "he would have trouble getting through to some of these people [the enlisted men in the regiment]."[47] Officers valued athletics for a variety of reasons. Sports helped keep officers physically fit, taught them lessons for their professional lives about leadership, built relationships between military personnel and local civilian communities, developed esprit de corps, and reinforced expectations of masculine behavior predicated on strength, aggressiveness, and competitiveness.[48] Sports were significant in the enlisted man's experience too. Apart from regular periods of mass athletics, most units maintained competitive athletic teams. Post and unit newspapers along with more widely available military publications such as the *Army and Navy Journal* and *Infantry Journal* consistently dedicated considerable space to covering the records and exploits of these teams.

Athletics also continued growing in popularity and importance at West Point during the interwar period. This growth occurred most explosively between 1919 and 1922 under the Academy's dashing young superintendent, Brig. Gen. Douglas MacArthur. A longtime sports enthusiast himself, MacArthur believed that sports were crucial to the preparation of junior officers, especially in developing "the coordination of mental and physical effort, an appreciation of the principle of cooperation, the development of hardihood and courage, and the inculcation of an aggressive and determined spirit."[49] Along with the Academic Board, MacArthur oversaw a curriculum reorganization that instituted a mandatory intramural program for all cadets on top of the foundational training all Fourth Class cadets received through Koehler's system. All cadets learned to play baseball, football, basketball, soccer, lacrosse, track, tennis, golf, and hockey in six-week periods that culminated in intramural competitions. Cadets received grades for their participation and performance that contributed to their all-important class ranking, thereby formally incorporating sport as a requisite and essential element of officer education. MacArthur also expanded the Academy's intercollegiate athletics program by adding several teams and taking controversial steps toward instituting the recruitment of athletes. Even Koehler endorsed the Academy's growing embrace of athletics as an adjunct to individual physical training, arguing that "participation in athletic competition is the best school for leadership, self-discipline and team work."[50] But as before, Koehler qualified his support on the basis of his belief that the Academy was more capable than other institutions of resisting the evils often associated with intercollegiate athletics.

However, athletics did not become an integral part of systematic physical training in the wider Army as they did at West Point. Echoing elements of the official physical culture existing before World War I, the two activities were generally considered to be associated and complementary, but they were not effectively integrated. Allen voiced this in his stadium dedication speech in 1925 when he noted that "official recognition" had long been given to disciplinary drill while athletics had "subsisted solely through the interest of its devotees."[51] Raycroft had explicitly recognized and encouraged the relationship between physical training and athletics, but the Army's physical training system in the interwar period did not. *Training Regulation 115-5* and the *Basic Field Manual* of 1936 recommended that leaders dedicate some time to mass athletics, which could include competitive athletics, but these manuals were primarily concerned with other forms of training. Athletics came under the purview of athletic officers, who were not necessarily the same individuals that led comprehensive unit physical training.[52] With the demise of the Physical and Bayonet Training School, no centralized institution certified individuals in the management of a comprehensive physical training program. Army policies also tended to regard athletics more in terms of recreation than training.[53] So while athletics remained a prominent part of Army life, the Army's official physical culture generally disaggregated training and sport. Raycroft and his team tried to harmonize physical training, athletics, combat sports, and more in a single program oriented toward maximizing the individual's combat efficiency. In the interwar years, this comprehensive program fractured. The bonds between physical training, sport, and activities such as bayonet training weakened. By the mid-1920s, the Raycroft interregnum in the history of the Army's physical culture closed.

While systematic training in the Army reverted to its nineteenth-century roots, other changes in the Army's physical culture were afoot. Unlike in earlier periods, much of this change is best understood by considering first what officers *were not* discussing—namely, the basic value of physical training. Between the last quarter of the nineteenth century and America's entry into World War I, professional military journals regularly featured articles or letters to the editor concerning physical training. Some reflected doubt in the force at large as to the desirability of regular, systematic training. Most made a positive case, often while positing a regimen or program. All implicitly or explicitly took a position on the value of exercise. After World War I, articles on physical training largely disappeared, even from the *Infantry Journal*, as the subject became more accepted and less controversial. Major General Allen's dedication speech for Fort Benning's Doughboy Memorial Stadium in 1925 illustrated this widespread acceptance throughout the Army: regarding physical training and athletics as "fundamental elements of all military training" was "no new doctrine," Allen asserted, and they did not belong among the "many fads that have sprung up in our service like mushroom growths."[54] Allen's comments directly contradicted the common assertion of an earlier generation that physical training was a dangerous fad best avoided. Though officers wrote less about whether to exercise or how to exercise, they did not forget physical training. Instead, they turned their attention to *who* should exercise and leveled a finger at the young American male. After World War I, a discourse of declension concerning the population's physical fitness manifested in American society. Associations between physical fitness and a concept of citizenship defined by obligations intensified. The Army's official physical culture became a part of this discourse. Its definition of fitness provided the ends for numerous physical training and education advocates, many of whom both inside and outside the military endeavored to appropriate the Army's methods for civilian use. In short, these advocates averred that America's youth must be "prehabilitated" for future service because the health and strength of the body politic depended upon the health and strength of the individual citizen.

The declension discourse largely emerged from concerns over draft rejection rates that were widely perceived, in both military and civilian circles, as being alarmingly high. The first thorough statistical analysis of draft rejections, authored by Charles Davenport and Albert Love under the surgeon general's supervision, appeared in print in 1920.[55] Both men had worked for the office of the surgeon general during World War I compiling anthropometric data on draftees. Using this data, which local draft boards and camp physicians collected on more than 2.5 million men enlisted during the war, Davenport and Love found that approximately 46 percent of the recorded population presented a defect of some kind.[56] The report's authors divided the deficiencies into eleven groups ranging from "mechanical" ones involving bones, joints, hands, and feet to "nervous and mental" issues and venereal disease. Recognizing that not all were equally important, Davenport and Love broke the defects down into five categories established by draft and military officials during the war, two of which totally prevented the draftee from serving in the military.[57] Counting only those totally rejected, and not those qualified for limited duties,

Davenport and Love found that about 12 percent of all men examined were rejected for military service.[58]

Prior to the Davenport and Love analysis, and as early as 1918, much larger draft rejection figures began circulating, which were often cited in the declension discourse over the two following decades. Most of these pegged the rejection rate at about one-third of drafted men, which clearly counted more than just those completely rejected for service.[59] Extrapolating from these rates, commentators alleged a serious problem in American society with national power implications that bordered on crisis. For instance, Walter Camp, the Navy CTCA's athletic director and "Father of American Football," wrote that the war revealed the "flower of our racial stock" to be largely "deficient physically when put to the test before examining-boards."[60] The most immediate concern was of a military nature. Great powers needed to be able to field armies numbering in the millions to fight and win industrial-era wars. The vast majority of those soldiers would be conscripts, and conscripts represented a broad cross-section of the nation's manpower. Nearly all men were liable for service and, as the logic went, therefore obligated to maintain a baseline of physical fitness. Additionally, commentators linked defects disqualifying men from military service to the quality of the nation's labor force and the individual's ability to live a full life.[61]

A guilt-laden sense of crisis was particularly acute in the civilian physical education community. Thomas Storey expressed these sentiments in an address to the American Physical Education Association in April 1919, claiming that the war had "heartlessly, relentlessly and with calculating accuracy" revealed the quality of America's peacetime physical education.[62] Noting the "army of young men" rejected for service, and using the 30 percent rejection rate, Storey harangued the American educational system for failing to teach hygiene and make students' bodies fit for the "supreme obligation of citizenship."[63] The University of Minnesota's John Sundwall advanced a similar argument about how the wartime experience demolished the myth of an America comprising a "superhealthy, superstrong, and superactive and vigorous people."[64] Sundwall, like Storey and others, laid much of the blame on the US educational system and urged colleges and universities to "accept their share of responsibility" and to "do their part in the physical regeneration of America."[65] Dudley Sargent, one of the venerable old fathers of physical education, lent his voice to the chorus too. In Sargent's opinion, schools had not done enough to develop in American youth the "physical, mental, and moral qualities" that make good soldiers. Echoing concerns that drove the development of physical training in the Army and university a generation earlier, Sargent argued that physical educators had a duty to offset the deleterious effects of urbanization, industrialization, and undesirable immigration.[66] They seemed to have fallen short.

Serious concerns about the educational system having failed American youth and the nation spurred searches for solutions. One set of solutions followed from a common critique about the narrowness of prewar physical education in terms of both populations and subjects. According to conscription statistics, some regions of the country produced more defective men than others. Statistical imbalances existed between socioeconomic classes as well. As a remedy, many educators called for making physical education more accessible to everyone and, if possible, mandatory. For instance, George Fisher argued during the Athletic Research Council's annual meeting in December 1919 that the physical education community had to capitalize on the "tide of popular sentiment" for physical preparedness. Harnessed, such a tide could bring compulsory training to all schoolchildren, and even to the workplace.[67] This movement gathered steam. States "vied with each other," in the words of one observer, through the 1920s to pass physical education legislation.[68] By 1934, thirty-seven states had mandated physical education as part of their students' general education.[69] Physical education advocates also argued for the broadening of curricula because many men were rejected due to venereal disease and other problems that could be reduced or eliminated through hygiene instruction.

Another point on which most critics of physical education agreed was that the military seemed to have succeeded where civilian institutions had failed. Such assessments tended to overlook the fact that the military population contained only those who had passed entrance exams. The military population would therefore naturally appear more fit than the wider population. Nevertheless, the military's training system came in for frequent praise. For instance, the YMCA's James McCurdy, who spent time overseas with troops during the war supervising and directing recreational activities, wrote that "no man could have observed the Army . . . without having a deep impression of, and an overwhelming pride in, the deeds of valor of the American soldier."[70] McCurdy credited much of this to the Army's ability to cultivate "physical efficiency" in its troops. In this, McCurdy believed that the Army "did a marvelous piece of work."[71] Similarly, Fisher claimed that the US Army deserved credit for producing between three and four million soldiers who were "in better condition than any similar number of men have ever been at one time in the United States."[72] Such sentiment existed in the popular imagination too. One ditty making the rounds in the nation's newspapers in 1921 promised not only that the Army functioned as a melting pot for ethnically diverse American youth, but that it built *men*:

> Have you heard of our Army's slogan? We shout it—THE ARMY BUILDS MEN! / We care not for features, they're all of God's creatures, they go to the "melting pot." Then / watch for the change that comes o'er them, / Are these the young lads whom you knew? / They are hearty and hale, each a red-blooded male, / That's what our Army can do. / Deep-chested, square-shouldered and active, / Erect and with twinkling glance, / Straightforward and true, we return them to you, / These boys but needed the chance.[73]

Reciprocal relationships between civilian physical education and Army physical training were especially evident during World War I and in the immediate postwar period. These relationships modified the Army's physical culture, but they also informed the search for solutions to perceived shortcomings in the physical education community. In 1917, the Army had called on civilian educators to help expand, improve, and man the institution's physical training system. In doing so, Raycroft and his peers advanced a concept of using multiple activities, ranging from hygiene training and recreational athletics to disciplinary drill and boxing, to achieve higher-order educational outcomes. A few short years later, civilian educators looked to the Army as a guide and inspiration, believing that the Army had achieved a remarkable success in rapidly building healthy young men. No sooner had the war concluded than civilian educators began discussing the application of the Army's model to improve childhood education. Given the distress over draft rejections, qualification for military service also became something of a standard for physical education outcomes. Wartime experience and Army successes also contributed to a renewed emphasis on training for citizenship within the physical education community.

Looking to the Army as a guide and inspiration for reforming civilian physical education convinced some educators and school administrators to borrow its pedagogies, but these efforts met with mixed success. In a positive example, systems created to train large numbers of recruits yielded effective practices for primary and secondary schools. The Commission on Training Camp Activities' (CTCA) boxing training program provided a particularly useful case study in this regard. Schools did not suddenly start teaching children to box, but educators derived methods of mass instruction to teach the fundamentals of other sports to large bodies of students.[74] However, not all attempts to align civilian and military practice were embraced as widely. A more controversial effort that arose from a misunderstanding of the Army physical culture's nature and context saw physical education replaced with military training, usually marching drill and the manual of arms, to prepare pupils for immediate service. After the war, some high schools and colleges continued permitting military drill in place of physical education.[75] The leading luminaries of the physical education profession opposed such policies, arguing that drill could not possibly replace the many activities needed to promote holistic student growth and development.[76] For instance, Springfield College's James McCurdy opposed drill because it was too narrow and did not address problems identified by examination boards that could only be remedied by health and hygiene programs. McCurdy also believed that drill did not promote all-round individual improvement or the cultivation of "vigor" needed to meet the demands of modern war.[77] Military authorities also opposed drill in school. Secretary of War Newton Baker did so explicitly in 1918, arguing that school-time drill contributed very little to the nation's military strength.[78] Echoing McCurdy, Col. F. J. Morrow, a General Staff officer responsible for education and special training, argued that drill alone could not "provide an adequate course of physical training."[79] Military training could supplement physical training, but not replace it. The positions taken by senior Army officials highlight how much the Army's physical culture had changed since the 1880s. Earlier, elder officers opposed systematic exercise and sport as wasteful—even dangerous—fads, and considered incidental training through drill and duty sufficient. By 1920, senior leaders had embraced the utility of systematic physical training, even if their conceptual horizons remained fixed along Koehler's lines.[80]

Resistance from physical educators to the use of drill and the manual of arms in schools also reflected how their wartime experiences reinforced earlier trends in physical education's prevailing philosophies. Specifically, these educators cautioned against blindly importing practices such as drill from one context to another when searching for solutions to American society's perceived declension dilemma. They urged peers and school administrators to instead consider the specific needs of a given population and the broad array of tools and practices available, and then tailor programs to those specific needs. A report authored by Raycroft in 1918 titled

Suggestions for Colleges from the Army Experience of Physical Training captures this approach perfectly. In it, Raycroft recalled that he and his team tackled the Army's physical training problem with open minds, seeking only "those things which would give results in training recruits."[81] The basis for such a search had to be "straight thinking" that discriminated between "*exercise* and *training or education*."[82] This differentiation was also key to making improvements in college physical education according to Raycroft. What he meant was that too often Army officers and college faculty members alike regarded physical training as either purely for exercise or purely for recreation, and thereby lost sight of the educational value possible with the proper utilization of physical training activities.

Physical educators aligned with this thinking tried taking to heart a lesson from the Army's wartime experience about the need for tailored, educative approaches. Raycroft exemplified this movement in seeking to maximize physical training's educational value by applying a broad range of means in new ways to enhance mental, physical, and character development.[83] He expressly advocated using intercollegiate athletics rather than abolishing them, for instance.[84] These ideas also reflected the powerful influence of educational developmentalism at the time, which endorsed holistic student growth in order to mold young pupils into creative and critically thinking individuals.[85] Educational developmentalists, like Raycroft, often critiqued ossification and narrowness in pedagogical practice and school curricula. One could nearly always identify and integrate new ways and means to educate students, they argued. In one discreet example, the National Education Association's James Rogers critiqued some educators of the postwar decade for placing too much stress on health education instead of integrating the many other activities residing under physical education's big tent.[86] What is notable here in respect to the reciprocal relationship between civilian and Army physical cultures is that the two moved in opposite directions in some ways during the postwar decades. While civilian educators looked to the wartime experience and saw cause to expand, enlarge, and integrate activities, the disaggregation of activities came to characterize the Army's interwar physical culture.

While physical education and the Army's official physical culture diverged in regard to system comprehensiveness in the years after World War I, they initially converged on the importance of training the American public for citizenship. At this time and in the declension discourse especially, military authors and physical educators defined citizenship mainly in terms of military service obligations.[87] Thus, citizenship was predicated to a large degree on fitness. In turn, fitness meant a baseline of strength and endurance, along with an absence of health-related disorders and deformations. In the immediate postwar years, educators and military leaders alike counted the population's physical fitness as a leading consideration in national preparedness and contended that improving the population's health and fitness could not wait for the emergency of a future war.[88] In such an emergency, limits existed on what the military could do with the material the nation gave to it, even with an excellent training system. Improving the military's raw human material before it arrived at examination boards was therefore crucial, and that improvement had to come through the education system or new programs targeting American youth. As Colonel Morrow had reasoned in 1919 at the APEA's national convention, no efforts directed toward promoting the "average citizen's" fitness could be successful "unless they begin with the boys and youth of the country, in order to mold them during the plastic period of life."[89] In short, building men's bodies for battle necessitated their prehabilitation years before they might be called to service.

Prehabilitation's prominence in physical fitness discussions within the Army signified a major change in the service's physical culture during the interwar years. Content with the sufficiency of their service's training system, Army leaders turned outward. Compared to previous decades, discussion in professional journals centered less on *how* soldiers should exercise. Instead, the matter of *who* should exercise arose most frequently, and the "who" were typically young American men and boys theoretically liable to render military service with little forewarning. Civilian educators agreed for a time. However, by the 1930s they rarely explicitly connected military service and citizenship, or military fitness standards and expectations for physical education. For educators, preparation for good citizenship lost its martial flavor over time and increasingly meant social development and the "health of the entire personality."[90] Participation in a democratic society required social skills, a capacity for "self-expression and self-realization," education to make the best use of increasing amounts of leisure time, and the vigor and health to be happy and productive in a vocation.[91] Military writers agreed with much of this, though they emphasized discipline and stuck to an explicit, direct, and close linkage between preparedness for service and citizenship.

Few sites provide better opportunities to observe this tight linkage and the consequent application of prehabilitation than the Citizens' Military Training Camps (CMTC) program's dusty fields. The CMTC program, comprising three progressive, month-long summer training courses run by active-duty service members at military posts, was charged with improving national military preparedness while teaching attendees to be better citizens. Specifically, the CMTC was supposed to bring together a diverse lot of boys and young men, develop them "physically, mentally, and morally," equip them with some basic military training, and "teach Americanism in its true sense."[92] Those few who completed all three courses could become eligible for a commission in the Reserves. The CMTC was a direct outgrowth of the pre–World War I preparedness movement. Its leaders traced their heritage directly to the "Plattsburg Camps," which had grown into a system of Officers' Candidate Schools that operated between May 1917 and November 1918. Though technically created by the 1916 National Defense Act, the CMTC was not implemented until 1921. It remained in operation until 1940.[93] Twelve camps made up the CMTC system in its first year of operation, and together they graduated a class of nearly ten thousand.[94] At its peak in 1927, the CMTC operated fifty-three camps and graduated more than thirty-eight thousand candidates annually.[95]

While the CMTC was a weak substitute for the universal military training advocated by many officers and by groups such as the Military Training Camps Association, it afforded the Army an opportunity to perform prehabilitation.[96] Take the Red Course, for instance, which was the first of the three courses and the only one completed by a vast majority of candidates. Its program of instruction focused on basic infantry training, but physical training featured as a prominent subject and often occupied several hours of every boy's day. This physical training served a dual purpose according to the CMTC's creators, directors, and political sponsors. First, training improved every candidates' fitness, thereby preparing them for service and correcting deficiencies that might otherwise "impair their worth as citizens of the nation."[97] Second, training produced fit candidates who would carry "right standards of physical life" back to their communities upon graduation.[98] Graduates inculcated with knowledge about and a proclivity for exercise could spread the gospel of physical training to multiply the effects of each camp's prehabilitation efforts. This latter argument had long been a common component in the linguistic toolkit of the military's systematic training advocates.

The rhetoric around physical training in the CMTC's programs of instruction illustrates dominant philosophies about prehabilitation's need and nature within the US Army. In the Red Course manual, the physical training chapter opened with an infographic map of the United States in which each state's shade corresponded to its percentage of drafted men who had passed entrance examinations during the last war. Some basic analysis accompanied the map, pointing out differences such as the relatively better health of rural populations, native-born youth, and the Midwestern states.[99] Though the manual's authors did not use the language of crisis when discussing draft rejection rates, they did make a point about the cost of wastage using a bit of sensational napkin math—a population of one hundred thousand native-born youth would yield thirty-five hundred more soldiers than an equivalent population of foreign-born youth, and a thirty-five-hundred-man regiment "stopped the last German drive on the Marne."[100] The logic may have been shaky, but the implications were clear: improvements in the American public's general fitness meant more soldiers for the battlefield, and even marginal change could make all the difference. The CMTC's textbook also echoed many ideas and much of the language from a small book from 1920 written by the textbook's lead author, Col. P. S. Bond. In that book, Bond made an even greater claim about the value of military prehabilitation: the nation's "wealth, . . . strength and . . . happiness" rested on the health and vigor of its citizens.[101] Physical training and health education for martial service therefore laid a foundation not just for national military power but for America's basic social, political, and economic well-being.

Comprehensive prehabilitation called for more than exercise, however, even if its promoters limited most of their rhetoric to the virtues of physical training. The CMTC and other prehabilitation efforts appear to have taken this into account. After all, many of the defects that had disqualified men from service during World War I were not remediable by way of exercise. A close examination of draft statistics reveals that at least 47 percent of all defects concerned sense organs, "disease-groups" such as tuberculosis and venereal disease, developmental and metabolic complications, nervous and mental issues, and diseases of the nose, throat, skin, or teeth.[102] Even defects of the "mechanical sort," which comprised the plurality of defects at 39 percent, often had little to do with a lack of proper exercise.[103] The problem seemed to be chiefly one of health and hygiene. The CMTC's health program addressed these issues in several ways. For instance, attendees received examinations to identify problems that might otherwise have gone undiagnosed. Many also received treatment for those problems.[104] Additionally, the CMTC curriculum included preventative health training on issues ranging from basic oral hygiene to venereal disease. Daily life in the camps also taught healthy habits such as smoking cessation, eating in moderation, and keeping to a regular sleeping routine.[105]

Although one could argue, given draft rejection statistics, that health and well-being issues constituted the primary problem a prehabilitation program needed to address, the CMTC's curriculum chiefly emphasized physical training. Explaining this apparent gap between statistical reality and the persistent desire to sculpt young attendees' bodies through exercise requires a return to the definition of and value placed on physical fitness within the Army's prevailing physical culture. Since at least the 1880s, advocates of systematic training claimed several functions for exercise. First, it strengthened and improved bodies. In this, there were assumed corollaries with the remediation of physical defects, even if the linkages were not explicit. Second, training developed qualities beyond the physical. Koehler's and Raycroft's cultures intersected on this, even if they differed on the qualities to be improved and the specific means to do so. Members of the Army therefore saw physical training as a potentially crucial tool in achieving prehabilitation's broader goal of making better citizens. The CMTC's overall mission was to develop young men "physically, mentally, and morally."[106] Physical training, as expressed and understood in the Army's physical culture, could address all three.

Beyond informing the purpose of physical training in the CMTC program, the Army's physical culture also informed the CMTC's system of physical training. That system largely mirrored practices in the Regular Army, though it differed on time allocation and some points of emphasis. Similarities included twice-daily sessions most days, one in the morning and one in the afternoon. As in the Army, morning sessions concentrated on calisthenic exercises and longer afternoon sessions afforded time for games or applied physical training. Morning calisthenics in the CMTC system simply combined the basic setting-up drill from Koehler's earlier manuals executed in formation with, if the instructor wished, quick-time marching. This corresponded with the Army's "Recruit Course," which was an introductory series of exercises that prepared soldiers for more advanced work.[107] Though the morning calisthenics were supposed to "accomplish an all-round development in which each muscle is properly developed," the CMTC curriculum allotted just twenty minutes to morning drill.[108] In reality, only minimal gains in muscular strength and endurance could be expected from such sessions. However, the stated object of physical training included three other goals that physical training simultaneously addressed: building mental alertness, filling candidates with "enthusiasm," and providing discipline.[109] These latter goals accorded with the aim of training candidates for good citizenship, which CMTC authorities associated with discipline and "habits of obedience, dependability, [and] respect for proper authority."[110] Koehler labored for decades to inculcate these qualities in soldiers and cadets. As he had often asserted, and as the authors of the CMTC textbook continued to assert, physical training was a means to those ends.[111]

Afternoon mass athletics and group games differed sharply from the practices of the Army's earlier physical culture. However, this unabashed embrace of sport aligned with Army life in the interwar years. A plethora of stadiums, gymnasiums, and playing fields sprouted at US Army bases in the 1920s and 1930s. Sports featured prominently in most soldiers' lived experiences.[112] Daily life in the CMTC was no different. In contrast to the twenty-five minutes allotted for calisthenics, the standard CMTC schedule included at least three hours of athletics daily when not on the range conducting target practice.[113] Off-duty recreational events offered even more opportunities to compete. According to the recollections compiled by historian Donald Kington, athletics were a highlight of many CMTC candidates' time in the camps—more candidates recalled their time on the playing field than in the morning drill formation.[114] The CMTC's leadership also seems to have viewed sports as an effective tool for marketing the program to potential candidates. For example, the vast majority of illustrations in Bond's promotional book *Your Boy & the Other in Universal Training* featured uniformed individuals playing sports or posing with sports paraphernalia.

In contrast with contemporary Army practice, diversity typified the opportunities available in these afternoon sessions. Many activities were of the sort organized by the CTCA's wartime athletic directors. In fact, the CMTC textbook directed instructors to use Raycroft's *Mass Physical Training* section on group games.[115] Such activities included variations on tag, relay races, and ball-throwing games. Mass athletics were even more popular than these group games. Units within each camp organized teams for baseball, volleyball, and other games that competed against one another in tournaments and, on occasion, against local civilian teams. Sports involving one-on-one competition were also available. Former candidates recalled boxing being the most popular, though more enjoyed spectating than fighting. Beyond its programs of instruction, the emphasis placed on athletics within the CMTC was also apparent in the large amount of space sports occupied in camp yearbooks and in the numerous medals and awards distributed at graduation to recognize accomplishments on the playing field.[116]

The privileged place of sport in the Army's premiere prehabilitation program deserves some extra elucidation, especially given the concurrent disaggregation of training activities in the Army's physical culture. One explanation has to do with timing. Movement toward creating the CMTC began in World War I's immediate aftermath. Its creators drafted much of the program's curriculum in 1920 and 1921 when Raycroft's training system still existed in institutional memory—*Mass Physical Training* was published in 1920 and the Physical and Bayonet Training Course at Benning had recently graduated two classes of instructors. Clearly the CMTC's creators knew of Raycroft's new manual because they cited it as a reference in their own text.[117] In its conceptual integration of athletics and other activities into a comprehensive system of training, the CMTC curriculum reflected the Army's prevailing physical culture at the time of its creation. Objectives sought by the CMTC program also provide an explanation. Because recruitment was an immediate concern, the CMTC's promoters used sports as a means to entice young men into the program. Sport's prominence also helped smooth concerns some parents felt about sending their sons to military training. Athletics haloed sites of combat preparation in a softer summer camp glow. As an officer familiar with the program observed, one of the CMTC's goals was to assure the American public that "military training does not mean militarism."[118] The CMTC's core mission of providing training in citizenship was more significant, however. The desired product was a good citizen eligible for service, not a soldier. Given prevailing ideas in military physical training and civilian physical education, sports were considered better able to cultivate the desired characteristics of a citizen than was drill, bayonet training, or gymnastics. Sports could make physical activity attractive in a way that drill could not. Athletics were more likely to encourage healthy lifelong habits, even after candidates returned home. Also, physical educators maintained that sports developed qualities beyond the physical. Through participation in organized athletics, candidates might also learn social skills and how to put their leisure time to wise use. According to this line of argument, "the man who goes in for sane, healthful and clean recreation is always a good citizen" because he "works the same as he plays—fair, clean and above-board."[119]

Beyond the CMTC, other prehabilitation efforts and citizen-making initiatives arose in the 1920s and 1930s that focused on different populations but pursued similar ends. One in particular responded to the ravages of the Great Depression, which created grounds beyond World War I draft statistics for concern about the health and vitality of young American men by the mid-1930s. The effects of the Great Depression were devastating for many Americans. Malnutrition and sickness took a heavy toll on the many unemployed families. The effects were so severe that even when given work through New Deal programs and other sources, many men had difficulty performing that work.[120] Perceiving simultaneous economic, masculinity, and ecological crises, President Franklin Roosevelt created the Civilian Conservation Corps (CCC) by signing Executive Order 6101 on April 5, 1933.[121] Over the following nine years, more than 2.9 million single and unemployed young men in the CCC would plant trees, build roads, fight fires, construct bridges and dams, and stock streams.[122]

Although explicitly founded as a civilian agency sensitive to the period's dominant mood of antimilitarism, the CCC became an unintentional site for martial prehabilitation. In large part, this owed to the War Department initially taking a lead role in organizing and administrating CCC camps. The Roosevelt administration tasked the War Department with inducting hundreds of thousands of CCC enrollees, screening them for medical conditions, and moving them to camps. Initially, Regular Army personnel also served as the camps' leadership cadre. By July 1933, more than three thousand officers and five thousand enlisted men of the Regular Army served in these capacities.[123] Subsequent concerns about this mission's impact on military readiness later led to a sharp reduction in direct military involvement. Within two years, officers of the Organized Reserve Corps acting in a civilian capacity had mostly assumed duties as camp commanders and CCC enrollees themselves took over the roles once held by Army noncommissioned officers and enlisted men.[124] Despite the War Department's declining involvement, the CCC bore many marks of military influence. For instance, enrollees learned to maintain neat uniforms and living areas, and to live in a regimented organization. The model of masculinity endorsed by the CCC was also highly compatible with military service.

At root, the CCC was, to borrow a term from Christina Jarvis, a "man-building agency."[125] Because the period's dominant form of manhood encompassed several ideals, man-building proceeded along multiple lines of effort. First, man-building taught the value of productive work and equipped men with the skills necessary to find such work in order to realize a bread-winner ideal. As the organization's second director remarked, when an enrollee planted twenty-five thousand trees, he "feels like a man."[126] Second, man-building taught proper social behavior and instilled desirable character traits. This line of effort's primary goal was to fashion better citizens and prepare men to become husbands and fathers. Traits targeted for cultivation included strong work habits, discipline, a love of clean living, self-reliance, tolerance, and attachment to family and religion.[127] Third, man-building involved health interventions and self-care education. For example, enrollees received immunizations and physical exams in addition to being taught good dental hygiene practices and how to avoid venereal disease, among other lessons. This emphasis on health education aligned well with concurrent trends in civilian physical education. Finally, man-building involved building up and sculpting men's bodies. The CCC celebrated changes in enrollees' physical appearances time and again through both text and photographs. Where more than 75 percent of enrollees entered the CCC at weights below Army standards, only 4 percent left a year later at substandard weights.[128] A year of hard work, clean living, and good eating sent men back into society with "more weight on their bones, more strength in their backs and arms, and more hair on their chests."[129]

Man-building in the CCC contributed to the project of prehabilitation desired by physical training advocates in the Army, even if direct Army influence on the CCC waned rapidly after 1933. As a site of prehabilitation, the CCC was less explicitly designed to prepare young men for military service when compared with the CMTC. Yet the CCC did seek to improve the physical, mental, and moral fitness of potential future soldiers along lines advocated by Army officers in prehabilitation programs. The CCC's physical culture differed from the Army's in the interwar period in that it put less emphasis on cultivating discipline and obedience. Instead of the hour of drill and physical training soldiers were supposed to experience daily, CCC enrollees performed for only fifteen minutes.[130] CCC enrollees were strongly encouraged to participate in afternoon athletics, however, much like CMTC attendees. This, combined with the strenuousness of their work, hardened bodies and imparted lifetime fitness skills.[131] Health education and character development similarly seemed to promise a way to raise more men to basic enlistment standards, thereby reducing draft rejection rates in a potential future conflict.

The Army's physical culture underwent change in the two decades following the First World War, but not necessarily in the way that its wartime athletic directors had hoped. In general, the Army's physical culture reverted to its prewar form as the dual pressures of institutional inertia and cultural memory squeezed out the CTCA-developed body of theory and practice. However, wartime experience had confirmed the value and utility of both systematic physical training and athletics. No longer did Army officers question whether or not soldiers should exercise. No more accusations of dangerous faddishness turned up in the discourse about physical fitness within military circles. Instead, conversations reoriented on new bodies outside the military in need of conditioning. New programs manifested in part from that discourse to export the Army's physical culture in the name of prehabilitation for potential soldiers.

Inside the Army, physical training remained a part of the daily experience for most soldiers during the interwar years, but the form it took hearkened back to prewar practices. The movement toward aggregation central to Raycroft's physical culture reversed course. While a central school at Camp Benning run mostly by former members of the defunct CTCA Athletic Division kept their pedagogy alive through 1919, it proved unable to survive the harsh budgetary environment in an era of normalization and antimilitarism. Even Raycroft's book, *Mass Physical Training*, succumbed to these pressures and failed to achieve official standing within Army doctrine. Though the Infantry School continued promoting an integrated system of physical training through the 1920s, neither it nor the Physical and Bayonet Training Course exercised sufficient influence to effect permanent change in the Army's physical culture. Instead, control of that culture's central texts reverted back to West Point, where Koehler's influence persisted even after his retirement in 1923. The resulting physical training regulations of 1928 echoed the *Manual of Physical Training* of 1914 in a remarkable example of organizational inertia's power. As a consequence, emphasis returned to drill and discipline. Athletics remained a major part of most soldiers' lives, but they were no longer integrated with drill and other activities into a coherent, overarching training system. In place of the individual warrior, the disciplined cog in a military machine returned as the physical culture's ideal product.

In contrast with the reversion to earlier philosophy and practice, prehabilitation was a new feature in the Army's physical culture and the discourse surrounding it. Prehabilitation seemed vitally important because of anxieties about the fitness of American men that spun out of unexpectedly high rates of draft rejections between 1917 and 1918. The seeming need for prehabilitation grew over time, fueled in part by beliefs held by members of the military and the civilian physical education community that the military had succeeded in sculpting fit bodies and minds where the educational system had failed. Warfare in an age of industrialization and mass conscription compelled states to maximize the percentage of their male population eligible for conscription. Especially within the military, citizenship came to be defined chiefly by the obligations one owed, especially military service. Given this schema, every male citizen had an obligation to become fit and healthy because every male citizen was theoretically liable for combat duty on short notice. Calls for universal military training to ensure that men met this duty withered on the vine in the years immediately following World War I, but other sites for prehabilitation emerged. One, the CMTC, connected directly with preparation for military service. Another, the CCC, was less explicitly militarized, though it touched the lives of many more men and ultimately served as an unintentional paramilitary training agent in the 1930s. The Army's physical culture influenced physical training in both. However, both emphasized athletics at the expense of more formal training in the interest of developing qualities associated with good citizenship and instilling a lifetime interest in healthy activity.

By the close of the 1930s, the men most responsible for shaping the Army's physical culture had jettisoned or forgotten most of the lessons learned through experience in World War I. Many military and civilian authorities had turned more attention to building up the bodies of American men in both real and symbolic terms, especially during the Great Depression's ravages. Yet as war once again loomed in 1940, concern resurfaced about the adequacy of Army physical training and the Army's organizational capacity for the production of trainers. That year, Brig. Gen. Lewis Hershey, director of the Selective Service, warned Regular Army officers to be prepared for an influx of draftees whose physical quality would be lower than that of the recruits they had been receiving.[132] A familiar challenge returned. In the event of a mass mobilization, could Army physical training prepare men for the demands of expeditionary warfare on the modern battlefield? Would the Army's physical culture and its associated system prove adequate?

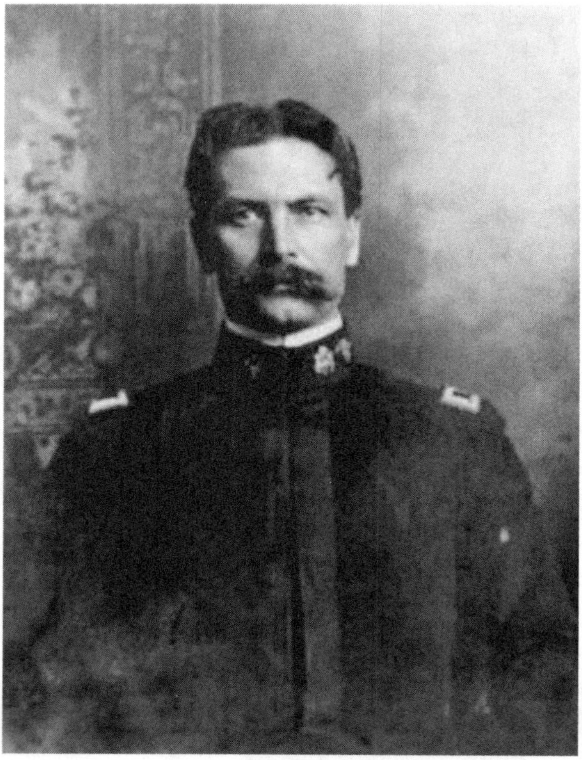

Herman Koehler, pictured in 1904 as a captain, became known as West Point's father of physical education. Arguably, he was also the US Army's. Courtesy of the United States Military Academy collection.

ARM. 17

3. Circle arm, or arms, inward. Fig. 17*a*.
4. Circle arm, or arms, outward. Fig. 17*b*.

5. Circle right arm backward and left arm forward.

6. Circle left arm backward and right arm forward.

Command: 1. *Arms forward*, 2. CIRCLE.

Execute from position of *arms upward*.

At command *circle*, swing the arms around in as large a circle as possible, keeping them fully extended and the hands tightly closed.

Continue by repeating *One, two*.

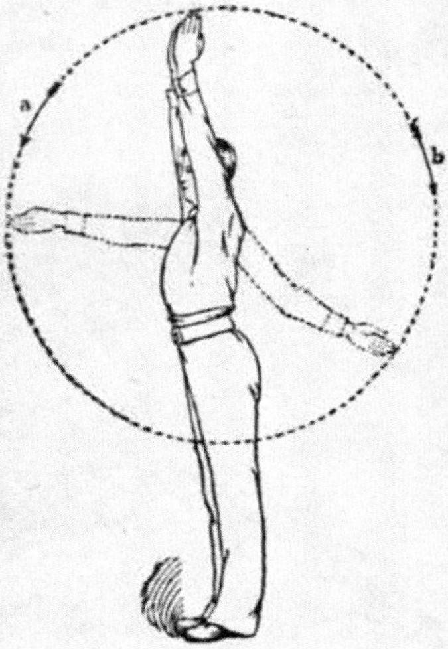

Fig. 16.

VII. FUNNELING.

1. Funnel arm, or arms, forward. Fig. 18.

2. Funnel arm, or arms, backward.

3. Funnel right arm forward and left backward.

4. Funnel left arm forward and right backward.

Command: 1. *Arms forward*, 2. FUNNEL.

Continue by repeating *One, two*.

16200——2

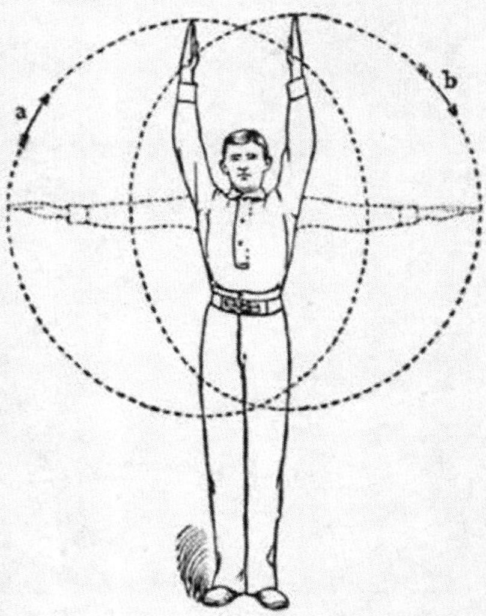

Fig. 17.

The light-work gymnastics system Koehler created for cadets appeared in his *Manual of Calisthenic Exercises*, published in 1892. This page is typical of the diagram-text pairing used to explain exercises.

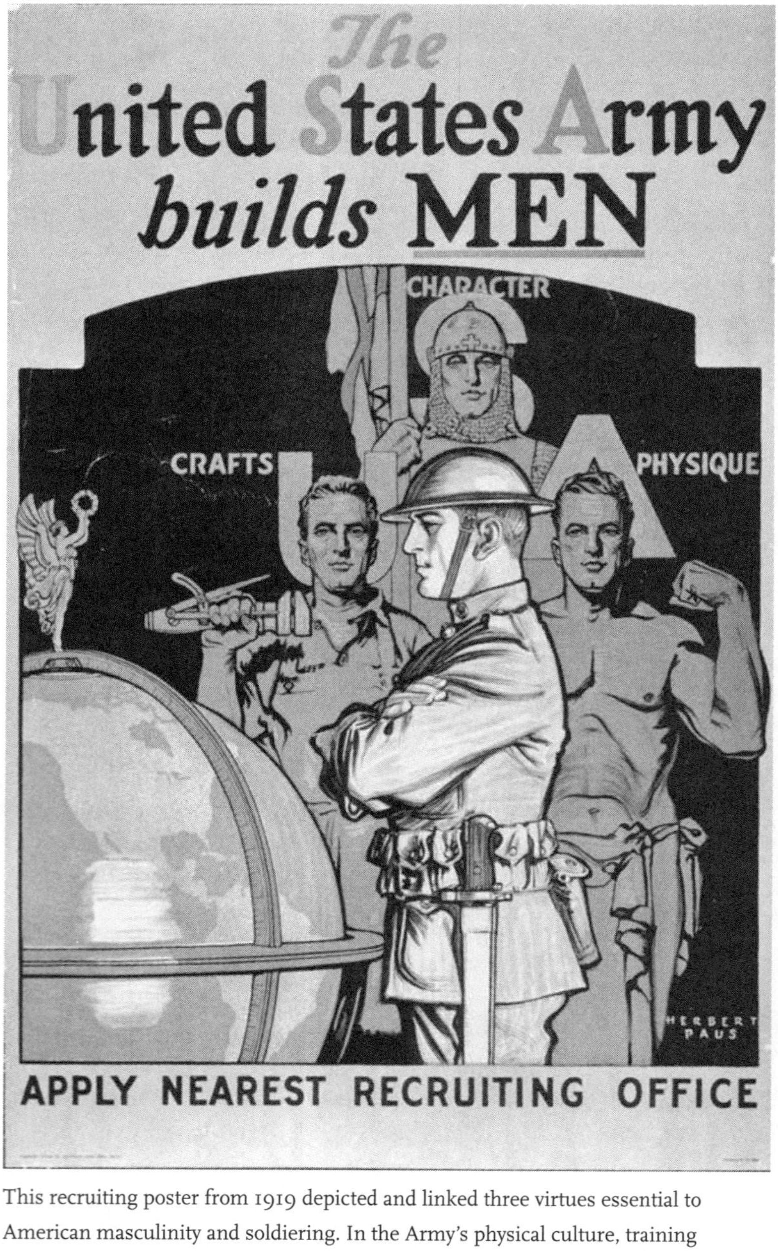
The
United States Army
builds MEN
CHARACTER
CRAFTS
PHYSIQUE
HERBERT
PAUS
APPLY NEAREST RECRUITING OFFICE

This recruiting poster from 1919 depicted and linked three virtues essential to American masculinity and soldiering. In the Army's physical culture, training supposedly cultivated character and physique. It addressed overlapping projects of man-, citizen-, and soldier-making.

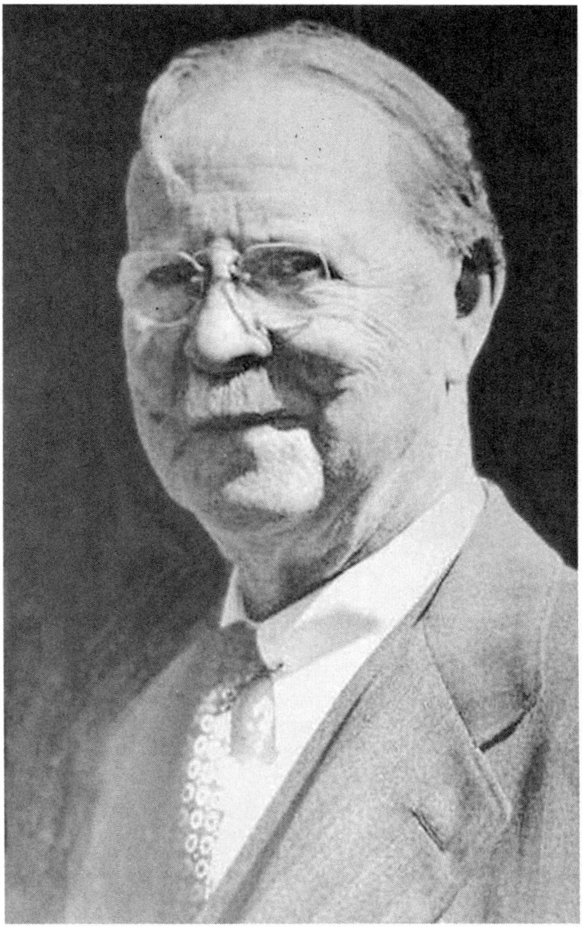

Princeton University's Dr. Joseph Raycroft led the Commission on Training Camp Activities' Athletic Division during World War I. Under his leadership, the Athletic Division's civilian members reshaped the Army's physical culture along functional fitness lines. Courtesy of the Seeley G. Mudd Manuscript Library at Princeton University.

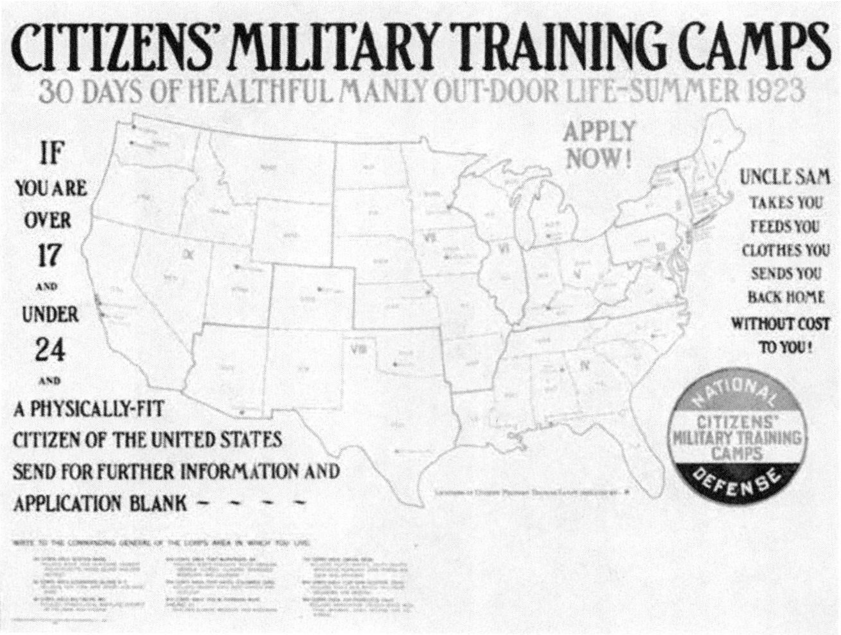

The Citizens' Military Training Camp program was an early prehabilitation effort that responded to the high draftee rejection rates during World War I due to physical shortcomings.

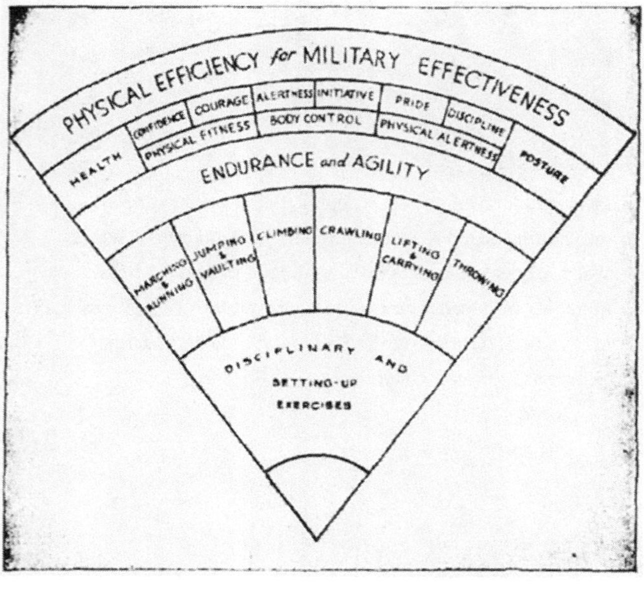

The Basic Field Manual 21-20 of 1941 visually depicted the Army's concept of fitness for the first time, but it differed little from Koehler's. Discipline was the foundation of fitness. Intangible mental qualities followed from physical exercise.

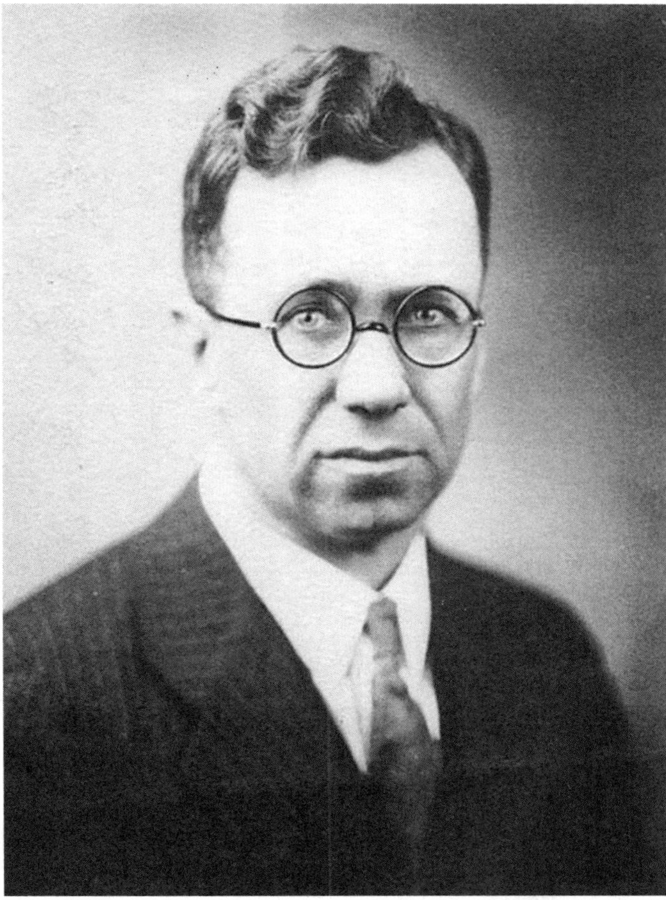

During World War II, the University of Iowa's Dr. Charles McCloy pioneered the use of individual physical performance standards derived from statistical analysis. Permission from Mr. William McCloy, grandson of Charles McCloy.

40 **PHYSICAL CONDITIONING**

1. GROUND EXERCISES

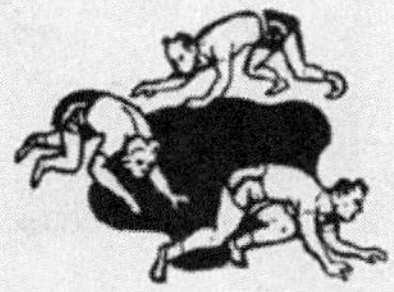

Fig. 23

a. **All fours.**—Face down on hands and feet, walk forward.

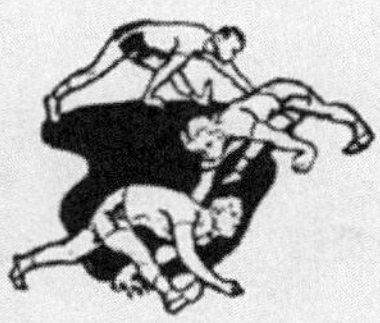

Fig. 24

b. **Bear Walk.**—Face down on hands and feet. Travel forward by moving the right arm and right leg simultaneously and then the left arm and leg simultaneously. Keep knees straight.

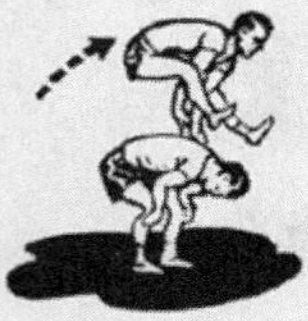

Fig. 25

c. **Leap Frog.**—Count off by twos. At start, odd leap over even numbers. At next start, even numbers leap over odd. The men go clear around circle until they return to original position. Men bending should face forward.

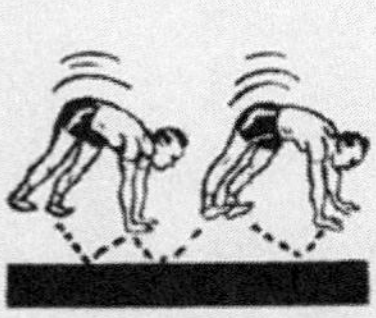

Fig. 26

d. **Bouncing Ball.** — Support body on hands at shoulder width, feet apart, back and legs in line, knees straight. Travel forward by means of series of short upward springs of hands and feet simultaneously. (Bounce hips up and down.)

Mass testing in 1942 revealed specific fitness needs. Theodore Bank, Charles McCloy, and their team addressed them with a revised system in *Training Circular 87*, published in 1942. Guerrilla drills were among the additions. Raycroft's manual of 1920 included similar exercises.

48 PHYSICAL CONDITIONING

2. **Go—stop.**—At the command **GO**, the men spring forward as a football team would do in running signals. At the command **STOP** they stop and drop to the lineman's crouch. At **GO**, they again sprint forward. This may be varied by the command **FRONT** which means to go to the ground on the stomach. If the command is **RIGHT**, they turn and spring to the right at an angle of about 45°. **LEFT**, in like manner, means to gō to the left. **GO** in each case means straight forward again. **TO THE REAR** reverses the direction. Keep this up for at least 5 minutes.

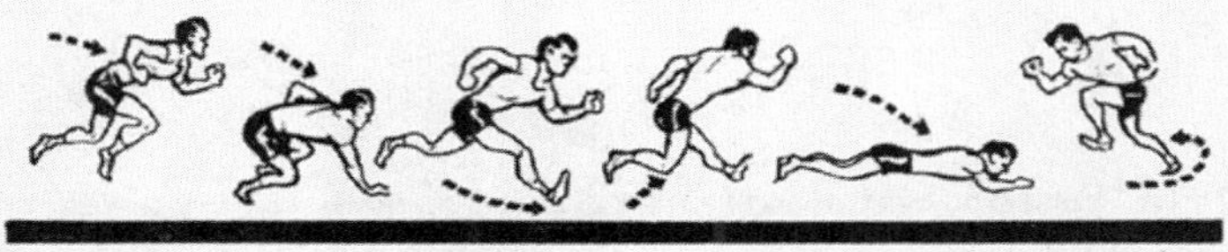

Fig. 53

3. **Zig-zag run and flop.**—The men, upon the signal to go, run fast about 45° to the right, and when the whistle sounds again, zig-zag 45° to the left, and on a second, or two blasts of the whistle, flop to the ground. Upon hearing the next whistle, they spring to their feet and run rapidly to the right, continuing as above until commanded to halt. This may be by a long blast on the whistle. Continue for 5 minutes.

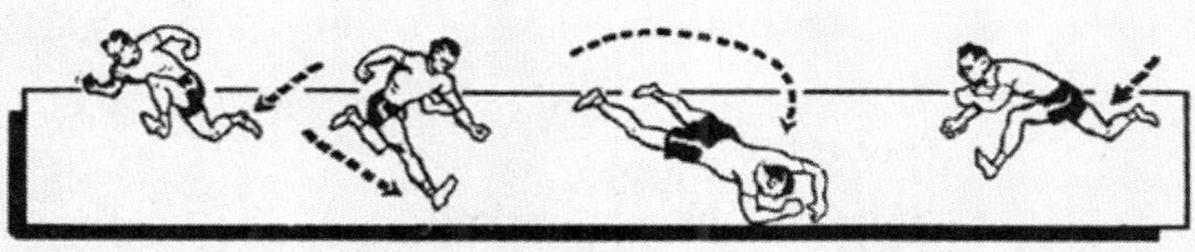

Fig. 54

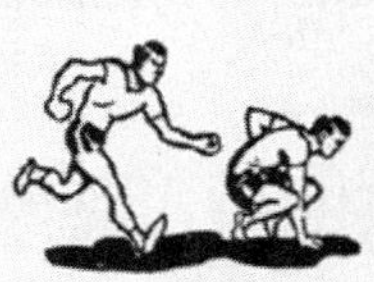

Fig. 55

4. **Zig-zag and squat.**—Same as (3) above, except on the whistle, instead of flopping to the ground, the men come to a full squat with hands on the ground. Continue for 5 minutes.

Grass drills, introduced in 1942, stressed soldiers' cardio-respiratory systems and trained them to move under fire.

2. BURPEE

a. Starting Position—Attention.
b. Cadence—Moderate.
c. Movement:
(1) Bend slightly at the knees and sharply at the hips; place hands on the ground in front of the feet in a squat position with the elbows inside the knees.
(2) Thrust feet and legs backward to a front leaning rest position with body straight from shoulders to feet, weight supported on hands and toes.
(3) Return to the squat position.
(4) Resume standing position.

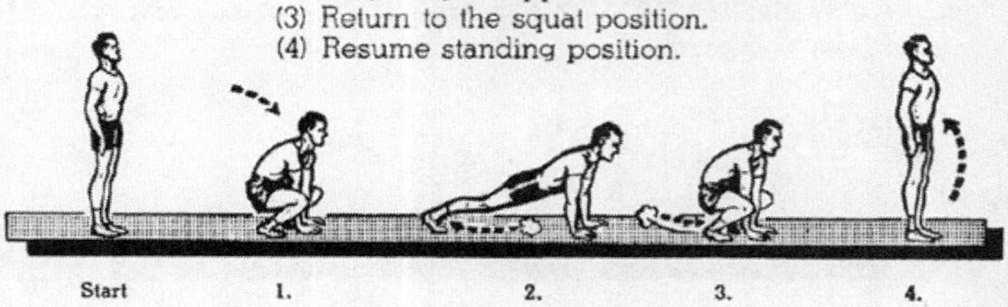

Fig. 8

The BURPEE is one of the best exercises to develop agility. It reaches and strengthens primarily the muscles of the trunk, thighs and hips. It also serves as an additional warm-up exercise.

3. SQUAT BENDER

a. Starting Position—Standing with feet slightly separated and arms in a loose thrust position.
b. Cadence—Moderate.
c. Movement:
(1) Full squat, thrust arms forward, fingers extended, palms down, keep trunk erect.
(2) Return to original position.
(3) Bend forward sharply, thrusting downward with fingers touching toes if possible, knees straight.
(4) Return to starting position.

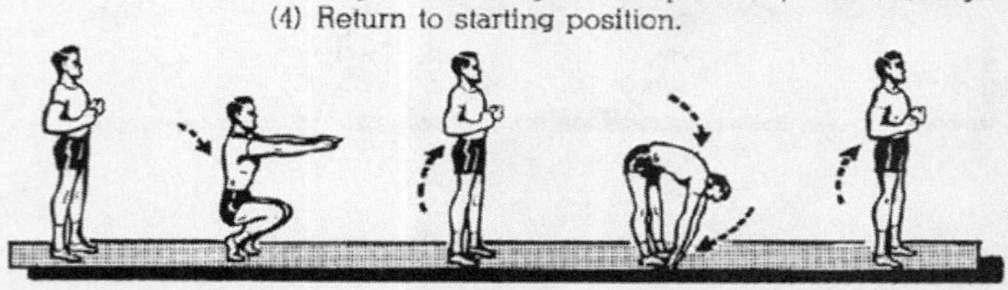

Fig. 9

The SQUAT BENDER strengthens the heavy muscles of the legs and thighs as well as the trunk forward-bending musculature. It has excellent postural benefits. When the knees are kept straight in the forward bend the exercise has a limbering and loosening effect upon the hamstring muscles.

Calisthenics remained fundamental in *TC 87*. Soldiers executed most of the same exercises in the same formations as had their forebears fifty years before.

74 PHYSICAL CONDITIONING

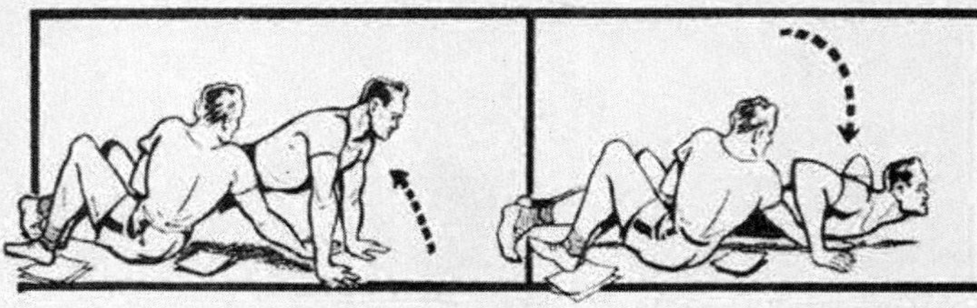

Fig. 96

5. **100 Yard Pick-A-Back.**—In this event, a person of approximately one's own height and weight is carried in pick-a-back fashion for a distance of 100 yards. A difference in weight of 10 pounds is permissible. After the men have been paired off, they line up with the one who is to ride immediately behind his partner. Upon the command "Get Set" or "Riders Mount," the rear man mounts astride his partner's back. The carrier **must** grasp and continue to hold his partner's legs with both arms from the outside. The rear man should keep his chest in close to his partner's back. He should avoid swaying to the side or leaning backward. If the pair should happen to fall during the first 75 yards of the race, they should not attempt to continue, but should run in a later heat. If they fall in the last 25 yards, the judge may estimate the time.

It is helpful to have the runners perform this event in lanes. Each runner must have a judge who records the time which is called out by the timer. Immediately upon finishing, the runner walks straight back to the finish line and gives his card to the judge for scoring. After the card is scored, the pair returns to the starting line (outside the running area) where they reverse their original positions. As soon as one heat crosses the finish line, the next should be started.

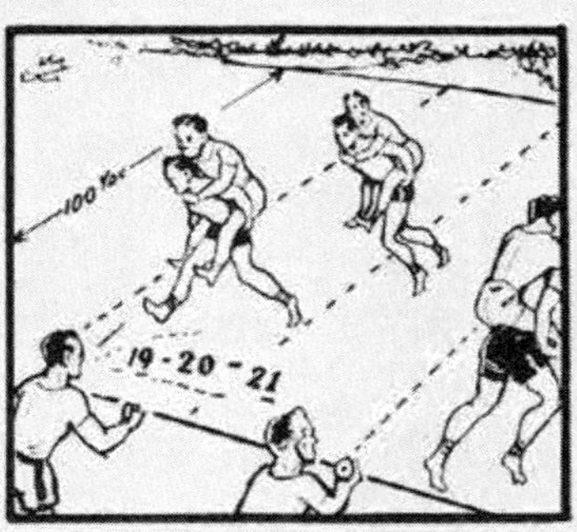

Fig. 97

In timing this event, the timer calls the seconds aloud, emphasizing the syllable marking the second; for example, eight**een**, nine**teen**, twenty-**one**, twenty-**two**. If the man crosses the line just as the second is called or immediately after-

Efficiency testing did not exist in the Army's physical culture apart from in Raycroft's system. That changed in 1942. *TC 87*'s authors labeled testing an "integral part" of any training program because it enabled leaders to diagnose shortcomings and prescribe remedies.

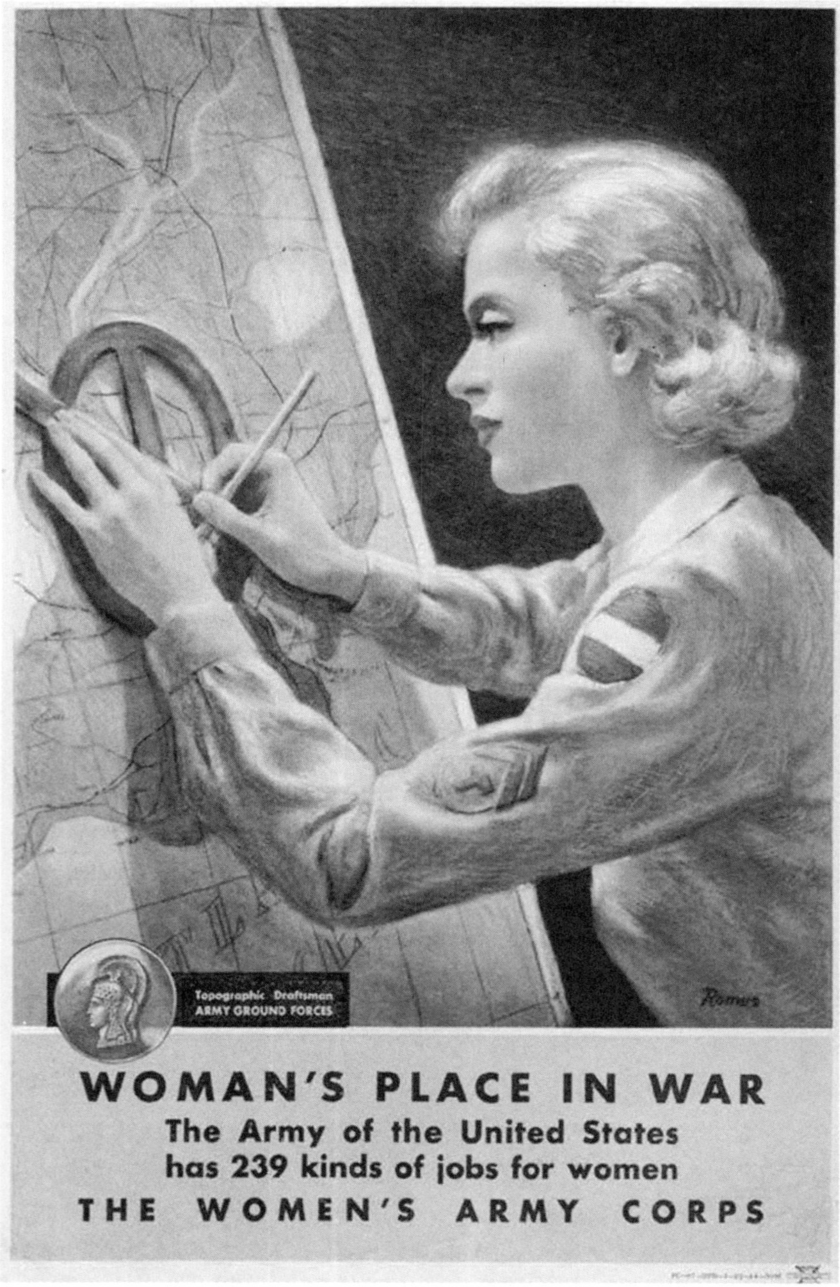
Topographic Draftsman
ARMY GROUND FORCES
WOMAN'S PLACE IN WAR
The Army of the United States
has 239 kinds of jobs for women
THE WOMEN'S ARMY CORPS

WAAC and WAC service members challenged the Army's physical culture because it centered on combat readiness and masculinity cultivation. This poster series made clear that a "woman's place in war" had nothing to do with combat or physically demanding labor.

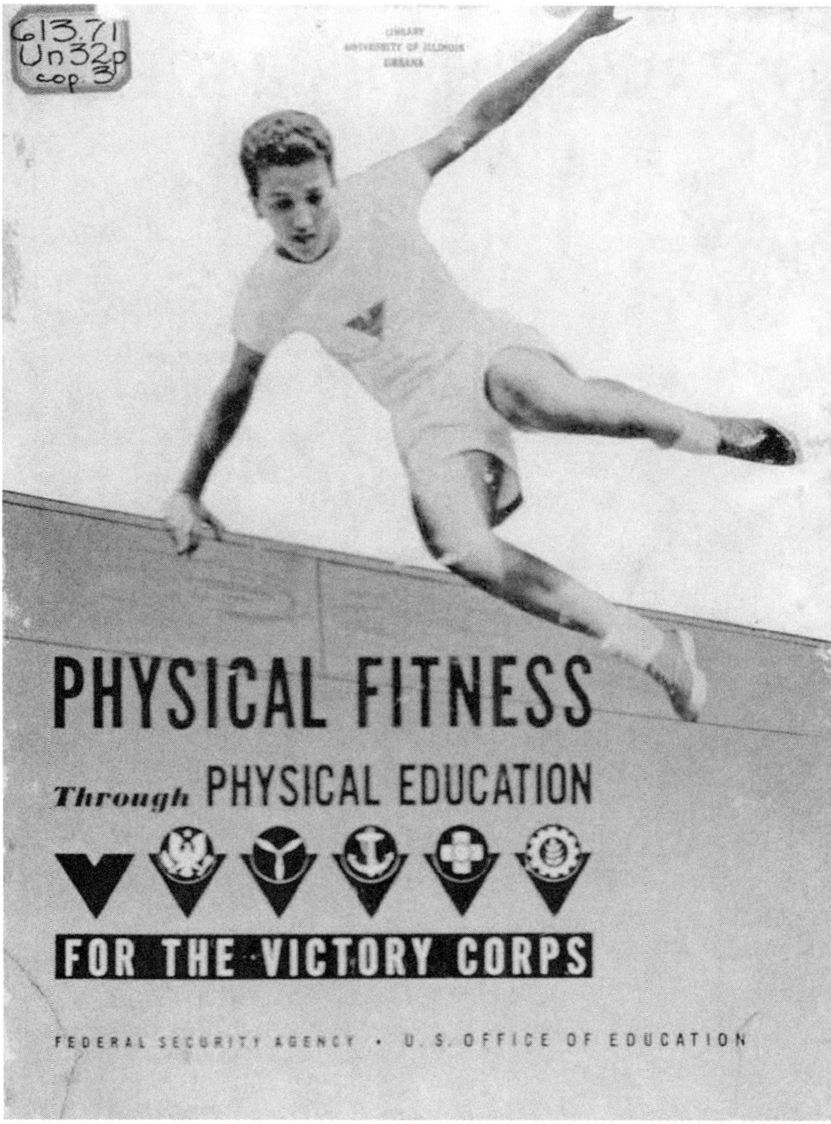

The Victory Corps aimed to improve the fitness of potential service members while in high school. This manual for educators offered guidance on systematic physical training and athletics.

OVERWEIGHT IN GRADE?

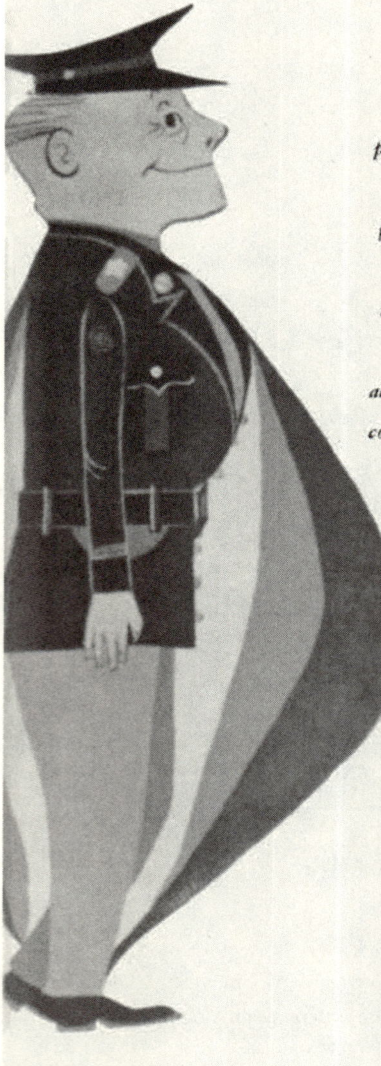

"It is a military duty for all officers and men to maintain a high level of physical fitness as a requirement of their profession. An Army man must be physically fit to perform his duties with maximum efficiency, either in peace or in war. He needs to be physically fit so that, by presenting the model of an alert, ready fighting man, he will inspire confidence as a leader in his subordinates and as a guardian of the peace in his fellow citizens."

General Maxwell D. Taylor

My name is Major Pear Shape. Yes, I'm overweight in grade. I am one of those miserable souls who converts all food to a bulge. I just naturally have difficulty keeping in good physical condition. I entered the Army as a private during World War II because no arm or service would commission a 24-year-old with my outsize dimensions. I remember overhearing the physical examiner (as I sat outside the thin partition with other perspiring would-be's), "I understand we have another obese one today. I want to have a look at him." One look was enough. "Lose 45 pounds and your other qualifications for a commission will be considered."

By Maj Albert E. Lockhart

Overweight and obesity were new problems in the 1950s. Consequently, nutrition and body composition became components of fitness. For officers, new policies required physical fitness evaluations in efficiency reports.

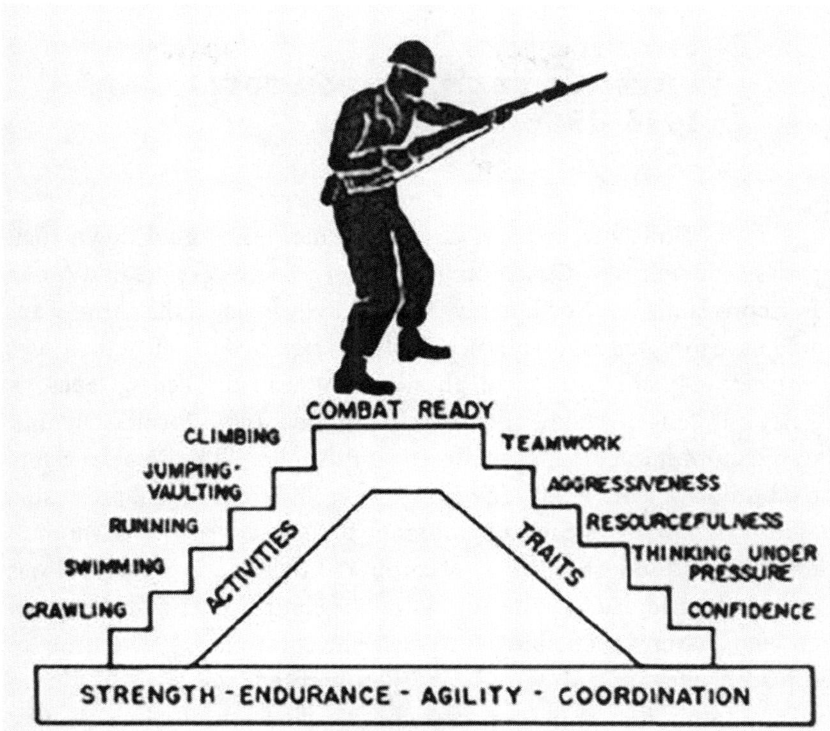

Technical Manual 21-200, published in 1957, framed fitness as readiness for infantry combat, deemphasizing athletics.

CHAPTER FIVE
PHYSICAL CULTURES FOR TOTAL WAR, 1936–1946

While American soldiers and marines ground down their Japanese opponents on Guadalcanal, and mere days before the first American troops landed in North Africa, John B. Kelly insisted that Americans would have to "toughen up physically" if they expected to defeat their Axis enemies.[1] Kelly, the director of physical fitness in the Federal Security Agency's Defense, Health, and Welfare Division and a former Olympic rower, communicated his desire to effect this toughening in a speech to the Columbia Teachers College's Institute on Physical Fitness, promising that his division's forthcoming program would make America's youth fit for combat and industrial work. According to Kelly, such a program was long overdue and had been delayed by public complacency and Congressmen who "haven't been able to see their shoes for years."[2] The time for complacency had ended. World War II's unprecedented scale and near-absolute nature demanded the extensive mobilization of whole peoples and economies. While the sheer quantity of manpower, materiel, and production mattered enormously in determining the war's outcome, quantity alone was not sufficient for victory. As historian Peter Mansoor writes, the "relative quality" of forces was "crucial to the ultimate outcome."[3] Systematic physical training appeared to Kelly and others to be a way of addressing both the war's quantitative and qualitative demands—better physical education and training made a greater proportion of the population fit to fight, and fitness enhanced the efficiency and effectiveness of military forces.

In seeking to improve American manpower, the nation's leaders faced many challenges in the realm of physical fitness that would have been familiar to their predecessors in 1917 and 1918. Beneath each challenge lay doubts about the quality of America's raw human material that had lurked since the late nineteenth century. Such qualms were seemingly confirmed by high draft rejection rates in World War I and then reinforced by millions of men falling short of Selective Service standards in the early 1940s. Consequently, when Kelly bluntly stated, "everybody is too soft," he gave voice to concerns shared by many American military officers.[4] Within the Army, the mechanisms available to address fundamental doubts about the population's fitness had originated in a physical culture chiefly attuned to the needs of a small, late-nineteenth-century force. That physical culture had changed little since Koehler's days at West Point other than the near-total acceptance among officers of systematic physical training's value. In fact, the Army's physical culture and associated training system had largely reverted to the old Turner model in the interwar years. Additionally, no central school had survived to research new practices or rapidly produce a larger pool of expert trainers. In short, the Army's physical training challenges resembled those it faced during mobilization for World War I: a huge influx of personnel deemed to be of lower quality because of state-determined physical defects or poor physical fitness, a physical training system best suited for maintaining minimum unit fitness and instilling discipline, and the Army's inability to rapidly expand its instructor corps.

As it had in World War I, the Army's official physical culture changed during World War II in response to that conflict's conditions and demands. A cadre of service members and civilians in the Special Services Division of the Army Service Forces chiefly drove this change. These reformers reoriented physical training with two objectives in mind. The first was practical preparation for combat activities, such as lifting heavy objects and moving rapidly over broken terrain. The second was producing measurable physiological outcomes while contending with the fact that mobilizing an army of millions inevitably depressed average recruit fitness levels. Although uniformed officers were responsible for physical training to a greater degree than they had been during World War I, civilian outsiders once again took the lead in reengineering the Army's physical training system. These civilians applied scientific methods, empirical data, and some of the latest trends in physical education to craft a system geared more than ever toward generating physiological outcomes alone. Meanwhile, a second official physical culture emerged with the introduction of women to military service through the Women's Army Auxiliary Corps. The perceived need for an alternative physical culture and its advent illuminated the fundamentally gendered, infantry-centric nature of the Army's primary physical culture. Consequences following from a gendered physical culture remain with the Army today, complicating the full integration of women into military service.

With war clearly looming in Europe, American political and military leaders in the late 1930s increasingly turned attention to planning for mobilization. Some of their efforts culminated in the passage of the Selective Training and Service Act in September 1940, which established the first peacetime draft in the history of the United States. The draft's induction processes applied physical standards as key screening criteria. In the Army, responsibility for determining those physical standards resided with the Surgeon General's Office, which drew on experiences acquired during World War I and subsequent planning for mass mobilization to craft Mobilization Regulations (MR) 1-9, "Standards of Physical Examination During Mobilization."[5] Issued on August 31, 1940, these regulations governed physical evaluations by draft boards until DSS Form 220 refined them in December 1941. MR 1-9 established high physical requirements because it was based on plans for an Army that was much smaller than that required by World War II.

High standards generated shocking shortcomings once inductions began. However, the depth of public anxiety does not appear to have equaled that of the period of 1917–1918, perhaps because the World War I–era shortfall still existed in living memory. The induction process included a layered examination scheme that applied the MR 1-9 standards, and later those of MR 1-9's successors, to identify men fit for service and screen out the rest. The Selective Service System, which Congress authorized on September 16, 1940, oversaw inductions, but local boards conducted the initial examinations. Men found fit for service then underwent examination by Army medical boards to receive a final determination of physical qualification. This system evolved between 1940 and 1945 to minimize the redundancy in dual examinations and to bring Army and Navy standards closer together, but the two-part process held throughout the war years.[6] Between November 1940 and August 1945, this system examined an estimated 17,954,500 for induction into military service.[7] The American public was surprised to learn that, prior to the United States entering the war in December 1941, rejection rates ran as high as 50 percent. Of the approximately two million men examined in 1941, nearly a million were rejected, and 45 percent of those were rejected for physical or mental defects.[8] Health authorities grew concerned with the "serious state of ill health among American youth" when statistics became public in late 1941.[9] Though few sounding the alarm over national physical fitness made note of it at the time, "physical defects" and "mental deficiency" were capacious categories. Many conditions ranging from musculoskeletal or cardiovascular defects to varicose veins or hemorrhoids could disqualify a man physically.

The significance of these rejection statistics was subject to some debate in the public discourse of the time. Some government officials were prone to stoke fears of national physical unpreparedness, echoing the post–World War I crisis engendered by draft rejection rates of around 30 percent. For instance, the Selective Service System's director, Brig. Gen. Lewis B. Hershey, declared that the rejection of approximately 45 percent of the first two million men examined for induction was "an indictment of America," and a "condition of which we nationally should be thoroughly ashamed."[10] Similarly, the Federal Security Agency's administrator and chairman of the Manpower Commission, Paul McNutt, opined that the proportion of registrants rejected for physical defects was "rather alarming" and that the "inevitable conclusion is that our reservoir of physically qualified man-power is disappointing."[11] Others sounded alarms outside the government, too. The *New York Times*'s Luther Huston, for example, wrote in April 1941 that the "outstanding lesson which the experience of six months has taught" was that "the collective health of young American manhood is not what it should be."[12] Different voices, especially those in the medical and physical education communities, expressed doubt about the statistics signaling a widespread crisis. Many skeptics pointed to the fact that American physical standards used for induction examinations in the early 1940s were more stringent than those of 1917–1918 and those used by other nations.[13] Critics also observed that detecting instruments had grown more effective since 1917, making the screen's filter finer than ever.[14] Hershey acknowledged these factors but argued that Americans still had cause for concern. Even considering the higher physical standards of 1940, Hershey claimed that "the fact remains that while we may be no worse now than twenty-four years ago, we seem certainly to be no better."[15]

The armed forces' voracious appetite for more and more men between 1940 and 1945 constantly pressured the Surgeon General's Office and Selective Service System to revise standards, examination procedures, and other elements of the induction process. Induction of "limited service" men was among the first steps taken in this direction. This policy took effect on August 1, 1942, and permitted the intake of men with physical defects in twenty categories, ranging from men with 20/400 vision that could be corrected to 20/40 with glasses to those with the loss of one or both external ears.[16] The limited service policy acknowledged that not all men rejected earlier were incapable of rendering military service. As one commentator put it in a marvelous machine-age metaphor, "only a small proportion of the rejected men were like jalopies which can only wheeze along a little longer before they stop for good." Instead, he maintained, most were "like cars in which the radiator is leaky, or the rubber worn off the tires in spots, or the battery low, or the valves pitted and noisy, or one of the sparkplugs cracked."[17] Cars with defects could still be of value, or, if repaired, driven for a time within a set of constraints. Similarly, men with defects could still be of value to the military. Downward revisions in standards and the introduction of gradations to those standards acknowledged that "fitness" was not a binary measure of fit or unfit.

Personnel policies further refined service classifications throughout the war years, thereby permitting the exploration of opportunities opened by discarding binary categorizations of ability. For example, Lt. Gen. Leslie McNair of the Army Ground Forces (AGF) championed a physical profile system beginning in 1943 that rated men in six elements of physical conditioning.[18] Reception centers began employing this physical profile system experimentally in February 1944, and it became fully operational in June 1944. Under this system, physical examinations rated men in each of the six elements along a four-point scale. McNair intended to use these physical hardiness measures as signs of fighting capacity, and then to make them the primary criterion of assignments as a way of improving combat troop quality. Accordingly, the AGF staff coded every enlisted job in the ground forces and related service branches based on physical requirements to set minimum physical standards for each duty position in each type of unit. For instance, a basic standard existed for all buglers, but buglers in infantry units were held to more stringent physical requirements than buglers in field artillery units. However, these standards were based on estimates generated by the AGF staff instead of quantified measures of combat's physical demands.[19] Standards also did not correspond strongly with conditioning, but were instead based on criteria that screened for physical defects. As always, the difficulty of quantifying combat's physical demands in a standard way challenged every measure of fitness, each of which was necessarily subjective. In addition to new service classifications, the federal government also explored opportunities following from broader conceptions of fitness by launching initiatives to rehabilitate some men. For instance, a major pilot program announced in October 1941 paid physicians and dentists to remediate physical defects found in two hundred thousand men identified by local draft boards.[20] A mounting shortage of civilian physicians killed this pilot program in 1942, but the Army pursued rehabilitation through the rest of the war years by inducting limited-service men and remediating shortcomings.

Other visible manifestations of anxiety over the nation's health also emerged in the early 1940s in the form of government-sponsored prehabilitation publicity programs. These programs began small in October 1940 when President Franklin Roosevelt appointed John B. Kelly, an Olympic rower and medalist in the 1920 and 1924 games, to head the Civilian Defense Physical Fitness Program. Kelly initially struggled to make headway without funding or a staff, but his situation improved in August 1941 when Director of Civilian Defense Fiorello LaGuardia appointed Kelly the assistant director of civilian defense in charge of physical fitness.[21] Kelly built two coordination committees by mid-1942, one for schools and colleges and another to target recreational groups. A second element of Kelly's program, the Sports Board, co-opted celebrities such as Jesse Owens to promote physical fitness initiatives.[22] On April 29, 1943, Kelly's influence grew further when Roosevelt established the National Committee on Physical Fitness under the Federal Security Agency.[23] In every incarnation, Kelly's organizations were charged with stimulating state and local efforts, developing and distributing information and exercise programs, and popularizing physical fitness. None had direct control over actual training programs, nor did they influence the Army's physical culture. However, they helped push physical fitness and national health to the forefront of national consciousness and participated in the wartime militarization of physical education in American schools.[24] Kelly's work ultimately enhanced the influence of military prehabilitation programs such as the Victory Corps and Universal Military Training while contributing to postwar concerns about the nation's health in a competitive world.

The spin that Kelly's committees, Selective Service leaders, and others put on available statistics also contributed to national anxiety over physical fitness. Most frequently cited statistics had little to do with the average American man's muscular strength and endurance or his cardiovascular health. In actuality, the most common problems identified in examinations were "static" medical issues involving psychological health, dental defects, venereal disease, illiteracy, and hernias.[25] Critics, especially in the physical education field, pointed this out in the public discourse. For instance, one educator argued that "physical unfitness" was really a misnomer and that a new term such as "militarily unfit" might be more appropriate because, as an example, a man with a "malocclusion [an imperfection of dental alignment, such as an under- or overbite] can hardly be termed, by any stretch of the imagination, physically unfit."[26] Yet Kelly, Col. Leonard Rowntree of the Selective Service, Hershey, and others presented the issue as one remediable by exercise. Rowntree observed that "many of the registrants were found to be pampered, soft, flabby and in need of conditioning."[27] Similarly, Lt. Col. Theodore Bank, who largely assumed responsibility for Army physical training policy in 1941, argued on the basis of physical efficiency test results that the "lack of strength, endurance, agility, and coordination" in America's newest soldiers was "shocking."[28] Bank also asserted that the Army had been "sadly handicapped" in preparing troops for combat "because of the physical weakness of the incoming men."[29]

Even if the nation as a whole was not as "pampered, soft, and flabby" as Rowntree and others alleged, the Army did face a fitness challenge. Between 1940 and 1945 the service grew from a force numbering about 270,000 to one numbering more than 8,250,000.[30] A higher personnel intake coupled with an easing of standards meant that the average recruit's fitness was bound to decrease. Critics may have been correct that the nation itself was at least as healthy as it had been in 1917, but fitness levels across the service decreased while the force expanded, just as they had during World War I. How well equipped was the Army's physical culture to prepare millions of new soldiers for the rigors of modern mechanized warfare? And how would the experience of preparing those men change the Army's physical culture?

Perceiving change over time starts with understanding baseline conditions, and then unpacking vital physical culture elements as they emerged and transmuted over the course of World War II. Between 1940 and 1946, definitions of fitness and approaches to exercise programming evolved. So too did the means of preparing physical training leaders, the relationship between sport and systematic training, and the role of efficiency testing. Initially, the physical culture manifested, with a strong hint of Koehler, as a training system in the *Basic Field Manual*'s (*BFM*) fourth chapter, published in 1936. The *BFM* chapter was little more than a reprinted portion of *Training Regulations 115–5* of 1928, itself only a marginal modification of the Army's original manual from 1914. However, Army physical training transformed in the decade following 1936. An older culture that emphasized discipline, morals, and obedience gave way to a more comprehensive training program predicated on scientific experimentation, empirical data, and physiological improvement.

Spring 1941 brought the first evolution in doctrine, though minor, with an updated version of the *Basic Field Manual*, designated *FM 21-20*. Reflecting the demands of mobilization, the new manual paid more attention to the task of speedily turning recruits into trained soldiers. Responsibility for the update fell to the US Military Academy (USMA), signaling that institution's continued dominance over the Army's physical culture. Prepared under the direction of USMA's superintendent, Brig. Gen. Robert Eichelberger, *FM 21-20* presented a familiar program of exercise. Its purpose centered on producing "a state of health and general physical fitness" that permitted a soldier to "perform the arduous duties required of him." The "ultimate goal" of physical training was thus the "physical efficiency which is essential to military effectiveness."[31] While the system itself differed little from those that preceded it except for Raycroft's, the simple statement about physical efficiency being essential highlighted the acceptance physical training enjoyed throughout the Army. In the 1880s, many officers regarded physical training dubiously as a fad of questionable value. By 1941, physical training was a vital element in the transformation of a civilian into a soldier.[32]

The authors of *FM 21-20* graphically depicted physical efficiency as resting upon multiple layers of other qualities, skills, and activities. Disciplinary and setting-up exercises composed the base layer. These were intended to prepare soldiers "mentally and physically" for training in basic skills such as marching, running, jumping, climbing, crawling, carrying, and throwing.[33] Training to become proficient in those basic skills supposedly produced endurance and agility, which composed the next layer. Physical improvement and the awareness of it cultivated less tangible qualities such as confidence, courage, alertness, initiative, pride, and discipline underlying physical efficiency for military effectiveness.[34] Though graphically depicted for the first time and slightly reworded, this physical efficiency concept was not substantially different from the pyramidal construct Koehler used in the 1880s. Keeping with Koehler's prioritization of psychological outcomes derived from physical exercise, the authors of *FM 21-20* promised that the development of such qualities was "a certainty" that might "equal, if not surpass, the purely physiological value of the training."[35]

In pursuit of developing physical efficiency for military effectiveness in new recruits, the authors of *FM 21-20* made four small changes to the Army's interwar training policy. First, they added "disciplinary exercises" as a precursor to the old setting-up exercises. Practicing facings, rests, hand salutes, mark time marching, the position of attention, and the starting positions of setting-up exercises all fell under this header. Disciplinary exercises had "no particular value in physical development" but were still of "great importance in instilling in the men that sense of discipline which is necessary for the efficient conduct of the physical training instruction."[36] Second, the authors of *FM 21-20* urged commanders to construct obstacle courses to help soldiers practice skills such as running, jumping, vaulting, climbing, and crawling. The recommended course included a hurdle, four-foot fence vault, panel dodge, seven-foot wall climb, low crawl, six-foot ditch broad jump, and a balance beam. This bore a remarkable resemblance to the course recommended by Joseph Raycroft during World War I as both a "group game" and a physical efficiency test.[37] As had Raycroft, *FM 21-20*'s authors recommended progressively more difficult obstacle course challenges intended to first build technique, and then work up to timed runs under light combat loads.[38]

In addition to disciplinary exercises and obstacle courses, the authors of *FM 21-20* recommended physical efficiency tests with minimum standards for average men. Commanders could use these tests at regular intervals to determine the "condition and aptitude" of their soldiers in order to design physical training programs based on their men's strengths and weaknesses.[39] The recommended test battery included a hundred-yard dash, running high jumps, broad jumps, and push-ups. Fourteen other test options with minimum standards ranging from baseball throws to half-mile runs also appeared in *FM 21-20*. Like obstacle courses, physical efficiency tests featured in Raycroft's program but not in the *BFM* of 1936. However, Raycroft's test battery was more explicitly concerned with practical combat skills. In addition to a hundred-yard sprint and running broad jump, Raycroft had included fence climbs, obstacle races, grenade throws, bayonet drills, hand-to-hand fighting, boxing, and a smattering of athletic events.[40]

Finally, the authors of *FM 21-20* added a major chapter on swimming and life-saving techniques. Swimming had been a staple of West Point's physical training regimen since Edward Farrow's program begun in 1882 and featured in the Army's original manual of 1914, but swimming instruction disappeared in the World War I–era training systems and in postwar manuals. Citing the prevalence of "sub-marine attacks on troops ships" and "battles over flooded areas, and across streams and canals," the authors of *FM 21-20* argued that swimming had become a crucial skill all soldiers should possess.[41] The manual of 1941 set three general swimming goals: the ability to ford streams, participate in landing operations, and survive emergencies in the water. Soldiers met these goals by practicing six recommended activities: fundamental strokes, short-distance swimming with arms or legs alone, short-distance swimming under light combat load, fundamentals of water safety, life-saving skills, and "elementary experience" in competitive swimming.[42] As with obstacles, the principle of progression was to be observed in swimming instruction. Soldiers first learned basic techniques, and then they crossed greater distances while wearing more and more clothing and equipment.

More substantive change in the Army's official physical culture began appearing in early 1942 owing to the work of the War Department's Joint Army and Navy Committee on Welfare and Recreation and the Army Special Service's Athletic and Recreation Branch. The former was established in February 1941, nearly ten months before the United States entered World War II, to plan welfare and recreation activities for the services and to coordinate those activities with civil agencies. The committee resembled the Commission on Training Camp Activities from World War I in some ways. However, its mission was to study issues and advise the services on the provision of activities, not to take direct charge of activities. From its inception, the committee looked with interest on the services' physical training programs.[43] Its first initiative in this area was an appraisal of the physical fitness program in use at the Naval Training Station in Norfolk, Virginia. A team of six physical education experts, including Joseph Raycroft as the committee's chairman, conducted the study.[44]

Between January 19 and 24, 1942, the survey team held conferences with the Naval Training Station's leadership and physical training instructors, inspected documents and facilities, and observed operations. The station's program originated in May 1941 with the induction of twenty men trained in physical education who developed an exercise and intramural athletics program, and then systematized it for use in the Navy's service schools. In July, the station formed a school to run six-week courses that certified instructors to teach this new system. Initially, classes of twenty men formed every two weeks, but the quota increased to fifty students per class, with new classes forming weekly, in January 1942.[45] The survey committee assessed this Norfolk system on its ability to produce the men that the Navy professed to need: those possessing not just health, strength, and endurance, but also "mental alertness, discrimination, initiative, determination and other like qualities."[46] Two months later, the committee issued an extensive report for the Navy. Among the many recommendations was counsel to incorporate mandatory athletics, recreational sports, and systematic physical training into a comprehensive program. In this case, systematic physical training included calisthenics, running, obstacle and apparatus work, "self-defense activities," group games, relay races, combative contests, tumbling, and life-saving.[47] Additionally, the committee recommended an enhanced testing program to assess fitness and the appointment of a director of physical training with an expert staff to organize and direct a physical training program for the entire Navy.[48]

These features are significant because the basic structure of the recommended Norfolk program also appeared in updated Army policy and practice in late 1942. For instance, the supplemental mandatory and recreational athletic programs became major features in the Army's suggested system of daily physical training. So too did the diverse offering of calisthenics, grass drills, and guerrilla drills in regular conditioning periods. Later, the Army introduced a more sophisticated testing regime along the lines recommended by the Norfolk survey group. Transmission of thought and practice occurred chiefly through the Joint Army and Navy Committee on Welfare and Recreation. Following its study of the Navy program at Norfolk, the committee consulted with the Army Air Forces (AAF) in developing their program. Next, they opened communications with the Army to assist the Army Ground Forces. This collaboration appears to have begun between March and April 1942 when the Joint Army and Navy Committee transmitted a copy of the Norfolk report to the Army's Special Services Branch.[49]

Of the joint board's members, the University of Iowa's Charles H. McCloy proved especially influential in changing Army physical training doctrine. Born in 1886, McCloy studied at Marietta College, the Johns Hopkins Medical School, and Columbia University, earning his PhD at the latter in 1932. Before becoming a professor of physical education at the University of Iowa in 1930, McCloy taught physical education and served in the YMCA in China and the United States. McCloy built a strong reputation in the physical education community through his contributions to the scientific measurement movement in the 1920s and 1930s.[50] This movement worked to enhance physical education's standing and respectability by producing a scientific body of knowledge derived from carefully constructed and validated experimentation and measurement. McCloy brought this empirical research methodology to his work with American military forces during World War II, first as a member of the Norfolk study team and later in 1942 as a lead technical advisor to the Army.[51]

McCloy's efforts and those of other joint board members dovetailed with a concurrent movement inside the Army advocating physical training policy reform. This movement originated within the Special Services Division and was spurred by concerns about the "combat physical condition" of ground troops expressed by senior leaders.[52] The Special Services Division was a component of the Army Service Forces (ASF), a new organization officially created in the War Department on March 9, 1942, as a counterpart to the Army Ground Forces, though the Special Services Division itself had existed since 1941.[53] The ASF's mission required it to "provide services and supplies to meet military requirements" and to relieve the fighting arms of "the distraction and effort required by supply, procurement, and general housekeeping duties."[54] While the ASF's chief function was the purchase, storage, and distribution of supplies, the ASF also assumed responsibility over many other functions such as premilitary training, manpower mobilization, and the direction of morale, welfare, and recreation activities. The latter fell under the purview of the ASF's Special Services Division (SSD).

Stimulus for investigation and reform of Army physical training came chiefly from Lt. Col. Theodore "Ted" Bank, the SSD's Athletic and Recreation Branch chief. Bank was a decorated combat veteran who had enlisted in the Army in 1916 at age eighteen, had fought along the Mexican border and in France, had received a wound in combat, and had been awarded the French Croix de Guerre for his bravery.[55] After World War I, Bank attended the University of Michigan, where he starred as the football team's quarterback in 1920 and 1921. Bank subsequently enjoyed a successful career as a football coach at Tulane University and the University of Idaho, but he remained in the Army Reserves. In February 1941, the Army ordered Bank back to service as a Captain.[56] By the time his plans for testing the physical fitness of ground troops gained traction in early 1942, Bank had been promoted to lieutenant colonel. Within two years he achieved the rank of colonel.

Apprehension about the physical fitness of American soldiers came to Bank's attention in the spring of 1942. His first step was to seek an explanation for why soldiers were apparently falling short. Whether this was a case of recruits coming in to the service below standards, as Kelly's committees, Rowntree, and Hershey claimed, or due to regression after basic training seems to have been unclear. Bank, in partnership with the Joint Army and Navy Committee on Welfare and Recreation, set out to answer this question by testing the physical condition of a cross-section of ground troops. Bank proposed testing newly inducted men, soldiers who had recently arrived in an infantry division from a replacement training center, veteran infantrymen and field artillerymen from eight different divisions, veterans in two armored regiments, and veterans from three different parachute battalions. Ten exercises ranging from chin-ups to zigzag runs composed the test battery, along with measures of height, weight, chest expansion, and abdominal girth.[57] Bank received permission to conduct the tests from Army Ground Forces in mid-April 1942 and brought in three other men to form his team: statistician Abram Jaffre of the Special Service's Research Division, Arthur A. Esslinger of Stanford University's Department of Physical Education, and Charles McCloy of the joint board.[58] Making use of his experience in scientific measurement, McCloy served as the experiment's general director.[59]

Findings produced by this team soon informed a major revision to Army physical training policy. Between May 10 and June 4, Bank and his fellows visited eleven Army installations across the country and administered tests to more than five thousand troops. McCloy completed a preliminary statistical analysis by the end of June and shortly thereafter proposed test standards for the wider Army.[60] The ownership of responsibility for physical training policy revision was unclear, however. In April, the joint board had recommended that this revision take the form of a manual to be used by the Special Services Branch School when training its athletic officers.[61] Bank disagreed, arguing that responsibility for the manual should fall to the chief of the Special Service instead of to the school, and that the manual should be published as a technical manual for general use.[62] Bank's argument ultimately carried the day. The discussion of ownership illustrates some problems resulting from the Army's continued lack of a central proponent for physical training policy. Mass mobilization in the early 1940s had again exposed the need for a center external to the USMA that could manage research, doctrine publication, and compliance inspections, or at least one that could produce an expansible instructor-training pipeline. As his awareness of existing conditions grew, McCloy pulled no punches in characterizing physical training in the Army as "a terrible mess" and in need of someone at the top to "get the thing straightened out." McCloy perceived "a lot of jealousies" and "ambitious strivings for position" that resulted in ground troops "really getting nothing."[63]

Resolution of the central proponent problem, at least during the war years, came in November 1942 with the publication of *Training Circular (TC) 87*. The circular, authored by Bank's Special Service Division, aimed to precisely address the needs of Army Ground Forces troops uncovered by the summer's testing and data collection efforts. *TC 87* was grounded in empirical data and brought cutting-edge ideas about physical training to bear on the specific problem of readying troops for combat. As historian Whitfield East observes, *TC 87* and its "outcome-based" program made *FM 21-20* and its "process-based" program look outdated, even though the field manual was little more than a year old.[64] With *TC 87*, Bank and the ASF's Special Service Division asserted their control over Army physical training policy, and ultimately over the official physical culture.

Bank's team continued refining the Army's official physical training system and the policies codifying it throughout the war. Taken together, the changes they made represented the second significant wartime evolution of the Army's systematic-training-based physical culture since its late-nineteenth-century inception. After *TC 87*, Bank and his team next published *War Department (WD) Pamphlet 21-9* in May 1944 as an "illustrated amplification" of *TC 87*.[65] The pamphlet added some commentary about *TC 87*'s history and the necessity of physical training, plus illustrations of a variety of activities, but it did not substantively alter any part of *TC 87*'s system. When *WD Pamphlet 21-9* entered circulation, its creators were already at work revising *FM 21-20* from 1941. Publication of the new FM, which superseded the old *FM 21-20*, *TC 87*, and *WD Pamphlet 21-9*, came in January 1946.[66] The new manual represented a fuller expression of the *TC 87* system, though it also reflected more of the USMA's influence than did its immediate predecessors. Taken together, the three documents published between 1942 and 1946 modified the Army's existing physical culture in many ways, including a revised definition of fitness, a combat-readiness orientation reminiscent of Raycroft's World War I–era physical culture, an emphasis on scientifically determined and measurable outcomes, an integration of training and athletic activities, and leadership by a corps of trained amateurs.

Much of the change followed from a revised definition of fitness championed by McCloy, Esslinger, and Bank. As noted earlier, *FM 21-20* from 1941 presented "physical efficiency for military effectiveness" as its goal. Physical efficiency sat atop layers of qualities such as health, confidence, courage, and alertness. Those qualities derived from the bodily endurance and agility built by practicing basic physical skills such as marching, jumping, climbing, and crawling. Below it all lay a foundation of disciplinary and setting-up exercises.[67] In contrast, the revised concept of 1942 situated physical fitness as a component of "total military fitness," which was a composite of technical, mental, emotional, and physical fitness. Technical fitness referred to basic tactical training and the ability to employ arms and equipment. Mental and emotional fitness, or morale, involved a sense of mission, a will to fight, and healthy habits of thinking.[68] Physical fitness, according to the authors of *WD Pamphlet 21-9*, was "evidenced by a body which can retain normal responses to stimuli in the face of fatigue and exhaustion" and continue to "function effectively" under the many stresses placed on it by the "routine and emergency tasks of war."[69] Such bodies manifested five elements: freedom from disease and defect, strength, endurance (both muscular and cardio-respiratory), agility, and coordination.[70] Physical fitness in turn complemented the other elements of total military efficiency, entwining physical and mental health.

Combat framed this new definition. Each fitness element related to battlefield or combat support tasks, whether it be lifting heavy objects, persisting through fatigue, or exhibiting sufficient speed, agility, coordination, and flexibility to "handle oneself in tactical operations."[71] This fitness concept aligned with experiences of soldiers who had experienced fighting. In one survey from 1944 of infantry combat veterans in the European Theater, 84 percent or respondents stated that "taking regular calisthenics and setting up exercises" in training before being sent overseas was either "very important" or "somewhat important." Of that population, 80 percent said the same about the importance of "plenty of practice in going through a hard obstacle course."[72] This physical culture did not concern itself much with discipline and obedience, which also reflected contemporary thought in the physical education profession and Army officers' experiences leading conscripted citizen-soldiers in World War I. Rather, it aimed to optimize the individual soldier's physical capacity. Indeed, *TC 87* and *WD Pamphlet 21-9* explicitly concentrated on cultivating and measuring the individual soldier's physical capabilities. While *FM 21-20* from 1946 revived a few reminders about the need to improve the mass's total military fitness and to measure a unit's quality by the "over-all picture" derived from the condition of *all* its members, it retained an emphasis on individual optimization different from most of its pre–World War II predecessors.[73]

Notably, this new definition of fitness only included measurable physiological outcomes. The earlier Koehler-based definition of fitness embraced qualities such as confidence, courage, discipline, and alertness as components of physical efficiency. By 1946, these qualities, along with basic military skills such as swimming, running, and jumping, were recognized as "valuable products" of a good physical training, but no longer as fundamental elements of fitness.[74] This change generated massive repercussions within the Army's physical culture. Perhaps the greatest was liberation of physical training from a dual mission of developing both discipline and physical capacity, which thereby opened new veins of activity to mine, both in the system as a whole and in the daily program. The authors of *WD Pamphlet 21-9* called for instructors to abandon the old "extreme formalism" that made the "chief objective" of physical training "discipline rather than physical fitness." Instead, the authors charged instructors with selecting conditioning exercises and conducting them "so that they impart the utmost physiological benefit." Insistence on accuracy and precision was only valuable if they assisted soldiers in deriving the "maximum physical benefit from the exercises."[75] Soldiers undergoing physical training must have appreciated the change. Instead of repetitively executing the same old setting-up exercises, they were supposed to experience a varied program of work intended to deliver bigger physiological results faster than ever before.

Proponents of the new program claimed that it produced much better results than did earlier systems. Unlike claims made by previous training advocates, these were supported more by empirical evidence than by reasoning and analogy. Between the time Bank's team collected its data in the summer of 1942 and *TC 87*'s publication in November of that year, four infantry companies piloted the *TC 87* program over a six-week period. Two companies used the new system under close supervision while the other two functioned as an experimental control group using "traditional calisthenics, jogging and obstacle-course running."[76] The companies tested their soldiers' strength, agility, endurance, and coordination at the beginning and end of this six-week period.[77] The results showed an improvement of only 3.5 percent in "total physical fitness" among the control groups, but an increase of 23.25 percent in those following the *TC 87* system.[78] Differences in outcomes were especially evident in the events of most obvious combat relevance such as the pick-a-back (piggy-back) and dodging runs.

Some threads of continuity persisted in the Army's physical culture. One was the argument that physical fitness, and therefore physical training, remained of the utmost value and necessity despite technological change. Indeed, the effects of new technology upon warfare may have even heightened and accentuated the need for physical fitness in this line of reasoning. As did early proponents of physical training such as Herman Koehler, Edmund Butts, and James Pilcher, the World War II–era authors connected military physical training to the practices of the ancient Greeks and Romans. Like their turn-of-the-century predecessors, the new authors also evinced some Social Darwinist belief in the strength of a people being dependent upon the strength of its military-aged males, and of the pernicious effects on that strength of "soft luxurious living."[79] Channeling many of their predecessors' concerns about weak men and widespread fear of the American man's decline revealed in draft rejection rates, the new authors assumed that the Army's raw material was of a less-than-perfect quality. For instance, *WD Pamphlet 21-9*'s authors asserted that physical fitness testing had revealed "clearly the declining strength, endurance, agility, and coordination of the past two or three generations" owing to the "weakening influence of our modern machine civilization."[80] Opinions shared by the propagators of Army training policy changed little by 1946, as shown by *FM 21-20*'s warning that "few recruits" would enter the service "physically fit for the arduous duties ahead of them."[81]

"Modern machine civilization" may have reduced the average American man's fitness in the opinion of the producers of the Army's physical culture, but they also believed that mechanization had "accentuated rather than minimized" the importance of physical fitness in war.[82] Authors of the Army's new manuals directly connected advances in the "strength, speed, power and endurance" of military machines to the physical demands placed on soldiers. Every technical improvement demanded a corresponding improvement in the quality of the humans operating the machines.[83] This argument echoed those made by proponents of the offensive in the years prior to World War I who asserted, in the words of historian Antulio Echevarria, "that the human element must be strong enough to provide a vigorous complement to the newfound power of military technology."[84] Bank and his team gave several explanations for such an association. First, mechanized warfare increased the tempo of combat, putting a premium on endurance. Second, most fighting still occurred between infantry troops. The "grueling ordeal" of war still involved making assaults, running and crawling, jumping in and out of "fox holes, craters, and trenches," and "lifting and carrying heavy objects."[85] Bank also often employed as rhetorical devices emergency situations that might confront even tank operators and pilots—tanks break down and planes crash behind enemy lines.[86] Finally, the new producers recognized a tight linkage between physical fitness, mental health, and morale. Troops in better physical condition were better equipped to withstand the stresses of war, and thus better equipped to sustain their will to fight.[87]

The perceived gap between declining fitness and increasing physical demands was a core feature of the Army's official physical culture between 1942 and 1946. The training system that the culture produced reflected the perceived gap. Bank openly blamed America's physical educators for the weak bodies entering service in the 1940s. Their shortcomings "handicapped" the Army in its efforts to make new recruits combat-ready.[88] Bank, McCloy, Esslinger, and their team envisioned overcoming this handicap with a more efficient training program. They also assumed that achieving the "total conditioning of all the men" required many different types of activities because no single one could adequately develop all components of fitness.[89] Their training program therefore integrated many activities into a comprehensive training program based on empirical research in an effort to rapidly produce specific, measurable physiological outcomes in men of varying states of fitness.

Measurement itself was not a wholly new or novel feature of the Army's physical culture, but the characteristics measured in 1942 differed from those measured in earlier decades. Koehler began collecting data on members of the US Military Academy Corps of Cadets in 1885 and continued to do so throughout his tenure. His measurements focused on anthropometric features such as height, weight, and waist size, although he also assessed strength by using pull-ups, dips, grip tests, and weighted back and leg lifts.[90] No absolute standards existed against which these measures could be compared. Instead, Koehler used data to track change over time for individuals and groups. Koehler's methods aligned with trends in physical education at the turn of the century. Dudley Sargent, a pioneer of physical education and testing alike, similarly tracked anthropometric data such as height and chest girth and measured strength with simple tests such as the vertical jump.[91] Testing and measurement recommendations did not appear in the Army's original physical training manual of 1914, but Raycroft championed individual efficiency tests beginning in 1917 to identify "weak and inefficient men."[92] Raycroft established minimum standards for his hundred-yard sprint, running broad jump, eight-foot wall climb, hand grenade throw, and standard obstacle course tests. Again, this comported with contemporary trends, this time emphasizing "physical efficiency" and "motor ability" over anthropometric measures.[93]

Testing disappeared from the Army's system in the interwar years but resurfaced in the edition of *FM 21-20* published in 1941.

While the Army's use of testing waned in the interwar years, civilian physical educators grew more interested in creating and applying research-based test batteries. Charles McCloy made one of the most significant contributions to this movement by publishing a widely used test battery in 1934 that measured athletic power with a focus on general motor ability and strength.[94] The differences between Koehler's measurements and McCloy's are noteworthy. The former measured body shape and size in the interest of promoting symmetrical development. The latter measured physical capabilities and charted performance on a graduated scale built upon empirical research. McCloy imported his approach into the Army's physical culture, initiating a transformation that increasingly oriented the culture on physiological outcomes such as strength, endurance, and efficiency instead of physical appearance and the moral qualities assumed to be connected with it.[95]

Between 1942 and 1946, the test batteries recommended in published training manuals remained consistent and focused on measurable physiological outcomes. Both *TC 87* and *War Department Pamphlet 21-9* proposed the same seven-event battery that four companies had piloted in 1942: pull-ups, twenty-seconds of Burpees, squat jumps, push-ups, a hundred-yard pick-a-back run, sit-ups, and a three-hundred-yard run.[96] *FM 21-20* recommended the same battery, but without the Burpees and pick-a-back run. Furthermore, *FM 21-20* offered an indoor test battery that was identical to its outdoor battery except that a shuttle run and sixty-second squat thrust test replaced the three-hundred-yard run.[97] These differed from Raycroft's in that they did not feature events that measured skills such as grenade throwing or obstacle course runs. Instead, in line with McCloy's scientific measurement work, the World War II–era batteries focused on various elements of physical fitness such as strength, agility, coordination, and endurance. These batteries also aligned with tests used by many physical educators in the civilian world, so "valid standards" were available by which soldiers might be evaluated and by which point scales might be formed.[98] Uniformity was essential to this testing regime because a lack of consistency compromised the value of collected data. Extensive instructions therefore accompanied each event and several paragraphs urged the use of impartial judges, a consistent order of events, and other methods of controlling variables external to the soldier's physical capabilities.[99] However, the manual's authors lacked the authority to mandate use of a standard test battery. The best they could do was strongly recommend theirs and provide some criteria for selecting a different battery if desired. The pamphlet's authors also made sales pitches to their readers, touting the bevy of benefits that testing yielded. Among these was a tendency toward intensification in training programs when commanders could compare the condition of their units with others using definitive measurements.[100] Here the pamphlet's authors likened physical directors to physicians. As the latter diagnosed patients before prescribing a course of treatment, the former could use measurements to tailor programs to the "physical assets and liabilities" a unit's men possessed.[101]

The system introduced by *TC 87* in 1942 provided Army leaders with many tools, such as the new testing regime, to leverage when crafting tailored courses of treatment. These tools were more diverse and easier to implement than those available in all previous systems except for Raycroft's. For instance, the original manual of 1914 put ten categories of activities at an instructor's disposal, but one differed little from the setting-up exercises except for the addition of weights, four others required gymnastic apparatus and advanced skills, and one was athletics (about which little was said and little expected in terms of systematic training).[102] In contrast, *TC 87*'s seven activity categories were more diverse and easier to execute in austere environments: calisthenics, guerrilla exercises, grass drills, combatives, running, relays, and marching.[103] To these *FM 21-20* of 1946 added log and rifle exercises, a "strength course" using machines that units could manufacture, and obstacle and confidence courses. No activity in *TC 87* required additional equipment or apparatus, which increased the likelihood of instructors actually using all of the manual's tools. While calisthenic exercises executed in formation, in response to commands, and with an emphasis on precision still formed the core of the program, these exercises were generally more dynamic than their setting-up drill ancestors.[104] Also, the authors of the World War II–era program did not claim that the calisthenic drill alone was sufficient to get men into fighting trim. Instead, calisthenics merely formed a foundation upon which other activities built. The interwar tendency had been toward the disaggregation of activities, but *TC 87* inaugurated a return to aggregation and comprehensiveness in training programs.

TC 87 also introduced more combat-oriented functional training in an echo of similar wartime trends between 1917 and the early 1920s.[105] Guerrilla exercises and grass drills, two of the manual's new exercise categories, illustrate the turn toward functional training. The former ostensibly were "designed to prepare and train soldiers for guerrilla warfare," though the actual connection to guerrilla warfare is unclear.[106] The drills did develop agility, coordination, and endurance by making men move in new and different ways, though. For instance, duck waddles, crouch runs, and various crawls built muscles and skills needed to move under fire. "Double exercises" such as fireman's and cross carries cultivated components of physical fitness and prepared men to move casualties. Grass drills, borrowed from football conditioning programs, similarly improved endurance and agility while teaching practical skills such as dodging, transitioning from the prone to standing and vice versa, and moving between sites of cover.[107] Running and swimming, two other major exercise categories in the *TC 87* system, were similarly justified by appeals to battlefield demands instead of discipline-building. On bayonet training, the new system departed from Raycroft's. In fact, Bank specifically excluded bayonet drill from the Army's physical training program.[108] Although Bank did not explain this decision, the focus he and his coauthors placed on measurable physical conditioning probably reduced the value of bayonet drill, which had been primarily intended to develop psychological qualities and specific skills.

Along with the new tools that *TC 87* and *WD Pamphlet 21-9* offered, the manuals also provided more guidance on combining activities into a comprehensive training program than did any previous Army publication. Apart from the strict order and composition of the calisthenic drill, physical training directors could use this guidance to tailor a program to meet their unit's needs by applying three principles: periodization, progression, and overload. The first was a familiar feature in Army systematic training, but its incarnation in 1942 was more specific and structured. For example, the manual of 1914 offered different setting-up drills for the "recruit" and "trained" soldier but did not explain the difference between these categories or give much guidance on modifying the program beyond employing a different setting-up drill.[109] In contrast, *TC 87*'s authors identified three stages in a conditioning program. They also gave specific advice on how to approach training in each phase in such a way as to put most men in good condition within twelve weeks. In the first stage, dubbed the "toughening phase," soldiers spent one or two weeks mastering good form between liberal rest periods inserted to remedy muscle soreness. In the second phase, which lasted between six and eight weeks, rapid physiological adaptation brought big fitness gains before plateauing at the end of the phase. In the final "sustaining phase," little improvement was thought possible, so instructors were supposed to spend most of their time and effort maintaining men at their "peak of physical condition."[110]

Similarly, the principles of progression and overload were not wholly novel, but *TC 87*'s precise articulation of them and the detail of the accompanying guidance signaled the system's greater sophistication and its application of practices from the fields of physical education and athletic training. Both the manual of 1914 and Raycroft's *Mass Physical Training* had urged progressive fitness development, but neither did more than advise instructors to tailor their daily routines to the condition and needs of their charges, or to make each day's work "dovetail into the next."[111] In contrast, *TC 87* gave specific guidance on increasing intensity and load over time across a training program and within each activity type. The manual's authors also defined the "overload principle," referring to the fact that muscles developed proportional to the demands placed on them. Unlike warnings against "overdoing" found in Koehler's manuals, *TC 87*'s authors asserted that there was "no easy road to the attainment of excellent physical condition" and that exercises had to be strenuous and repeated "until it hurts."[112] For example, instructors might increase the number of repetitions conducted or reduce rest periods as a means of progressively overloading the troops under their ministrations.

Unit trainers received much more specific direction on incorporating periodization, progression, and overload into their programs than had their pre-1942 predecessors. *TC 87* contained a twelve-week model schedule that allotted minutes to various activities on a day-by-day and week-by-week basis. With the exception of the calisthenic drills, instructors could select which exercises to do in each activity category with reference to the manual's insights into the relative intensity of exercises and how to best increase intensity over time.[113] The quality and quantity of program construction guidance continued growing in the version of *FM 21-20* from 1946. In it, McCloy, Bank, and company expanded on earlier ideas, gave more specific examples of how to apply progression, addressed the problem of maintaining physical fitness in combat areas, and offered a second model schedule for a unit's maintenance phase.[114]

Such highly detailed guidance reflected movement in the Army's physical culture toward a more scientific basis and the influence of McCloy and his fellow physical education professionals, but it also helped offset the lack of a qualified physical trainer corps. The problem of producing and maintaining a corps of qualified instructors runs as a thread of continuity throughout the evolution of the Army's systematic training-based physical culture. Koehler had put forward West Point as an Aldershot alternative, but no "postgraduate" program ever materialized. Raycroft maneuvered between 1917 and 1920 to establish a school that would certify physical trainers, but his pilot program fell victim to interwar budget reductions. In contrast, Bank seems to have accepted this state of affairs. Writing in 1943, Bank characterized the Army physical training program as "decentralized." Physical training specialists simply did not exist. Even if they did, Bank calculated that not even ten thousand would be enough to meet the needs of the growing Army.[115] Thus, ownership by commanders and amateur-led training were, by necessity, features of the Army's physical culture in the World War II era.

As Bank noted, Army policy as expressed in *FM 21-10* and elsewhere made commanders responsible for the fitness of their men. Usually this responsibility devolved to company commanders.[116] However, most officers had little experience in planning and executing a physical training program beyond their physical education as youth, participation in athletics, and exposure to the subject during commissioning training. West Point graduates would have been relatively advanced amateurs in this area, as Koehler had originally intended. All would have undergone rigorous training and most would have led training sessions during their cadet careers, even if they had not planned a program. Similarly, Reserve Officer Training Corps (ROTC) cadets would also have participated in a physical training program, though likely not in one as comprehensive as the Academy's. Enlisted men converted to officers by way of Officer Candidate Schools (OCS), which commissioned more than 150,000 between 1942 and 1945 in the Army Ground Forces alone, received only rudimentary training.[117] The curriculum governing these schools' operations provided only general training geared to produce competent platoon leaders within, at most, seventeen weeks. Physical drill, which candidates executed daily, was a part of that curriculum, but it involved little more than a few candidates from each platoon in an OCS class leading drill daily using *FM 21-20* as a reference before receiving peer critiques on their performance.[118] OCS, ROTC, and the USMA all provided experience in physical training as session leaders or participants, but none qualified men to build programs from scratch. The manuals published between 1942 and 1946, with their detailed guidance and user-friendly system, were thus keystones in the Army's physical culture. They were crucial to both the provision of consistent, effective, and efficient training across the Army and the culture's propagation.

While physical training was a commander's responsibility in the Army's World War II–era physical culture, and while minimally trained amateur officers planned and executed most of that training, some specialists were available to assist. These specialists came from the Special Service, which was organized under the Army Service Forces and held responsibilities once apportioned to the Morale Branch and Commission on Training Camp Activities (CTCA) in 1917–1918. Specifically, the Special Service was responsible for "thoroughly planned and systematically promoted" initiatives to sustain good morale and a healthy sense of duty in Army commands.[119] This diverse portfolio ranged from library management and theater performances to soldier publications, educational activities, and athletics. The Special Service's Athletic and Recreation Branch, headed by Bank, provided trained athletic officers and enlisted assistants to field army, corps, division, and often regimental headquarters staffs.[120] By 1944, Special Service companies extended these services to forward echelons by supplementing organic Special Service staff with additional technicians and equipment.[121] Whether assigned to headquarters staffs or Special Service companies, Athletic Officers and technicians usually possessed both a background in athletics and training in implementing the Army's physical training system. The Special Service companies in particular were capable of taking charge of physical training programs and executing them in line with *TC 87*.[122] Essentially, Special Service officers were uniformed versions of the CTCA's athletic directors, similarly able and willing to "give help and leadership" to officers responsible for physical training.[123] However, the availability of Special Service officers was never so great as to relieve most commanders of responsibility for planning and leading physical training, and many of them focused chiefly on organizing morale-building athletic competitions.

That the Army's only body of physical training specialists actually had the specified mission of planning, developing, stimulating, and supervising athletic events illuminates the entwinement of athletics and systematic training, which was a key feature of the Army's World War II–era physical culture. Like the incorporation of combat-oriented activities, the reemergence of athletics in systematic training illustrates aggregation's return to the Army's physical culture. Sport, once considered a potentially dangerous distractor, assumed a central role in the Army's physical culture by 1942, thereby culminating a movement characterized by a historian of martial athletics as one from "indifference to obsession."[124] In examining the latter years of that movement, historian Wanda Wakefield posits that by World War II sports were even "intended to permeate the lives of the off-duty soldier or sailor."[125] According to Wakefield, ubiquitous sport served four functions: a distraction for soldiers, an assurance to civilians and soldiers alike that America fielded an army of citizen-soldiers, a tool for identifying and selecting the "best men" in the military's hierarchy, and a means of entertaining large populations.[126] Bank would have added a fifth—building and sculpting soldiers' minds and bodies in a way that enhanced work done by systematic training.

Bank envisioned athletics and systematic physical training as coequal parts of a larger "total physical conditioning program" for the Army. He held that adding sport enabled the physical training program to "contribute substantially to mental and emotional fitness."[127] Strictly defining physical fitness as being able to retain "normal responses to stimuli" and function "effectively" under great stress focused the physical training program on generating empirically measurable physiological outcomes.[128] However, earlier beliefs in the ability of exercise to develop less measurable mental, emotional, and character traits had not disappeared. They just mostly migrated to the domain of sport. Thus, sport in Bank's construction was an amplifying adjunct in the pursuit of physical fitness, but a critical line of effort in developing the "mental and emotional" components of "total military fitness."[129] Neither systematic training nor athletics could replace the other, but they synergized. Bank's explanation of the Army's physical training program to civilian educators illustrated his concept of exercise-sport harmony. Where he pitched the value of exercise in terms of raw performance on a test battery, Bank framed athletics' value as a crucial "morale-building" activity and as a way of training soldiers "in the elements of combat."[130] The "intangible benefits" of sport included characteristics familiar from earlier formations of the Army's physical culture: comfort with bodily contact, confidence, aggressiveness, initiative, determination, and teamwork.[131] Furthermore, Bank and his team believed that sport's popularity helped cultivate soldier interest in the physical training program. Soldiers would "gladly engage" in purely conditioning activities, according to *FM 21-20*'s authors, if "they know they will be able to play speedball, soccer, touch football, or push ball afterwards."[132]

Training Circular 87's system and that of its successor, *FM 21-20*, operationalized the balanced value placed on systematic exercise and sport. Both manuals' recommended programs began with a heavy emphasis on basic calisthenics and conditioning exercises. But by the twelfth week of the program, games occupied more than 55 percent of the total time allotted to physical training weekly under *War Department Pamphlet 21-9*, and 38 percent under *FM 21-20*.[133] Not all of these games were of the popular spectator sport variety owing to the need of justifying games "in terms of the contribution they make to physical conditioning."[134] Yet many were, and the training system also strongly encouraged participation in recreational athletics outside of programmed training time.

Bank's insistence that athletics serve the masses instead of the elite few was consistent with earlier formulations of sport's value in the Army's physical culture, if not always with actual practice. In Bank's case, he made "Athletics for All" an explicit goal for his Special Service division and for the physical training program.[135] While Athletic Officers were supposed to organize some competitive teams, mostly for the purposes of building esprit d'corps and providing men with heroic examples, they were chiefly charged with maximizing participation. This emphasis increased throughout the war as illustrated by the revision in September 1944 of the Special Service Officer technical manual, *TM 21-205*. That manual dropped the assumption that all men were familiar with athletics. Instead, it urged athletic officers to conceive of their mission more broadly: to welcome newcomers to sport, to offer alternative activities to the major sports, and to incentivize participation with prizes.[136] Ultimately, the physical culture that emerged during World War II combined sport with traditional systematic training and combat-oriented functional training in response to demands for rapidly preparing hundreds of thousands of new soldiers. While that culture incorporated more scientific measurement, data-informed design, and other trends imported from the world of civilian physical education, it also displayed many continuities such as traditional linkages between mental, physical, and moral fitness.

Change in the Army's physical culture during the World War II era was generally moderate and much of it called back to similar change between 1917 and 1920, but one development required a fundamental reevaluation of fitness definitions and practices within the service—the inclusion of women. The creation of the Women's Army Auxiliary Corps (WAAC) in May 1941, renamed the Women's Army Corps (WAC) in July 1943 when the WAC became a part of the Regular Army, prompted questions about physical training. For instance, how should fitness for women be defined? Did "fitness" mean something different for men and for women? How should women exercise? To what ends should women's minds and bodies be sculpted? The solution, a wholly separate physical training system, illuminates the balancing act involved in leveraging women's service without severely destabilizing gender roles, and it reveals that the Army's physical culture was fundamentally rooted in traditional visions of gender. Women could not fit into the existing physical culture because they were women.

From the WAAC's inception, the idea of simply adopting the existing physical culture seems to have been beyond consideration. For example, the process of crafting a physical training program for the WAAC's new inductees differed from the process used to create other training programs. Typically, the WAAC's leadership and staff borrowed an existing course as a template, and then substituted "practical courses" designed to address likely duties in place of men's "combat courses."[137] Physical training was an exception. Partly out of concern expressed by the WAAC staff that men's physical training might be harmful to women, the WAAC's leadership opted to fashion a unique system from the ground up. The nature and character of such a system proved to be contentious topics.[138] Physical cultures help explain the prickly quality of this debate. After all, members of the WAAC staff and leadership were not just debating the most efficient and effective way to improve the physical capacity of their organization's members. They were also struggling over the very definition of fitness, along with its purpose and value. Physical training in the US Army had pursued objectives beyond simple physical conditioning since its inception. Character traits, moral qualities, and a man's identity as a soldier and member of a unit were widely regarded as valid physical training outcomes. Civilian physical educators had also sought to use exercise and sport as a means of socialization and of educating the whole person through the body. Similar entanglements and intersections informed the creation of the WAAC's physical training system. In this case, exercise and fitness conformed to extant social mores and gender norms. To illustrate, the larger Army's physical culture did not distinguish between a clerk and a rifleman. Both clerks and riflemen ostensibly exercised in the same way in pursuit of the same ends. Yet the distinctions between male and female clerks were apparently so great as to require wholly different physical cultures and attendant training systems.

Fort Des Moines's parade ground was the primary workshop on which a series of trainers constructed the WAAC's distinct physical culture. Credit for the first comprehensive effort to define both a culture and an associated system belongs to Catherine Van Rensselaer. Appointed the WAAC's director of physical education in 1942, Van Rensselaer brought to bear professional credentials and more than twenty years of experience as a civilian physical educator.[139] Her task was to create a physical training system, implement it to train the WAAC's first few officer classes at Fort Des Moines, and then hand the program off to graduates who would staff the school's physical training section. Assisted by three other civilian instructors, Van Rensselear developed an exercise regimen chiefly comprising rhythmic exercises in the Danish gymnastics mode complemented by a smattering of games and sports.[140] According to Van Rensselear, nothing in her system was "strikingly new."[141] Very little differentiated these exercises from the old setting-up drill or even the new calisthenic drill in terms of format. Instructors led formations of inductees through a series of bodyweight exercises executed in response to commands. However, the exercises were not especially vigorous. The goal was to strike a balance in ensuring that inductees were "properly trained but not overtrained." Trainees needed to develop stamina, endurance, the flexibility "to work complex machines," "sound" bodies, and an "outlook for a new life." Underlining the importance of balance, Van Rensselear stated that she and her trainers wanted "the girls to have fun" but at the same time "remember that we are in a war."[142]

Many inductees who trained in Van Rensselear's system were critical of it. Historian and WAC officer Mattie Treadwell divided critiques into two categories, one alleging that the exercises were "positively harmful to women over the age of 18," and a second that charged Van Rensselear's system with not being strenuous enough.[143] Many of the voices advancing the latter position, characterized by Treadwell as the "strength-building school," belonged to newly commissioned officers with backgrounds in physical education.[144] Chief among them was Capt. Donna Niles, a former physical educator at Northwestern who possessed a master's degree from Columbia and additional education from the University of Wisconsin and Northwestern.[145] After graduating from the WAAC school in its first officer class in August 1942, Niles became chief of the school's physical training section and, six months later, director of the WAC's Well-Being Division. Owing to Nile's power, the strength-building school's influence on the WAC's physical culture remained dominant throughout the war years.

Behind the disagreements over how women should exercise lay a fundamental disagreement over the nature of and need for physical fitness in the WAAC. What did fitness mean? Fit for what? Both the early and later cultural producers mainly approached answering these questions and defining fitness along functional lines. Van Rensselear conceived of a woman's duties in the narrowest sense. Assuming that most of the work expected of a woman would "be the desk variety of job," Van Rensselear rejected strength training. Instead, she aimed to "keep them fit" for their duties.[146] The exact nature of that "fitness" is unclear, but recreation, endurance, flexibility, and mental well-being seem to have been key components. Niles similarly approached fitness from a functional perspective, but she set the bar above desk work to account for more rigorous requirements and the possibility of emergencies.[147] According to Niles, the nation was engaged in a total war, which demanded that women replace men so the latter could join the fighting ranks. Women had to be ready to take on most noncombat military duties "alone and unaided" at any time. A woman who "lacks strength, who tires easily, whose mind and body do not work in swift accord, and who is constantly prey to illness and moods" could not fulfill these obligations.[148] A fit female soldier in Nile's schema was not an "Amazon," but she had the physiological foundation needed to accomplish any job, appeared competent, possessed "mental, emotional, and physical stability," and took ownership of her physical development.[149]

Niles vividly expressed her concept of fitness and cemented it as the WAC's dominant definition in 1943 in the physical training manual for the Women's Army Corps, *FM 35-20*. From its first page, the manual argued that women must be fit to "perform a soldier's noncombat duties."[150] A fit woman needed a "strong body and steady nerves," plus an "appearance" that gave "assurance" in her ability.[151] Ultimately, a WAC service member's fitness was contingent on three basic areas: physical, mental, and appearance. In the physical realm, strong bodies exhibited the qualities of strength, stamina, coordination, and stability.[152] These corresponded closely with *WD Pamphlet 21-9*'s constituents of men's physical fitness, though the WAC's "stability" emphasized daily performance and presence to a greater degree than did *WD Pamphlet 21-9*'s "freedom from disease and physical defects."[153] Training these physiological characteristics by way of systematic exercise was also supposed to cultivate muscular tone, stability, "efficient elimination," resistance to illness and deprivation, improved posture, stamina, and general well-being.[154] Hence, physical exercise simultaneously addressed mental health by relieving tension and generally toughening women to meet the daily grind of office work and light labor.

Foregrounding appearance, the third constituent of WAC fitness, broke significantly from the wider Army's physical culture and helped make the WAC's distinct. For men, appearance was a minor consideration and a by-product of exercise by 1942. Physical fitness was supposed to make them capable of marching long distances, driving vehicles over rough terrain, making assaults, fighting in hand-to-hand combat, carrying heavy objects, and maneuvering across broken ground.[155] *WD Pamphlet 21-9* briefly addressed posture, justifying its importance as giving "the impression of strength, control, confidence and vitality," but made little other mention of appearance.[156] However, appearance was front and center for women. According to the WAC's physical training manual's authors, *being* fit was not enough—women also had to *appear* fit and capable. Appearing fit and capable required clear complexions, healthy facial coloration, no excess fat, toned muscles, poise, and grace without reliance on "synthetic beauty" products.[157] "The Army will judge you by your appearance," advised the manual's authors, because "a smart, soldierly carriage usually means smart, soldierly performance."[158] Similarly, the WAC's later introductory handbook for new service members, *WAC Life*, advised that while "soldiering is a grim business, and your job may be on the messy side," this was "no reason" to "overlook the little things which contribute to attractiveness." According to the handbook's authors, other men and women would "judge your personality by the old standards," which included neat hair, makeup, tidy uniforms, fresh breath, and the absence of body odor. Maintaining "feminine appeal" was key to sustaining morale and happiness.[159] In short, they needed to be Hollywood starlets, or at least models of middle-class, college-educated respectability.

FM 35–20 summarized WAC physical fitness with a negative example and cautionary message accompanied by photographs: "don't be a Josephine Jerk."[160] Josephine Jerk was the "limp number in every outfit" who dove into her daily exercises with "the crisp vitality of a damp mop." Her joints were "all limber in the wrong places" and she was built unlike other women in that her body had "a posture all its own." Because of weak muscles and bones, Josephine counted on "her girdle to hold her up" and could not sustain effort in a tough activity such as mopping for more than ten minutes. Josephine Jerks were downright dangerous because they "hinder[ed], rather than help[ed], the war effort."[161] Here were all the features of WAC physical fitness on display in a negative example. Josephine lacked strength, stamina, coordination, and stability of both mental and physical varieties. Her mental well-being was simply not suited to enduring the long haul of a total war. On top of it all, Josephine *appeared* comically incompetent more often than not.

Similar to the Army's *TC 87* system, the WAC system divided physical training into the two categories of systematic conditioning exercise and recreation. Unlike in the Army's *TC 87* system, the two activities were not equally valued in the WAC. Niles characterized the former as the "vitamins" of the system and the latter as the "dessert."[162] Niles conceived of her mission as bringing "huge numbers of women" to fitness by the "quickest and most direct means."[163] Sports did not meet these criteria because she believed few women had much knowledge of or experience in athletics; thus they were unlikely to get much exercise out of play. Furthermore, the nonphysical qualities sport was supposed to develop in men such as aggression and leadership held little value in the WAC's physical culture.[164] Hearkening back to the Koehler era, the producers of the WAC's culture accordingly viewed sport mostly as a site for recreation and incidental development, but not as a crucial tool for developing fitness. Differences between sport's place in the WAC's and in the wider Army's physical cultures provide further evidence of both being gendered constructs.

The WAC's physical culture stressed systematic conditioning most. Niles and her fellow authors organized conditioning into three phases that dictated the amount and type of exercise service members performed: basic, specialist, and field training. In the basic and specialist training phases, which might last as little as five weeks, the system introduced women to the essentials of physical conditioning and was supposed to "throw the responsibility for maintaining physical fitness squarely up to each woman."[165] Between forty minutes and one hour daily were to be spent in training and recreation, totaling five hours per week. In this time women learned the four basic cadence series (which were sets of warm-up exercises), began mastering levels of the strength progression series, executed a foot-strengthening exercise, and played various games to develop agility, balance, and coordination. The strength progressions composed the bulk of a daily training period. Each series targeted a different area of the body: shoulders and arms, abdominal, back and neck, and legs. Seven progressively more difficult exercises made up each series, culminating in four exercises: full-dips (push-ups), sit-ups, wing lifts, and running.[166] With the exception of wing lifts, these culminating exercises were all basic exercises every male recruit was expected to be able to execute in the *TC 87* system. A WAC spent nearly her entire period of service after initial entry training in the field training phase of physical conditioning. Here, officers were responsible for ensuring that women spent fifteen minutes daily on conditioning exercises, specifically the cadence series and strength progressions. This aligned with the daily fifteen minutes of calisthenics required of men, though the *TC 87* system also called for thirty-five to forty-five more minutes every day of rigorous athletics and games.[167] Tension release activities, unarmed self-defense, and functional swimming were also recommended as part of the WAC physical training system, especially during the field training phase, but they were largely optional except for in deploying units.

Notably, the WAC system put the onus for physical fitness on the individual to a much greater degree than did its Army counterpart. While the *TC 87* system sought individual physical optimization far more than did earlier systems, it did not pin responsibility for fitness on the individual soldier. The manuals discussed ways to get men to buy in to the training program and participate, but commanders and physical training instructors were responsible for maintaining their men's interest and for the overall fitness of their units.[168] This was a thread of continuity that ran back to the earliest days of systematic physical training in the Army —fitness ultimately mattered because it made units more efficient and effective in battle, even if the relative value of the individual's warrior qualities changed over time. In contrast, the WAC system's authors never wrote on the importance of unit fitness. Instead, what mattered was the individual woman's readiness to take over a man's noncombat job. Though company commanders and school cadres bore responsibility for training programs, every individual woman was "responsible for her own physical fitness" in the "final analysis."[169] Charging women with responsibility sidestepped concerns that military service might somehow impose masculine characteristics or make women less feminine. It also echoed hopes expressed by the Army's earliest systematic training advocates and by World War I–era social reformers that service members would go on owning their physical fitness after their terms of service. Women might take their new knowledge, training routines, and appreciation for the benefits of exercise home to their families to become "more useful and happier member[s] of tomorrow's world."[170] Niles went further, giving voice to a dream that the WACs might totally change America's cultural views on women's physical fitness.[171]

The degree to which women actually took ownership of their physical fitness or tried to maximize their speed, strength, or endurance is not clear. Some WACs certainly realized Niles's best hopes. However, the value of physical fitness in the WAC's passive culture at the unit level does not seem to have aligned in most cases with the official physical culture. Many company-level WAC officers complained that the exercises were "too strenuous" and not as valuable as recreational activities for desk-bound workers.[172] Company commanders also complained bitterly about the requirement for fifteen-minute daily drills, mostly citing difficulties with finding suitable training spaces. When the Army's Military Training Division mandated physical tests every three months to enforce training, complaints came from as high as the WAC's director, Col. Oveta Culp Hobby. Complainants alleged that men had no similar requirement for regular testing, that standards were too high, that women's bodies were not suited to perform these exercises purportedly designed for men, and that women simply did not need strenuous training to execute their duties.[173] A poll of WAC company commanders found 95 percent opposed a systematic training program, preferring recreational sports to strength-building calisthenics.[174] Niles and some allies in the Surgeon General's Office continued pushing systematic training and ultimately won the debate. Through the end of World War II, the Military Training Division continued requiring daily calisthenics and regular testing.[175]

Taken together, the WAC's official physical culture and the system of exercise supporting it represented a fundamentally gendered project. The system was ostensibly designed to prepare women specifically for their duties, but job requirements alone were insufficient to explain the need for a totally separate system of exercise. After all, many more men than women served in the same rear-echelon support roles that the WAC was meant to take on. More than 1.7 million men served in the Army Service Forces at the ASF's peak strength.[176] Adding to this the number of men in the Army Ground and Army Air Forces serving in support roles with a marginal likelihood, at best, of seeing combat takes the sum above one-third of the Army's total strength in World War II. Yet no similarly duty-specific system emerged for this population. Instead, the Army's physical culture treated every man as a potential combatant, and so officially maintained a single system of exercise that was historically centered on the infantryman.

A better explanation for the existence of an alternative physical culture for women comes from historian Leisa Meyer. In her book *Creating GI Jane*, Meyer argues that the creation of the WAAC crystallized public fears about undermining the "established sex/gender system."[177] Difficulties in constructing the new category of "female soldier" in American society provoked grave concerns about military service depriving women of their femininity, turning them into victims, or encouraging sexual deviance. These anxieties manifested in a slander campaign against the

WAC spread by word of mouth and the mainstream press in 1943 and 1944.[178] At root, the smear campaign rested on an assumption that the military was, in the words of historian Janann Sherman, "'unnatural' for women and that only those with base motives could wish to serve."[179] Thus, women who joined the military must have been deviants of some kind. Meyer argues that the WAC's leadership, and especially Hobby, developed a strategy of attempting to comprehensively control the construction of the "female soldier" in order to safeguard both the organization and individual women. Respectability and minimization of fears over sexual, gender, race, or class hierarchy subversion were central narrative elements of that strategy.[180] The WAC's physical culture and the internal disagreements over its systemization, especially discontent over Niles's emphasis on strength-building and strenuous work, support Meyer's conclusions. Physical training was meant to literally sculpt female soldiers in line with a desired model—respectable, capable, and feminine. Stressing individual ownership and meeting the individual woman's needs elided concerns about the organization forcibly reshaping women along undesirable lines. Underscoring training for desk work reassured audiences that women would not be masculinized in preparation for combat. Even Hobby's resistance to strenuous exercise and testing—"Are they trying to make Amazons of our women?"—reflected a concern with keeping the female soldier feminine.[181]

Simply in existing, the separate WAC physical culture and its associated training system revealed the degree to which the wider Army's physical culture was gendered. Building men had been a central element in the discourse around systematic physical training in the Army since the earliest advocates and cultural producers began beating their drums. Much of the impetus for physical training had emerged from fears about the ability of modern man to meet the evolving demands of the modern battlefield. Early advocates framed many of the expected benefits of systematic physical training in terms of improving American society by way of improving men's bodies, minds, and characters.[182] Women could not participate in a physical culture that evolved in response to what might be termed a persistent martial masculinity crisis without becoming more masculine, or so the reasoning went. Thus, when the existence of women in the military posed questions about definitions of fitness, the means of pursuing it, and the ends toward which minds and bodies should be sculpted, the answers required a separate physical culture.

The perceived need for a separate physical culture for women highlights one of this work's central themes: namely, that much more was always at stake in physical training than simply maximizing the physical performance measures of individual bodies. In this case, physical training helped reinforce gender hierarchies and define the idea of a "female soldier."[183] The gendered nature of the Army's physical culture in 1942 has ramifications today. Since women entered the Army, ideas about fitness and exercise have been framed in terms of what men and women could or should do, not what soldiers could or should do. Historian D'Ann Campbell arrives at similar conclusions in her comparative study of gender-integrated antiaircraft units in World War II, noting that decisions about roles for female soldiers usually had more to do with social values than with efficiency and performance.[184] This mode of thinking buttresses perceptions of women as second-class or less capable soldiers. Such perceptions are an obstacle to the integration of women into combat arms roles. Though the Army's physical culture has propped up this obstacle since 1942, the culture's present movement toward duty-position-defined fitness standards may be a powerful means of reducing that obstacle's stature in the future.

Between 1942 and 1946, the Army's physical culture underwent notable change. However, that change was not as shocking or revolutionary as were developments between 1917 and 1920, and much of it aligned with existing trends or had precedents in earlier periods. For instance, definitions of fitness oriented more toward combat efficiency and the system of exercises created to develop that fitness became more combat-oriented as they both had before. The Army's physical culture moved in a similar direction during World War I under the guidance of Raycroft and his CTCA team. Sport's contentious place and value in the Army's physical culture also followed a familiar trajectory toward a more formal, entrenched role in developing "total fitness," if not physical fitness. However, some irony exists in the fact that parties responsible first and foremost for athletics, such as Colonel Bank of the SSD's Athletic and Recreation Branch, assumed control of systematic training when athletics had once been considered an adjunct to, and possible distraction from, physical training in Koehler's original formulation. Still, many of the basic concepts that had framed sport's value in those early days continued to do so in the 1940s: maximum participation, emphasis on the average many rather than the elite few, and development of nonphysical characteristics and qualities.

A familiar sense of crisis at the intersection between perceived masculine decline and growing combat demands continued informing the way producers of the Army's physical culture viewed their challenge. Bank's judgment that World War II–era recruits were "not physically fit" and that they manifested a "shocking" lack of strength, coordination, agility, and endurance echoed nineteenth-century warnings about masculine decline in American and European societies.[185] Yet this time, Bank and others like him read revelations about the high rates of rejection in both world wars' drafts as validations of such concerns. A familiar sense of crisis produced a familiar mission—to rapidly bring vast classes of low-quality recruits and conscripts up to a standard of fitness sufficient for competition against veteran opponents in mechanized combat in a conflict approaching absolute war, even if relatively few soldiers would engage in combat. At the same time, continuity in the purpose of physical training, which responded to concerns about masculine decline in male soldiers, spurred the creation of a wholly separate physical culture for women when they entered the service.

More novel change came in the form of an increasingly scientific approach to defining, building, and measuring physical fitness. Studies conducted by McCloy, Bank, and their team leveraged empirical research to produce a precise definition of physical fitness based on five purely physiological factors: freedom from disease, strength, endurance, agility, and coordination.[186] This culture's producers reoriented physical training to "impart the utmost physiological benefit," largely omitting immeasurable qualities such as general health, self-reliance, and courage.[187] Cultivation of such qualities did not completely vanish from the list of systematic training's promised outcomes, but it was a task mostly left to sport. As in World War I, outsiders drove this change. Uniformed officers owned physical training policy to a much greater degree than they did in World War I. However, some like Bank were just called to temporary service and the people most responsible for crafting the new training system were civilian experts. Men like Charles McCloy brought the latest methods and ideas in civilian physical education to bear on the problem of military fitness as they understood it and a reformulation of the Army's official physical culture resulted.

Ultimately, cultural change during World War II echoed change during World War I, although the relative magnitude of difference between the 1940s wartime culture and its prewar culture was smaller than in the case of World War I. In the years after 1946, cultural reversion would also prove consistent with the reversion that followed World War I. However, that reversion could not be wholesale because the Army's physical culture also had to adapt to new expectations of combat in a nuclear world.

CHAPTER SIX
HARD BODIES FOR A COLD WAR
CONDITIONING AND PREHABILITATION, 1945–1957

The Cold War's advent brought with it an abundance of reasons for sustained interest in the bodies of the United States' youth, uniformed or otherwise. At first blush, the awesome destructive power of nuclear weaponry might have implied the irrelevance of the individual soldier's strength and endurance. Every service's pursuit of high-tech weapons, advanced platforms, and space-age gadgets may likewise have suggested the soldier's diminishing relevance. However, the Army's senior leaders did not forget the flesh-and-blood sinews of warfare. Warfighting concepts, revised doctrine, and new force structures, such as the Pentomic Division, consistently emphasized the necessity of fitness on nuclear battlefields. There, success was thought to depend upon dispersion and rapid, aggressive maneuver. Actual combat experience on Korea's battlefields also reinforced the importance of physical fitness. At the same time, the Korean War seemed to reveal the modern American man's shortcomings once again. Other national fitness red flags, such as the Kraus-Weber report, published in 1955, also appeared to expose an emergent "muscle gap" with the Soviet Union and the pernicious effects of easy living in a mass-consumer society. Because the Army's manpower policies relied heavily on conscription, soft citizens meant soft soldiers. Youth and soldier physical training alike thus remained subjects of public and expert interest.

Throughout this period of turbulence, the Army's physical culture remained consistent. Cultural inertia and institutional continuity minimized change, generally restraining it to the trajectory set between 1942 and 1945. Writing in 1957, Gen. Maxwell Taylor, the Army's chief of staff and a principal promoter of technology-centric modernization, illustrated the endurance of cultural values and beliefs: "It is a military duty for all officers and men to maintain a high level of physical fitness . . . to perform [their] duties with maximum efficiency," he wrote, and then claimed that fitness inspired confidence in subordinates and fellow citizens alike by "presenting the model of an alert, ready fighting man."[1] Taylor conceived of fitness in physical terms and as an external manifestation of intangible inner qualities. He also prioritized the average soldier's fitness, not the "development of muscle men or record-breaking athletes," while emphasizing the individual before the unit.[2] Taylor's definition of fitness, valuation of exercise, and focus on the individual all aligned with the Army's World War II–era physical culture despite a decade of technological, doctrinal, structural, and political ferment throughout the service. Institutional continuity complemented cultural endurance in minimizing change. Although responsibility for physical training research and doctrine development changed hands several times between 1945 and 1954, ongoing studies sponsored by Army Field Forces and the US Army Infantry School's influence kept the physical culture oriented toward basic preparation for infantry combat and responsive to data-driven research. When concerns about soldier fitness arose, cultural inertia and institutional continuity encouraged a doubling-down on the existing physical culture instead of substantial revision.

Much more change occurred in the US government's approach to prehabilitation. The military's continuing reliance upon conscription to fill its ranks fixed attention on young, male American bodies. Many of the Army's senior leaders opined that those bodies tended to be inadequate for modern warfare's demands and that they needed to be improved before entering military service. In the words of Brig. Gen. Stanley Larsen, the assistant commandant of the United States Army Infantry School (USAIS), the "era of exertion and hardship" of America's forefathers had given way to "an age of ease and comfort" enabled by technology and consumerism.[3] Contrary to Larsen's interpretation, anxieties over national fitness were not new or novel. They were persistent, but were amplified by new evidence that emerged throughout the 1950s. The government's responses to these anxieties changed over time, though. During World War II, prehabilitation's chief vehicles were explicitly martial programs, such as the Victory Corps, in the mold of the interwar Citizens' Military Training Camps. After the war, prehabilitation advocates attempted to expand mandatory training in a military format through Universal Military Training (UMT) legislation. The Victory Corps and UMT achieved few lasting successes, but they both generated significant resistance, especially among educators. In 1956, the Eisenhower administration introduced a new prehabilitation model with its "advisory state" approach, which the President's Council on Youth Fitness (PCYF) exemplified. Neither mandatory nor militaristic, the PCYF used public relations and advertising to market and popularize a fitness concept that aligned with the Army's physical culture. This approach proved more successful and durable, and more palatable to the public, than any that came before, and it remains the government's preferred approach today.

Between the end of World War II and 1957, the Army's physical culture changed little despite a larger politico-military context that could have de-emphasized the significance of the individual soldier's physical fitness. Debates about ground forces' relevance and utility played out regularly during the Cold War's first two decades. At least until the Korean War, public opinion inclined toward doubt over the need for maintaining large conventional forces. After all, new wonder weapons capable of destroying whole cities had ended World War II. The desire to cash in on a peace dividend in combination with the allure of a new high-tech, push-button concept of war seemed to signal the Army's limited utility both as a tool of national policy and in any future war.[4] To counter this narrative, the Army generally pursued two lines of effort. One sold the service's relevance to lawmakers and the public while staking out claims to resources in fierce interservice competition through organizational and doctrinal changes aimed at restructuring ground forces around nuclear weapons. The other involved establishing the enduring value of the Army's core competencies. For instance, Army doctrine writers retained an emphasis on maneuver, decisive engagements, destruction of enemy forces, and the offense in general throughout the 1950s.[5] Both lines of effort asserted the soldier's centrality in warfare, even in an age of missiles and mechanization. In fact, this line of logic often led to the conclusion that soldiers needed to be *more* fit than ever before to meet the demands new technology imposed.

The means by which the Army sculpted soldiers' bodies and kept them fit reflected a continuity of thought on the qualities of a "good" soldier and his role in warfare. The edition of *Field Manual (FM) 21-20: Physical Training* published in 1946 laid out these means and elucidated the Army's official physical culture at the dawn of the Cold War. Assembled under the direction of the Office of the Surgeon General, *FM 21-20* superseded the manual of the same title from 1941 and the wartime publications *Training Circular (TC) 87* and *War Department Pamphlet (WD Pam.) No. 21-9*. The majority of the manual recapitulated the work of Charles McCloy, Theodore Bank, and company. Compared with the wartime manuals, *FM 21-20* advanced the same definition of fitness (itself a factor of total military fitness), the same rationale for fitness's value in an age of mechanization, and a very similar training program in terms of scope and organization.[6]

FM 21-20 also included an identical testing regime based on data collected by Bank's team in 1942. However, *FM 21-20* also recommended activities that had not been part of physical training doctrine for years. Some, such as boxing and hand-to-hand fighting techniques, reflected historical tendencies during war to incorporate practical combat skills into physical training. The reappearance of tumbling is more puzzling. Cartwheeling and back somersaults had last appeared in *Training Regulations 115-5*, published in 1928. Even then they were relics of the earlier Koehler culture. Gymnastics' temporary return illuminates the enduring influence of the Army's original systematic training culture and of West Point's physical education department. Gymnastics' return also indicates difficulties in forming coherent doctrine when responsibility for it did not consistently belong to a single body of subject matter experts. Bank, McCloy, and company had crafted a research-based training system during the war. In contrast, responsibility for the new *FM 21-20* formally belonged to the US Army's Surgeon General's office, which had not been involved with physical training previously and did not utilize specialized physical educators.[7] The result was an odd amalgamation of old and new activities.

Despite covering additional activities, *FM 21-20*'s actual training system and the definition of fitness on which it was oriented tracked very closely with what Bank and McCloy created during World War II. None of the additional activities was allotted time in either the recommended twelve-week introductory schedule or the maintenance program.[8] Drill Number One, known as the "Army Dozen," and its lesser known sibling, Drill Number Two, remained the foundational set of conditioning exercises. Guerrilla exercises, grass drills, rifle and log exercises, and running added interest-sustaining alternatives and supplements. Likewise, *FM 21-20* continued spreading the physical education world's gospel of overload and progression as introduced in *TC 87*. Specifically, it advised that strenuous exercise should continue "until it hurts" and that work should intensify over time in a program.[9] Likewise, *FM 21-20*'s definition of fitness adhered strictly to the World War II model, which included five measurable, physiological components: freedom from disease or anatomical defect, strength, endurance (muscular and cardio-respiratory), agility, and coordination.[10] These factors differed significantly from the abstract qualities and traits such as smartness, activity, precision, self-respect, neatness, and grace sought in the physical culture's earlier forms. Development of basic military skills, self-confidence, and a will to win remained likely and valuable by-products of physical training, but not goals in and of themselves.[11] Where earlier forms of the culture had emphasized unit discipline as a product of physical training, this one concentrated on the physiological components of fitness belonging to the individual soldier. Focus on the individual was most explicit and visible in the manual's rejection of "extreme formalism" in training, which was supposedly productive of discipline alone. Instead, the culture promulgated in *FM 21-20* of 1946 prioritized "the utmost physiological benefit."[12]

While little about the Army's official physical culture changed between 1946 and 1950, in practice tactical-level organizations increasingly preferred recreational athletics to systematic training. Doctrinal revisions tracked somewhat with this preference. The revision of *FM 21-20* published in 1950, still authored by the Office of the Surgeon General, offered no innovation, but its creators removed hand-to-hand fighting techniques, wrestling, and tumbling while adding a chapter on "mass games."[13] The addition of mass games reflected general trends at the small-unit level between 1945 and 1950 that, as one later analyst put it, allowed the "recreational tail . . . to wag the physical conditioning dog."[14] In part, these trends began when units hemorrhaged many of their veterans and shifted to a peacetime footing. They also partly resulted from deliberate policy decisions that originated in a conference in August 1944 called to develop plans for an Army athletic program that would support postwar demobilization. Representatives of the Special Services Division's Athletic Branch and several civilian sports authorities recommended that programs be put into place that were chiefly designed to help commanders maintain a "high state of morale." Furthermore, they recommended that "purely military instruction" be reduced to the bare minimum necessary and that as much of the training day as possible be devoted to "comprehensive educational, athletic and recreational programs."[15] The turn away from physical conditioning coincided with declining soldier quality in physical and mental terms (the Army being characterized in one War College study as representing "the bottom of our manpower barrel") and with the need to address problems of low morale across the service.[16] The general preference for recreational athletics over conditioning persisted until at least the Korean War.[17]

Incidentally, a central school existed that could have facilitated innovation had rigorous conditioning remained an Army priority and had the school been sufficiently empowered and properly oriented. Yet the aptly named Physical Training School (PTS) stayed out of doctrine development and concentrated instead on producing athletic officers through the mid-1950s. As of 1946, when the school moved from Lexington to become a component of the Quartermaster School at Camp Lee, Virginia, the PTS's mission was twofold.[18] First, it trained nearly twelve hundred officers annually as "Physical Training and Athletic Directors" capable of "organizing and administering efficient programs" in their units centered on organized athletics, as had the Special Service officers of World War II. Second, it trained an equally sized pool of enlisted men as "instructors and assistants" to Physical Training and Athletic Director officers.[19] The school's leadership conceived of their mission narrowly. The school trained officers and assistants, but it did not provide input on physical training doctrine or policy revisions, nor did it conduct research. The school's mission began slowly broadening after September, 1946, when the Army Ground Forces (AGF) assumed responsibility for the PTS and directed another move in search of better facilities, this time to Fort Bragg, North Carolina.[20] Simultaneously, AGF reoriented the PTS toward training and conditioning over recreation and expanded its mission by assigning the PTS responsibility for collecting and maintaining data pertaining to "methods of unit physical training and conditioning." The data was intended for use in preparing material on conditioning for Mobilization Training Programs, and in preparing students to supervise unit-conditioning programs.[21] The school did not control physical training doctrine and policy, which the Office of the Surgeon General still owned. However, AGF's changes positioned the PTS to potentially become the Army's repository of specialized knowledge on physical training and conditioning, and consequently a major player in the production of the Army's physical culture.

But before the PTS began exerting its influence, US intervention on the Korean peninsula started catalyzing change in some aspects of the Army's physical culture. Combat on Korea's rugged terrain demanded that soldiers be well conditioned, causing officers at every level of command to perceive gaps between battle's demands and the average soldier's physical fitness.[22] American setbacks on the battlefield, discipline problems throughout the force, and prisoner of war behavior interpreted as inappropriate came to be attributed inside and outside the Army to soft soldiers drawn from unworthy youth. Furthermore, decreasing troop quality accompanied increasing rates of conscription, as it had during both world wars, at a time when the Army already struggled to attract and retain high-caliber manpower.[23] Among the many pieces of evidence cited by critics of America's soldiery in the ideologically charged Cold War environment, perhaps the most unsettling concerned prisoners of war. Numbering more than seven thousand in total, American prisoners held by North Korean and Chinese forces suffered a mortality rate of approximately 38 percent. This far exceeded the rate of prisoner deaths in previous American wars. Furthermore, approximately a third were found to have collaborated with their captors. Few escaped, few resisted, and twenty-one even chose to remain in North Korea after the war.[24]

In trying to rationalize early failures and ugly reports, an explanatory narrative developed among government officials, senior military leaders, and veterans' organizations that assigned blame chiefly to junior soldiers and leaders at the regimental level and below.[25] According to that narrative, a high standard of living, rampant "mom-ism," and a mass-consumption society had ruined the young generation fighting in Korea. They had been pampered into failure. America's fighting men suffered from "give-it-upitis" and were soft, deficient in grit and ingenuity, effeminate, selfish, and so lacking in character as to be susceptible to "brainwashing."[26] This narrative differed slightly among analysts who treated the young generation more fairly and who instead stressed failure to properly train for war.[27] But whether America's "soft" youth or poor training were to blame, explanations nearly always involved critiques of physical fitness. This interpretation of the Korean War experience became a hallmark of arguments for the importance of physical training. For instance, when the authors of the later *Field Manual (FM) 21-20: Physical Training*, published in 1957, urged units to develop "vigorous and continuous" training programs, they pointed to the "alarming number of casualties" in Korea that they attributed to "the inability of the U.S. soldiers to physically withstand the rigors of combat over rugged terrain and under unfavorable climatic conditions."[28] Four decades later, the authors of the *FM 21-20* published in 1998 still referenced American failures in July 1950 as a reason to prepare soldiers for the physical demands of war.[29]

Whatever the narrative, complaints filtering back to the Infantry School from the front through 1952 suggested that commanders "deplore[d] the physical condition" of men arriving in theater.[30] Among the numerous lessons to emerge from Korea, many concerned deficiencies in "combat skills, physical conditioning, and fighting spirit." When combined with the demands of the future nuclear battlefield predicted by Army concept and doctrine authors, these lessons pointed to a need to get back to "tough training."[31] Additionally, a study of World War II physical training programs released by the American Association of Health, Physical Education, and

Recreation (AAHPER) in 1951 even challenged memories of high-quality training between 1941 and 1945. Zeroing in on a lack of command emphasis, the study's authors found that commanders during World War II had offered "much 'lip service'" to the importance of conditioning, but little supervision or direction. By and large, company commanders, who were usually inadequately prepared to organize a physical training program, had been "free to carry on whatever activities they desired." The result was a program inferior to the Navy's and Army Air Force's in many ways, according to the study.[32] Combined, this study and Korean War experiences resurrected concerns in the Army about declining national fitness and insufficiently rigorous conditioning practices, while turning attention back to combat-oriented physical training. Army leaders and physical culture producers alike sought explanations for the failings. Was the physical training program itself inadequate, or was proper implementation of it a bigger concern?

The latest edition of *FM 21-20*, published in November 1950, seems to have fueled some dissatisfaction with the program. As noted earlier, the manual was virtually identical to the version from 1946 with two exceptions. First, its authors cut sections on hand-to-hand fighting, wrestling techniques, and tumbling. Second, they added a new chapter on "mass games," such as kickball, and recommended a "prominent place" for them in any training program.[33] These games were different from organized athletics in that they could be played with large numbers of participants, required no advance organization, and needed very little equipment. Few required vigorous activity either. The manual perfectly captured major trends in the Army's physical culture between 1945 and 1950: torpor, a growing preference for recreational activities over conditioning, and the declining significance of combat-oriented training. Its release four months after American forces entered combat in Korea helped throw questions about the adequacy of the Army's physical training program into sharp relief.

The Army's top leadership initially responded by reaffirming support for the existing physical training system, but also by stressing to commanders the importance of rigorous, methodical conditioning in the Army's physical culture. This dual-track approach was most visible in the issuance of the highly directive *Training Circular No. 27* (*TC 27*) in August 1951, which addressed concerns that *FM 21-20* might not provide "adequate guidance and direction" for properly structuring a three-phase conditioning program.[34] Issued over Army Chief of Staff J. Lawton Collins's signature,

TC 27 enunciated the physical training mission, policy, doctrine, and tenets of the Army's official culture—but it did not change anything. *TC 27* declared conditioning the key task in the service's "physical training mission" and its authors identified three mission objectives. First, to "indoctrinate all personnel regardless of branch of service or present duty assignment" with the need for and importance of a "high standard of physical fitness and good posture." Second, to develop the "highest possible degree of physical fitness" in each individual soldier to adequately prepare him for his duties. Finally, to produce visible outcomes of a "well-conducted physical training program." While these outcomes included qualities such as self-confidence and the will to win, measurable improvement in the five physiological components of physical fitness received emphasis.[35] Ultimately, the circular reiterated every commander's responsibility for physical training, focused attention on systematic conditioning, and mandated adherence to existing policy.[36]

Beyond this immediate reaction, Army Field Forces also laid groundwork for mid- to long-term responses by initiating studies based on complaints from the field to evaluate the physical training program.[37] The Office of the Chief of Army Field Forces (OCAFF) turned to its specialists at Fort Bragg's Physical Training School (PTS) in April 1952, who had already undertaken preliminary research, to conduct the study.[38] Most of the complaints the PTS specialists considered related to the physical fitness test as prescribed in *FM 21-20*. Commanders in the field provided plenty of criticisms: scoring the test involved too much "subjective judgment," the test did not measure "combat related physical skills," men lacked motivation to complete maximum repetitions in some events, and the scoring table did not "accurately indicate physical capabilities and stamina" of personnel.[39] Several of these complaints reflected long-standing tensions within the Army's physical culture, such as balancing between developing combat skills and foundational physical, mental, and character qualities. On this specific issue, the complaints and study exposed the continuation of a historical divide between commanders and physical training experts. Commanders had tended to favor activities with obvious combat relevance since the 1880s. Physical training experts typically preferred activities geared toward enhancing specific physiological characteristics in accordance with their concept of fitness.

Conducting the study required a massive data processing effort. Between eight thousand and ten thousand cards capturing individual performances on conditioning tests needed tabulation.[40] Interpreting and analyzing the information contained in the resulting mountain of IBM punch cards represented the largest data-driven analysis of fitness practices in the Army's history. This research project catalyzed an expansion of the PTS's purpose and capabilities beyond its emergent responsibility for developing physical training policy and doctrine, which had grown out of initiatives by Devers and his AGF staff in 1946 that started recasting the PTS as the hub of the Army's official physical culture production. The testing study accelerated that reformulation. However, such an outcome was not initially intended, as evidenced by OCAFF's refusal to authorize new funds and personnel for the school.[41] Conditions began changing when complications made meeting the study's deadline of August 31, 1952, impossible. Initial card screening identified discrepancies, requiring units to administer additional rounds of testing and data reporting. Accepted and corrected cards had to be punched on IBM cards that were in turn outsourced for tabulation and analysis.[42] The sheer amount of data processing required and the expertise needed to do it correctly eventually justified the creation of the short-lived Research and Analysis Department at the school in the summer of 1953.[43]

While the Korean War had created conditions in which the PTS began to flourish, the war's termination rapidly pared growth. In August 1953, less than a month after the United States signed an armistice in Korea, the Army decided to shutter the Physical Training School and reactivate it in a truncated form under the Ground General School at Fort Riley on January 1, 1954.[44] In 1949, a PTS staff study had narrowly averted a similar fate by arguing that the school had too much value as a professional physical training nucleus, as a crucial interface with the civilian physical education community, and as a more economical alternative to decentralized training.[45] In 1953, similar arguments bolstered by ongoing projects such as the testing study, *FM 21-20* revisions, and a training aid film failed to buy the PTS even a few extra months of life.[46] Pursuit of "economy of manpower and funds" chiefly decided the school's closure, which illustrates the Army's austerity impetus under the Eisenhower administration, given that the school's forecasted budget for 1954 was a mere $300,000, and its leadership had offered to slash that in half.[47] Two years later, analysts studying the physical training program also suggested a cultural explanation. According to them, the move signaled a return to "recreational type" activities reminiscent of trends after both world wars, but at odds with the school's intensifying association with systematic training and its focus on conditioning.[48]

Closure of the PTS could have substantially altered the Army physical culture's evolution, especially if it had led to the erasure of the institutional knowledge and expertise built since 1942. During World War II, the team led by Bank, McCloy, and Esslinger reengineered physical training, grounding it in scientific, empirical study and gearing it to produce specific, measurable outcomes. The PTS staff began reviving this approach after the doldrums between 1946 and 1950. When the PTS officially closed on January 1, 1954, these projects were still ongoing and were therefore transferred to the new General School section.[49] However, none of the experts transferred with their projects, except for a single civilian training instructor, Mr. James Dawson.[50] There existed a high likelihood of returning to the doldrums without a central body of expertise. Also, closure of the PTS eliminated the Army's sole mechanism for training and certifying specialists capable of advocating, planning, and executing physical training in accordance with published doctrine. Without these specialists, efforts to align unit programs with the official Army physical culture and administer them optimally would suffer.

However, damage from a loss of expertise was partially averted in the fall of 1954 when the rump General School's Physical Training Department, including Mr. Dawson, packed up and moved once again, this time to the US Army Infantry School (USAIS) at Fort Benning. Unsurprisingly, the USAIS leadership took its renewed ownership of physical training doctrine and policy seriously. Infantry branch members had long been among the most vocal advocates of systematic physical training. Infantry officers wrote extensively about physical training in service journals around the turn of the century. An infantry-centric conception of combat demands had tended in most periods to dominate discourse within the Army's physical culture. After World War I, the USAIS had even been home to the short-lived Physical and Bayonet Training Course administered by former members of Raycroft's organization. When it acquired doctrine and policy responsibility in 1954, the school delegated responsibility for monitoring and implementing physical training Army-wide to the Combat Conditioning Committee under its Ranger Department and assigned it five functions: preparing and delivering training at the USAIS, preparing materials for nonresident instruction, preparing staff studies for the Army, authoring Department of the Army physical training publications, and conducting continual evaluation, research, and development of the physical training program.[51] Though the committee lacked the PTS's robust staffing, its resources were superior to the General School department's resources and it enjoyed the active support of the influential USAIS. Because of the infantry's understanding of combat and its relationship to physical fitness, the USAIS's ownership of policy and doctrine also helped tilt the Army's physical culture away from recreation and back toward conditioning and combat applications.

The sudden increase in the USAIS's control of physical culture production coincided with converging concerns in the Army and in wider American society over soldier and citizen fitness. This convergence spurred renewed interest in assessing the state of the Army's physical training system. A lodestar for such worries, the Kraus-Weber report, reached President Dwight Eisenhower's attention in the summer of 1955.[52] Its central claim was that American youth compared very unfavorably with their European peers in measures of strength and flexibility. Eisenhower's concern spurred several government and private initiatives to address the nation's apparently flagging fitness levels. Echoing the president's alarm, incoming Army Chief of Staff Gen. Matthew Ridgway expressed his suspicion in August 1955 that the Army was "not conducting a realistic physical conditioning program" and that insufficient emphasis was being placed on "soldierly posture and correct dietary habits."[53] Ridgway therefore directed the Continental Army Command (CONARC) to study the adequacy of the existing physical training program and its execution in the field. CONARC in turn assigned responsibility for the study to the Infantry School. Simultaneously, CONARC also directed its six Army Commands to conduct similar studies and forward their results to the USAIS.[54] The resulting study, issued in October 1955 along with the long-delayed physical fitness test report, was a sweeping reassessment of the Army's physical culture.

In the end, the USAIS researchers returned a full-throated affirmation of the Army's official physical culture as it existed in 1955. With the exception of "certain modifications," researchers determined that the existing physical training program and physical fitness test were "adequate for the attainment of proper physical condition."[55] Findings related in the study's final report reinforced central tenets of the existing culture. Conditioning came before all other activities, for instance. Measurable physiological outcomes were valued most, while traits such as self-confidence and discipline remained preferable by-products. Sport endured as a crucial part of the culture, but was secondary and supplemental to systematic training. Proper training required specialist instructors versed in the system, or at least competent amateurs able and willing to follow a program set down by experts. Conditioning could not be left up to individuals because expecting them to build and adhere to a rigorous, progressive program was "unrealistic and ineffective."[56] Instead, conditioning had to be a unit activity under the direction of trained specialists. Finally, the findings stressed maximizing the individual soldier's physical condition over unit fitness or discipline.[57] As with the valuation of outcomes, this focus on the individual reflected continuity with programs developed during World War I and World War II, but broke from the original formulation of the culture that Koehler dominated.

Yet not all was well with the Army's physical training program according to the report. Its authors did not dismiss concerns about the fitness of the average American or statements of dissatisfaction from the field. However, in allocating blame for perceived problems, the USAIS researchers pointed a finger at the population making many of the complaints. "The major barrier to the attainment of sound physical condition throughout the Army," they concluded "is the lack of continued command interest."[58] While the report's authors acknowledged some underlying causes for deteriorating fitness, such as a tendency during peacetime to "fail to realize the need for a high state of physical fitness" and a "growing national tendency to avoid muscular activity both in our work and recreation," they argued that commanders bore ultimate responsibility.[59]

The USAIS researchers expanded their case against unit commanders in blunt terms throughout the lengthy report. Physical training was a command responsibility according to Army doctrine and policy.[60] Yet too often commanders failed to prioritize training, organize it in a productive way, or hold their trainers accountable for proper implementation. As a result, unit programs were often too easy and did not follow the core doctrinal principles of progression and overload. Consistency across a unit program was often problematic. For example, commanders might run a vigorous conditioning program for three months, and then almost completely ignore it for the rest of the year.[61] Competing requirements tended to impinge on training time, which was already inadequate according to the report's authors and remained so according to 60 percent of officers surveyed in 1958.[62] Physical training sessions also regularly departed from doctrine. Instructors, whose lesson plans were apparently rarely subject to inspection, tended to improperly arrange activities. For example, they might schedule an hour of guerrilla exercises when ten minutes was the recommended maximum, or spend a whole week doing nothing but Drill One followed by a week on the obstacle course and so forth.[63] At the level of unit commanders and their staffs, inadequate knowledge and training exacerbated the problem of insufficient command emphasis according to the USAIS researchers. Guidance and planning had to be "based on scientific knowledge" and come from "technically trained leaders," but senior commanders typically left physical training completely up to company commanders, who often lacked "the proper concept of physical conditioning."[64] Furthermore, the prevailing "jockstrap culture" exacerbated competing demands between athletics and physical training by favoring the former over the latter.[65] Graduates of the PTS could have offset commanders' unfamiliarity with the program, but researchers found that these specialists were rarely utilized appropriately.[66] The quickest fix, according to the study's authors, was to sell commanders on the physical training program and convince them of its necessity "despite the fact that, like taking medicine, it is somewhat disagreeable."[67] Unit commanders who insisted "on superior care for the mechanical implements of war" and who knew that entering battle with "rusted, dilapidated equipment" would be "suicidal" needed to be convinced to place equal emphasis on their human implements of war.[68] Some irony exists in these findings because the USAIS itself had apparently failed to sufficiently indoctrinate its graduates in the importance and proper execution of a physical training program.

According to the USAIS report, skepticism and ignorance fueled the problem of the physical training system's insufficient implementation. Skepticism arose from what the authors called an "improper" or "inadequate concept of physical conditioning." Researchers found that many commanders simply did not know the principles underlying an effective program. Other leaders confessed faith in the old alternative to systematic conditioning—the belief that "ordinary tactical training activities" provided sufficient exercise.[69] This latter concept might have seemed especially attractive because, according to the study, commanders faced an enormous number of competing demands when building their training calendars. Achieving two objectives with one event would be appealing. Researchers also found that senior commanders rarely inspected their subordinates' physical training programs. This sent a message that physical training was less important than other competing demands and allowed company commanders to deviate from the standardized conditioning program without correction.[70] On top of all this, existing Army regulations did not require units to conduct or document standardized physical fitness tests, so few mechanisms existed to enforce compliance. Researchers recommended numerous solutions. The most straightforward was to simply insist on command emphasis from the top down. Others involved improving training and access to specialist knowledge, such as increasing time spent in advanced courses on teaching officers to develop and supervise conditioning programs.

One of the most powerful approaches to creating buy-in for physical training among commanders was to force officers to invest personally in their *own* physical fitness. To accomplish this, researchers proposed that raters and endorsing officials comment on an officer's "physical condition for combat service" when completing his annual evaluation. Researchers also counseled making these comments part of every officer's permanent record.[71] These recommendations became requirements a year later through a revision of *Army Regulation 623-105*.[72] The Army also issued *Army Regulations 600-160: Maintenance of Physical Fitness and Detecting and Correcting Physical Abnormalities among Officers* two months later on Chief of Staff Maxwell Taylor's authority. Although concerned chiefly with "physical or mental abnormality" that might disqualify an officer for "full military duty," the regulation required officers to exercise regularly and commanders to examine their subordinates. Being "physically incapable of performing the duties of his office, rank, grade, or rating" exposed an officer to risk of separation from the service for physical disability.[73] Although the regulations stopped short of mandating that officers participate in systematic conditioning programs, they directed weekly exercise and reemphasized the significance of fitness to individual officers. Officer fitness as a vector for stressing fitness throughout the force echoed turn-of-the-century initiatives from President Theodore Roosevelt and Gen. Franklin Bell, but this time disciplinary measures and regulations took precedence over inspiration and exhortation.

While command emphasis could do much to align unit practices with the Army's official physical culture, researchers also argued that trained specialists were necessary to advise commanders, design unit programs, and inspect organizations for compliance. The PTS's closure in 1953 therefore received heavy criticism in the study of 1955.[74] In the short term, the Army could leverage its existing specialist corps, certified by the PTS before its closure, if units took time to identify them and assign them appropriate additional duties. But this was not a long-term solution. Once again, producers of the Army's physical culture argued that a central school was necessary. The USAIS could build cultural continuity and develop doctrine and policy, but the probability of disconnect between policy and practice remained high without certified instructors to implement policy or officers qualified to plan and supervise unit programs.[75] In lieu of a PTS-style central school, the study's authors offered a compromise in the form of Army Area physical training courses. Pointing to a one-week course operated by the Fifth Army at Fort Riley and another at Fort Belvoir's Engineer School, researchers suggested that such courses could at least prepare unit personnel to lead physical training sessions.[76] Yet such schools would eventually run out of trained staff without a central school, and they did not prepare leaders to develop or supervise programs. The central school argument failed to gain traction, however. Comprehensive, skill identifier–granting training for specialists by a central agency would not return until the creation of the Army's Master Fitness Trainer program in 1983.[77]

The study's authors also addressed widespread dissatisfaction with physical fitness testing. Specifically, they reasserted the need for tests even though none was mandatory, revised scoring tables, and provided a new combat-focused test. To revise scoring, researchers completed a long-delayed study, initiated in 1953, that had been plagued by data tabulation challenges and disrupted by moves between Forts Bragg, Riley, and Benning. An updated set of scoring tables resulted that established more realistic expectations, particularly in the three-hundred-yard run event.[78] Researchers also responded to the "discontent of combat unit commanders" who felt that a "test better related to combat skills" was necessary by providing a new examination tool—the Physical Achievement Test (PAT).[79] Five events made up the PAT: a five-second rope climb, a seventy-five-yard dash, a triple broad jump, a 150-yard man carry, and a one-mile run. The first four events were to be administered on a single testing day, with the mile run conducted the following day or within four days if delayed by weather. Except for the man carry and rope climb, the PAT's events came from the extended battery that Drs. Charles McCloy and Arthur Esslinger piloted in 1942. The climb and carry events were borrowed from the British Battle Physical Training Test.[80] By design, the PAT was supposed to measure combat-related skills in addition to the basic components of physical fitness. Its USAIS creators promised that combat unit commanders could, "with some degree of confidence," be sure that soldiers were well conditioned if they scored above average on both the standard fitness test and the PAT.[81] The PAT subsequently entered doctrine in 1957 and reflected an infantry-centric focus that had long been a dominant strain in the Army's physical culture, and that had only intensified under the USAIS's influence.

Finally, the adequacy study's snapshot of the Army's physical culture highlighted a noteworthy new element—weight control became a concern to be addressed as part of a physical conditioning program for the first time. Sculpting appropriately sized and shaped bodies had been part of the Army's physical culture since its inception. Early cultural producers such as Herman Koehler and Edmund Butts had celebrated the masculine, disciplined, uniformed body in their writings. Koehler was especially concerned with sculpting balanced bodies in the late-nineteenth-century mode and measured cadets under his charge to track their progress. Height and weight standards were part of induction exams during both world wars, though cases of underweight recruits were more prevalent than overweight recruits. Induction exams during the 1950s also applied height and weight standards. However, the discourse around physical training policy and doctrine had rarely touched on the problem of *overweight* service members, or at least male soldiers, before the mid-1950s. The main exceptions to this were members of the WAC who had come under scrutiny for being overweight and had become subjects of diet experiments during the preceding decade. WAC weight issues had been primarily nutritional, having had much to do with the types and portions of food on offer in mess halls and post exchanges. These offerings were calibrated to the needs of young men engaged in physically strenuous daily activity, not to the needs of women performing more sedentary duties.[82] But by 1955, obesity was common enough across the entire service to warrant opening new fronts in the fight against fat.

Conceiving of obesity as a problem to be addressed through physical training increasingly gained traction within the Army's physical culture in the 1950s. Ridgway specifically expressed concern about "correct dietary habits" in initiating the study of 1955.[83] Discourse about fat also appeared in service journals. In one example, Maj. Albert Lockhart's *Infantry Journal Quarterly* article "Overweight in Grade," published in 1956, offered advice to the "large segment of the Army engaged in sedentary duties" on a "chairborne tour" about how to lose weight and avoid a negative evaluation per *AR 600-160*. Writing as Maj. Pear Shape, a self-confessed "Fatso," Lockhart related the trials and tribulations of an officer desirous of fitness but hamstrung by a packed schedule and competing demands. After an encounter with a general who informed him that "there's a weight limit for jeeps," Pear Shape found ways to get fit and shared them with his readers: train on your own schedule, seek competition, eat sensibly, stick with consistent and moderate exercise, and consult a doctor in case of concern.[84] Escalating apprehension over weight put the Army at the front end of an American dieting movement in which men increasingly participated in the 1950s. Since the 1890s, dieting and slim bodies had come to be seen in wider American society as a sort of moral compensation for consumerism and a way to display virtue. Overweight bodies became associated with more and more negative issues and qualities in the 1950s: psychological problems, heart disease risk, "softness," and feminization.[85] Because physical training in the US Army had always included moral and gendered aspects, weight control fit naturally as an objective worth pursuing through exercise.

Some harsh words, self-motivation, and a "custom-made conditioning program" of his own design might have been thought sufficient to remedy Maj. Pear Shape's condition, but the average soldier or noncommissioned officer with whom the Army's physical culture had long been most concerned could not be entrusted with such responsibility. Accordingly, the adequacy study's authors recommended that the Army systematically identify and correct obesity in the force. Their prescription was highly individualized and premised on a nuanced reading of the obesity problem. Noting that "true obesity" was "not too common" and difficult even for a physician to diagnose, the researchers recommended thorough evaluations of soldiers thought to be obese rather than simply relying on the height-weight tables.[86] Assessing body structure was the first step in such an evaluation. Some soldiers might exceed weight standards but be "heavy muscled, heavy boned," and without excess body fat. Others of a lighter build might be within the weight table standards, but not "considered as normal in the true sense of the word" owing to "relaxed musculature and disposition of fat."[87] After body build, consideration was also to be given to a soldier's obesity history, disabilities, and habits of eating, drinking, and exercise. Only after a full evaluation were commanders to prescribe a remedial program that targeted the problem's roots without endangering the soldier by demanding too much strenuous exercise too quickly.

Researchers endorsed several existing programs as models. They praised one in the Fourth Army that involved close coordination between commanders and installation surgeons, but they explicitly recommended another, developed by the Eighteenth Airborne Corps in 1953, for Army-wide adoption. The Airborne Corps's program required commanders to send overweight soldiers to the hospital for evaluation, and then enter them into a weight reduction program supervised by the unit's medical officer. Every month, commanders reported to the commanding general the number of pounds lost by each soldier on their weight reduction programs.[88] The report's authors declared that "the smaller the waistline, the longer the life-line" and that the "degree of over-weight" was "directly proportional to an individual's efficiency, namely his physical stamina and mental alertness."[89] In doing so, they made a case for a soldier's weight to matter, just like his strength, endurance, agility, and coordination. Surveilling and slashing excess fat became one more tool for strengthening a commander's "control over the physical state of his command."[90] Within a decade, the Army endorsed this concept by institutionalizing a weight control program and linking weight to measures of soldier and unit fitness.[91]

While the adequacy study addressed fallout from the Korean War experience, the *FM 21-20* revision cycle moved forward and senior leader dissatisfaction with a younger generation of soldiers simmered. Larger ongoing projects within the Army also continued concentrating attention on soldier fitness. Chief among them was the service's initiation of a major restructuring of its combat divisions. Labeled the pentomic concept, the reorganization was supposed to give the Army a modern face-lift and prepare it to fight either on an atomic battlefield or in response to limited aggression.[92] Army Chief of Staff Gen. Maxwell Taylor (1955–1959) in particular viewed the restructuring as a means of improving the Army's relevance vis-à-vis the nuclear-capable Air Force and Navy.[93] The Pentomic Division, created essentially by Taylor's fiat in October 1956, replaced the Army division's traditional regimental combat teams with five battle groups. Each battlegroup contained four or five maneuver companies, each comprising five platoons.[94] Theoretical research and highly controlled exercises informed this organization. Army theorists concluded that, generally speaking, nuclear weapons did not revolutionize the battlefield. Maneuver and conventional fighting remained necessary. As the authors of one widely circulated text for mid-career officers asserted, "No weapon, or system of weapons, can ever be a complete substitute for combat units. 'War without men,' 'pushbutton war'—all false shibboleths purporting to wage war without manpower—receive no support from atomic tactics."[95] However, using nuclear weapons and minimizing the effects of enemy weapons required new approaches to maneuver and organization. The Army emphasized three concepts in its adaptation to "atomic tactics": dispersion, flexibility, and mobility. Dispersion on a nonlinear battlefield to deny the enemy quality targets, flexibility to sustain losses and still operate effectively in chaos, and mobility to rapidly mass and disperse.[96]

If this was the future of general war between nuclear powers, then the soldier's physical fitness remained valuable according to the Army's top officers. Ridgway repeatedly predicted that wars would still be won by men instead of machines, even in the face of unimaginably powerful weapons.[97] So long as armies met in conflict and war did not escalate to an exchange of strategic nuclear weapons that would deny all parties victory, soldiers still needed to maneuver as part of units to defeat enemy forces and seize terrain. If anything, the atomic battlefield might demand *more* in terms of physical endurance. The Infantry School's assistant commandant, Brig. Gen. Carl Fritzsche, made this case in an article published in 1955. Fritzsche argued that soldiers and their leaders had to be prepared to "operate independently and at great distance" from bases and other units. They would also need to be able to operate for "extended periods under conditions unknown in the past," which in turn demanded the "confidence necessary for success" that came through good health and physical conditioning.[98] Furthermore, Fritzsche predicted that tactical nuclear weapons would accelerate the pace of hostilities, denying commanders the time to recondition men who had "grown soft."[99] Members of the Infantry School's staff studying the pentomic concept buttressed Fritzsche's prediction. By 1958, the school's combat conditioning committee had concluded that the pentomic soldier would have to "move farther, faster, oftener" than his predecessor, yet retain a "reserve of strength from which to destroy or pursue enemy forces."[100] A survey of Army units conducted in 1958 reflected similar sentiments in the field. Of eighty-three units surveyed, leaders in 75 percent of them felt that the pentomic concept increased physical requirements.[101] In short, physical fitness in this imagined future conflict remained imperative, and its development could not wait until that war commenced.

In the midst of this organizational and doctrinal ferment and two years after the adequacy study of 1955, the long-delayed, USAIS-led revision of *FM 21-20* went into print. Breaking from previous practices, a new technical manual, *TM 21-200*, accompanied the field manual. Field manuals were high-level guides that presented principles, tactics, techniques, and procedures that were widely applicable. Technical manuals provided very detailed and specific information about the operation and maintenance of a particular piece of equipment, or about the performance of particular tasks. *FM 21-20*'s target audience comprised commanders and staff officers responsible for planning, preparing, supervising, and inspecting physical training programs. The manual therefore covered subjects such as program planning and construction for various types of units, general human physiology, and fitness evaluations. In contrast, *TM 21-200* targeted instructors and provided detailed information about performing exercises.[102] Except for a formal weight control program, the new manuals converted into doctrine many features of the physical culture expressed in the adequacy study of 1955. The twin manuals of 1957 reflected a physical culture premised on conditioning, focused on individual fitness over unit fitness, rooted in empirical research, and oriented toward preparation for infantry combat.

In another novel move, the manuals' authors explicitly framed their system in a historical context and, knowingly or not, engaged in some historiographical interpretation. In relating a brief history of physical training between 1885 and 1957, the specialists at the PTS and at the USAIS who authored the manuals identified trends and turning points, criticizing some and praising others. Critiques and praises provide additional insight into the physical culture these authors belonged to and helped shape in the 1950s. Their history began with the US Military Academy's hiring of Herman Koehler in response to a perceived glut of physical deficiencies among the men enlisted to fight the Civil War. Every conditioning initiative through World War I was, in their words, Koehler's "personal endeavor."[103] Between 1914 and 1957, the manual's authors identified a boom-and-bust cycle. During World War I, World War II, and the Korean War, commanders specifically and the Army in general awoke to the need for rigorous conditioning through combat experience and to encounters with an American populace made soft by "leisure living." After each war, the Army drifted into complacency and prioritized recreation over conditioning. The authors characterized the need for individual soldier fitness as constant, perhaps even growing, throughout this period despite mechanization and technological advances. Sports also featured prominently in this short history. When praised, sport was employed as a "supplement to the conditioning of soldiers," as in World War I. When criticized, it competed with and eclipsed systematic conditioning. Other subjects for criticism included the old-fashioned brand of "formal calisthenics" that returned between the world wars, the dangerous practice of letting commanders design their own programs, the inadequate corps of specialists available to support mobilizations for both world wars, and repeated failure to sustain "vigorous and continuous" programs at the unit level.[104] On the other hand, the use of military and civilian specialists to craft a "modern program" during World War II earned acclamation, though the work of Raycroft and his team between 1917 and 1920 went unmentioned. The manual's authors identified strongly with the World War II–era specialists responsible for the third watershed in the history of the Army's physical culture—creating the first doctrine that "could be scientifically justified by testing procedure."[105]

Claiming to be heirs to this "new physical training concept," the manual's authors launched into the most technical treatment of physical training to appear in doctrine yet. Based on the premise that the human body, "like weapons and machines," must be "understood before proper techniques and care can be employed in conditioning it," nearly a quarter of *FM 21-20*'s pages were dedicated to a synopsis of body structure and functions.[106] Readers could learn about anatomical terms (medial, lateral, superior, inferior, and the like), the body's major bones, types of joints, muscle actions, major muscles, the functioning of the cardio-respiratory system, and more.[107] Beyond the principles of overload and progression that had propelled the training system since 1942, the manual introduced a slew of new technical terms such as *hypertrophy*, *crest loads*, and *stroke volume*.[108] One of the theses underlying this highly scientific approach to conditioning was that the system could build bodies better and quicker than could incidental or improvised training. Efficiency and effectiveness were especially valuable given the average recruit's level of fitness, which was assumed to be very poor. Just as their predecessors had six decades earlier, these new advocates of systematic training guaranteed a rational and rapid path to making bodies, which had grown soft in civilized life, ready for battle.

However, the manual's highly technical treatise was something new, and it seems to have served two purposes. First, it was an educational tool meant to bridge the gap between a commander's responsibility for and his ignorance of his soldiers' physical conditions. Second, the treatise reinforced the expertise of its authors because its content would have been daunting for lay readers, and may in that way have been intended to help sell the system to commanders. After all, could the average commander come up with something better if the human body was so complex?

Selling the program was important, given the adequacy study of 1955's finding that the system itself was sufficient, but that it was compromised by a lack of command emphasis. As observed before, top Army leaders and physical training advocates alike agreed in the 1950s that physical training was extremely relevant for the atomic battlefield of the future. Given the Korean War example and expectations of future conflicts, commanders would not have time to bring their units up to sufficient levels of fitness before entering combat. Thus, conditioning programs had to be consistent and continuous. The authors of *FM 21-20* worked to communicate this need and to make it easy for commanders to establish such programs. Dividing the system across a field manual and a technical manual is one example of this effort. Another can be found in the definitions of fitness each manual offered. Where the technical manual retained the five World War II–era components of physical fitness, the field manual simply located physical fitness as a constituent of total military fitness and made a case for its importance.[109] *FM 21-20* advanced an argument that commanders should care about conditioning because it prepared troops to meet the demands of combat, improved an individual's sense of well-being, cultivated an appropriate soldierly appearance, and enhanced soldiers' mental and emotional fitness, and hence also unit morale.[110] After making the case to commanders that they should care, the manual provided examples and guidance for tailoring their own programs to meet a wide range of needs. Individual and unit training both received coverage. So too did programs for specialists and staff personnel, which were often trusted to develop and maintain their own fitness—a practice proven to be "unrealistic and fallacious."[111]

Another aspect of the Army's official physical culture that the system of 1957 reflected was its infantry-centric character. In short, the ability to engage in infantry combat defined fitness at its core. Though notable throughout both the field manual and technical manual, this focus is especially visible in sport's place within the training system, the technical manual's revised depiction of fitness, and the Physical Achievement Test's addition. In regard to sport, the manuals' authors pushed back against the eminence of recreational athletics in the force. In the 1950s "jockstrap" culture that glorified sport across the service, interunit, interpost, and Army-wide competitions boomed. Commanders often placed athletically gifted troops and conscripted athletes on special duty and on traveling teams, denying them training as soldiers and corrupting unit training in many cases.[112] Stewards of the Army's official physical culture, which was premised on systematic training and conditioning, acknowledged the value of sport in building esprit de corps and as a "laboratory" for character development.[113] The manual even included new information about organizing leagues and tournaments in off-duty hours. However, the manual's authors maintained that athletics should be tightly controlled. Sports should "supplement the more vigorous conditioning type activities, rather than replace them."[114] The primary purpose of physical training was conditioning for combat, not recreation. This position was reflected in a new-but-familiar triangular depiction of fitness capped by a "combat ready" state. Basic military skills, such as crawling and climbing, and traits, such as aggressiveness and confidence, composed the triangle's two sides and supported combat readiness. Strength, endurance, agility, and coordination formed the foundation atop which everything else was built.[115] Physical training purportedly addressed all three sides of that triangle. In discussing "combat readiness," the Army's chief physical culture producers tended to frame it in terms of being able to maneuver dismounted on the battlefield. Evaluating combat readiness could be accomplished through the PAT. First proposed in the adequacy study of 1955, this battery tested skills such as rope climbing and partner-carries in addition to raw physical fitness.[116] To a degree, the PAT was a concession to commanders who were unconvinced that the regular physical fitness test measured a soldier's preparation for combat.[117] It also helped center the definition of fitness on readiness for infantry combat. Rope climbing, dashes, and mile runs were hardly relevant to tank or gun crews, much less to clerks. This orientation represented less a change and more an intensification of long-term trends favoring infantry-centric fitness and exercise concepts in the Army's training system. A widely held conception of the infantry soldier as the Army's basic element enabled the infantry branch to bolster these inclinations as it gained organizational dominance over physical training doctrine.[118]

A final, notable aspect of the Army's official physical culture reflected in the system of 1957 was the continued, if gradual, elevation of the individual over the unit as the locus of concern. Contrasting the *FM 21-20* of 1957 with its earliest predecessor underscores this trend. The *Manual of Physical Training* of 1914 ostensibly prioritized the "development of the physical attributes of every individual to the fullest extent of his possibilities," but only in order to make the soldier into a more effective cog in a larger machine.[119] Highly prized traits included discipline, precision, and subordination. As Koehler himself wrote, soldiers needed a spirit that reached "out beyond the individual" to make him "think of himself only in connection with the obligations" that the nation laid upon him. Physical training pursued physical and psychological objectives to render the soldier a "disciplined, interdependent and dependable" component of a larger unit.[120] Unit readiness was certainly still an element of the physical culture in 1957, but measurable individual fitness loomed larger than before. According to the field manual, commanders should care about fitness chiefly because it made the soldier better prepared for combat, not just because it made for a more disciplined unit. The technical manual's continued use of the five physiological components of fitness introduced in 1942 prioritized individual readiness over unit readiness, as did its fitness tests. Similarly, the manual's caution against extreme formalism was premised on formality's tendency to stifle a soldier's spirit and interest, and thereby his physical development.[121] Individual health considerations such as proper diet and weight control also moved toward the foreground. In part, concentration on the individual resulted from a more scientific approach to physical training that lent itself to measuring and maximizing a single body's capabilities. The move also aligned with tactical developments. Supreme valuation of discipline and unit effectiveness derived from the demands of linear warfare that informed military thinking up to World War I. However, dispersed formations and individual movement techniques became more important as new weapons made the battlefield deadlier. By World War II, small-unit success depended far more on the *individual's* ability to move and fight under fire than it had in the late nineteenth century, and the individual gained proportional significance within the Army's physical culture.

Less than a year after the publication of the new *FM 21-20*, the USAIS convened a physical fitness seminar at Fort Benning to evaluate the suitability of Army physical training doctrine in preparing soldiers for the future atomic battlefield. The seminar provided an opportunity for a wide range of stakeholders to weigh in on the state of Army physical training and to validate the adequacy study of 1955's findings and their incorporation into the *FM 21-20* revision of 1957. Seminar attendees included senior officers from field units and Army headquarters, representatives from various service schools, members of West Point's office of physical education, civilian physical education specialists, and those USAIS officers most responsible for crafting training doctrine. Specific objectives for the gathering included evaluating how civilian fitness affected the Army, determining relationships between physical fitness and total military fitness, determining the level of fitness needed under the new pentomic concept, and considering the best means for measuring fitness.[122] Opening remarks by Brig. Gen. Stanley Larsen, the USAIS assistant commandant, made clear that the whole official Army physical culture was under consideration. In asking, "what should we be fit for?," "how do we attain fitness?," and "how do we measure fitness?," Larsen asked attendees to grapple with the meaning, value, and methods of achieving fitness.[123]

Few revelations emerged from the briefings and committee reports. Most reaffirmed core beliefs within the culture or were predictable given extant trends, signaling the unlikelihood of significant change in the near term. However, four of the final report's most prominent ideas help refine our understanding of the Army's official physical culture as it existed at the dawn of a possible era of warfare defined by nuclear weapons. First, the attendees agreed that individual physical fitness was more important than ever despite technological advances and increasing mechanization. Briefers repeatedly asserted that victory on the battlefield might come down to relative advantages in foot mobility, the soldier's ability to "outmove and outfight" his opponent in adverse conditions, and characteristics such as self-confidence, aggressiveness, and a will to win.[124] Furthermore, *everyone* needed to be fit to fight because the Korean War experience and the pentomic concept suggested that the "rear area" had "been eliminated" in modern war.[125] Second, seminar attendees agreed that the training system expressed in *FM 21-20* and *TM 21-200* was fundamentally sound. A survey of organizations in the field revealed that units agreed—95 percent responded that the existing literature was "excellent" or "good."[126] Yet not all was well. Those same surveys revealed that as many as 72 percent of units felt that their programs were inadequate for mobilization or combat training. A sampling of responses from a survey of individual officers produced a similar finding. Insufficient time allotted to training was most commonly cited as the reason for unsatisfactory programs.[127] The cultural producers at USAIS recognized this gap between doctrine and implementation, the third prominent idea, as had their predecessors in the adequacy study of 1955. In the words of Lt. Col. James Reilly of the combat conditioning committee: "without effective implementation, strong command support and equally strong command supervision the program will fail in achievement of mission and objectives."[128] Remediation recommendations once again included more command emphasis, more "positive control" through supervision and inspections, and specialist training for instructors and program managers.[129]

Finally, seminar attendees agreed that the "Nation must be awakened to the necessity of youth fitness." American youth, specifically young men, needed to be "conditioned to meet all demands of citizenship."[130] These demands were manifold, and they included possible military service. However, conference attendees fretted that American youth might not be up to soldiering's demands. Giving voice to these concerns, Larsen claimed in his opening remarks that the "era of exertion and hardship" of America's forefathers had given way to "an age of ease and comfort" enabled by technology and consumerism.[131] Army leaders again turned their collective gaze externally to prehabilitation when confronted with perceived asymmetries between the demands of war and the ability of America's youth to meet them. Yet conditions had changed since the time of readiness camps and the Citizens' Military Training Camps (CMTC). Examining the development of federal prehabilitation programs since the interwar CMTCs shows how fears of totalitarianism and militarism, especially in the early Cold War years, reduced the appeal and utility of martial physical training for youth. Over time, the government had to devise new means and methods for sculpting young American bodies for battle.

Prehabilitation programs changed considerably between 1941 and 1957. The concept of prehabilitation was not new in 1941, but American entry into World War II heightened the perceived need for it. Afterward, Cold War concerns ensured that prehabilitation retained a place in American political discourse, in part because many cultural elites and political leaders intuited a growing "muscle gap" and dangers inherent in a "depleted manhood."[132] Additionally, widespread fears throughout the 1950s about a juvenile delinquency epidemic added a new dimension to the perceived value of prehabilitation. Physical preparation for military service might strengthen and discipline character even as it strengthened and disciplined bodies. Before 1941, initiatives such as the CMTC program and Civilian Conservation Corps (CCC) were martial in character and pursued both citizen- and man-building goals.[133] World War II and post-war-era efforts initially followed similar paths, but they encountered more limits. Examining how these efforts changed over time and the boundaries each encountered reveals some constraints on federal power to control and shape citizens' bodies. Analysis also reveals that while civilian physical educators easily and decisively influenced the Army's physical culture at key points in its development, the Army proved much less able to influence physical educators and wider American society's popular physical culture.

In 1940, the urgency of prehabilitation surged as the country moved toward war, largely because Selective Service boards rejected approximately 45 percent of the first two million men to be examined for physical or mental issues. While the Selective Service's director, Brig. Gen. Lewis B. Hershey, scolded Americans over their softness for which they "should be thoroughly ashamed," the presumed condition of Axis bodies also heightened anxieties.[134] Militaristic German, Italian, and Japanese cultures had spawned youth training programs that appeared to discipline, harden, and toughen future soldiers. In fact, some explanations for early German and Japanese successes circulating in the United States and Britain hinged on perceptions of superior soldiers conditioned for modern combat. Intentionally preparing America's youth for tomorrow's battlefield or factory therefore seemed necessary. The US government encouraged the idea of "crisis" spurred by the "deplorable conditions in physical fitness which imperil our Nation."[135] John Kelly's physical fitness organizations and his "Hale America" campaign were key sources for federal endorsement of the crisis narrative. From its origins in late 1940 to its sponsorship by the Federal Security Agency in 1943 and beyond, Kelly's organization gradually acquired more resources and influence to advance its mission of promoting fitness. Kelly's initiatives were always voluntary and advisory, but they sustained national attention on the bodies and minds of American citizens, and especially on young men of military age.[136]

Stepping beyond awareness and concern generation, the federal government unveiled its main prehabilitation effort, the Victory Corps, in September 1942. A joint effort of the Federal Security Agency (FSA), Office of Education, and armed forces, the Victory Corps aimed to prepare teenagers "for service tomorrow in the armed forces by preparing for service in the high school today."[137] Leaders in each sponsoring agency, such as the FSA's Paul McNutt, expected the Victory Corps to turn high school students into a trained reserve.[138] Interested students enrolled first as general members and later transitioned into one of five special service divisions if they met certain qualifications. Each division aligned with either community service, wartime industry, or a branch of military service.[139] Students could display their membership by wearing special Victory Corps caps, which they had to make themselves, or armbands emblazoned with division-specific patches. Regardless of division, the Victory Corps provided training in a variety of areas such as citizenship education, competence in science and mathematics, community service, and more. Nonetheless, one of its most "basic objectives[s]" was to "make the greatest possible number of pupils physically fit to carry on as members of the armed forces or as efficient workers."[140] Physical educators had repeatedly requested guidance from the government to best align their instruction with national needs. The Victory Corps responded by defining the citizen's obligation to contribute in total war as the rationale for youth fitness, and then suggesting a prehabilitation training system. That system found full expression in the manual *Physical Fitness through Physical Education*, published in 1942.[141]

The Victory Corps's system was a physical training regimen designed to prepare young bodies specifically for military or industrial service. According to military authorities, this approach was necessary owing to the shortcomings of physical education. Col. Theodore Bank, one of the chief agents of change in the Army's World War II–era physical culture, repeatedly and bluntly spoke about existing shortfalls. In one talk in 1942 to Midwestern educators, Bank told conference attendees that schools had "done a poor job of conditioning the youth of American during the last 20 years." They were responsible for producing too many "puny" recruits when the military needed young men "with the muscles of a blacksmith, the agility of an acrobat and the stamina of a marathon runner."[142] The Victory Corps program aimed to close this gap with a holistic approach to fitness involving conditioning, education on healthy lifestyle choices, medical intervention to remediate physical defects, and the cultivation of character traits such as a "spirit of aggressive attack" and a willingness to "take physical punishment without flinching."[143] Most youth of either sex could participate in the Victory Corps, but the program concentrated on producing "strong and rugged boys who [could] become excellent soldiers or sailors promptly after entering the armed services."[144]

Participation in the Victory Corps introduced boys in particular to the Army's World War II–era physical culture. Its system included both conditioning activities and athletics, specifically the "vigorous and rugged" instead of the "recreational" varieties. As in the Army's official physical culture, athletics held value mostly because they were thought to develop certain character traits such as the "spirit of competition" and the "will to win."[145] However, the system's emphasis was on conditioning exercises. Consequently, most of the manual's pages were filled with activities designed to improve muscular endurance, strength, and agility while teaching skills such as grenade throwing and basic drill. The Army's *Training Circular 87* directly influenced the Victory Corps's prescribed running, relay, conditioning, grass drill, and "ranger" exercises.[146] Indeed, most exercises came straight from the Army system. A year later, a related manual targeting colleges and universities also extended this physical training and acculturation system to the older brothers of prospective Victory Corps members.[147] The Victory Corps physical training system ultimately informed some revisions to school instruction, and the government's emphasis on fitness resulted in more hours dedicated to physical education courses and increased enrollment in those courses.[148] Nevertheless, the Victory Corps did not fundamentally modify physical education thought or practice to the degree that civilian educators had altered the Army's physical culture in the past.

In its close alignment with the Army's physical culture and its intervention in America's schools, the Victory Corps represented the most direct and comprehensive federal attempt at martial prehabilitation to date. And yet, despite great wartime pressures and anxieties about poor national fitness, the Victory Corps floundered. Within a year, surveys revealed that only 22 percent of eligible students were enrolled. Most enrollees remained general members or participated in the community service division. Of this population, the three armed-forces-aligned divisions each claimed less than 2 percent of total membership.[149] No federal funding proved forthcoming and the Office of Education considered the whole program a "dead duck" by the summer of 1944.[150] Postmortems emerged as early as 1943: some students considered the program childish, others preferred making immediate contributions to the war effort through community service, and many school administrators had too much pressing work and too little incentive to justify reforming curricula that seemed sufficient. Damningly, many educators and administrators also feared that the Victory Corps exemplified the "Great Intrusion of the Federal Government" into education.[151] Concerns about the "great intrusion" dovetailed with fears of militarism sparked by the Victory Corps, an organization to which comparisons with the Hitler Youth tended to adhere. Author E. B. White voiced this unease in arguing that "war itself is a Nazifying process," so dressing students in uniforms seemed "somehow a symbol of defeat, not victory."[152] Even with the unusual demands on society imposed by fighting World War II and anxieties about national fitness, Americans rejected a prehabilitation program premised explicitly on preparation for military service for being too martial in character and purpose.

Universal Military Training (UMT), the next major federal prehabilitation effort, came into being even as the Victory Corps withered and World War II ground toward a conclusion. President Franklin Roosevelt first publicly urged a program of mandatory training in a speech to Congress in January 1945, though at the time his was more an idea than a plan.[153] Roosevelt's successor, Harry Truman, continued his advocacy after the former's death in April. The Truman administration also began filling out the details of a compulsory service program during its campaigns with

Congress and the public between 1945 and 1948, and between 1950 and 1952. The proposed program would require nearly all young men to spend a year undergoing military training after graduating from high school. Advocates of UMT, many of whom were Plattsburgers or members of the interwar Military Training Camps Association, such as Henry Stimson and Robert Patterson, advanced two general arguments about its value. First, the possibility of conflict with the Soviet Union demanded constant preparedness to avoid a disastrous opening campaign in a future war. Universal training could improve preparedness and create a large reserve without incurring enormous expenses.[154] A second argument highlighted social benefits for American society in general and young men specifically. Training could impart useful skills, improve health, develop discipline and morality, and deepen citizens' commitment to their civic duties. In the words of historian Michael Hogan, young men would emerge from the "democratic crucible" of UMT with "bodies hardened, skills honed, minds steeped in republican virtue, and values attuned to the defense of democracy in a dangerous, Darwinian world."[155] This narrative was especially prevalent in the campaign of 1945–1948 for UMT.

Of all the social benefits that advocates claimed UMT would yield, physical fitness was among those cited most often. Military officers frequently pointed to a need to enhance the conditioning of potential soldiers, usually with reference to high inductee rejection rates in the past. As it had since the late nineteenth century, when the US Army discovered systematic physical training, convergence between the deep mobilization required to fight modern wars and the tacit obligation of citizens to be prepared for such service helped fuel the focus on fitness. Commentary from Maj. Gen. Lewis Hershey, the director of the Selective Service during and after World War II, typified this position. Hershey argued that there was no time to waste in remedying physical, educational, and moral deficiencies because future mobilization periods would probably be short due to new technologies and a shrinking world. Furthermore, he alleged that existing educational systems were inadequate, given "public indifference and apathy" and how badly they had failed before World War II, a war in which, "roughly, 30 percent of American young manhood . . . [had] been found physically unfit to bear arms in the national defense." Because the ability to "carry his full share of the responsibility [of defending the country] efficiently and effectively" was a requirement for every citizen, a mandatory period of service in which young men could be made physically, mentally, and morally ready to meet that requirement was essential, according to Hershey.[156] President Truman similarly emphasized improving the physical standards of the nation's manpower in his messages to Congress beginning in 1945.[157] Like Hershey, Truman sold mandatory military service as a way to prehabilitate men before they might be called upon in war. Truman had been shocked as an officer in a National Guard field artillery regiment and later as a US senator to discover just how many Americans were physically unfit or lacked access to health care or physical education. Thus, he resolved to act in order to help Americans "make the greatest machine—the machine that God made—work as he intended."[158] Teaching the nation's youth "what it means to take care of this temple which God gave us" was among Truman's top priorities for UMT.[159]

Despite the Truman administration's efforts, UMT floundered in Congress against opposition spurred by concerns over costs, militarization, and the injustice of compulsory service. UMT died its first death in 1948 after a blue-ribbon commission in 1947 and an experimental Army UMT program failed to meaningfully advance Truman's agenda in the legislative branch.[160] The Korean War resurrected the idea of UMT in 1950, this time focused more on military need and less on civic improvement. However, an absence of public support and the incoming president Dwight Eisenhower's antipathy to the program culminated in a vote of 236–132 in March 1952 against UMT in the House.[161]

Outside Congress, educators composed one of the groups most vocally opposed to UMT. According to one survey of professional groups in 1947, as many as 75 percent of educators were against any program of obligatory training.[162] Many physical educators opposed UMT despite their relatively greater embrace of prehabilitation through the Victory Corps system, their profession's history of involvement with the military's physical training programs, and their acceptance of partial responsibility for so many rejected inductees. Some of the reasons for this opposition can be gleaned from a series of articles published in 1945 in the *Journal of Health and Physical Education*. In them, authors took issue with the implicit assumption that one year of exposure to the Army's physical culture could fix all the nation's fitness shortcomings. The authors also argued that money for UMT could be better spent in primary and secondary schools by increasing access to physical education, improving and adding facilities, and hiring more faculty.[163] Others expressed wariness about militarism and linked UMT to compulsory service in the German military, echoing similar critiques of the Victory Corps. New York University's Jay Nash expressed this disquiet when he contended that America should not "experiment with the beginnings of a nationalized youth movement." Instead, he reasoned, the nation should foster fitness, discipline, and citizenship in local communities to preserve the "grass roots of democracy."[164] Americans rejected a martial prehabilitation program even with Cold War tensions, recurring anxiety about American society's physical decline, Korea's sharp reminder about the continuing need for fitness in modern war, and a political culture that still defined citizenship reciprocally based on obligations. Both the Victory Corps and the proposed UMT program felt too militaristic and seemed to pose too many threats to American liberties by way of control over young bodies.

Still, interest in prehabilitation of some kind persisted into the 1950s. A general explanation for this persistence exists in the space where the perceived consequences of material affluence and suburbanization overlapped with broad Cold War fears. This combination created a moment of cultural anxiety that one scholar has dubbed the "muscle gap."[165] Historians have shown that Americans in the early Cold War period typically understood the consumerism, abundance, and easy, sheltered nature of suburban life both as symbols of national success and as vectors for effeminizing the nation's youth.[166] John Kelly, the famous Philadelphian who raised concerns about men in World War II, certainly thought as much. He claimed in an article published in 1956 that the United States had become a "nation of weaklings." "Already today's youngsters are softer, weaker, and flabbier than the youngsters of certain foreign countries," Kelly asserted, "and it is obvious that they are growing still softer every year."[167] These allegations of "softness" carried multiple meanings. In one sense, weak youth meant weak soldiers, which constituted a real problem when the nation contemplated a possible future war with the Soviet Union. In another, "softness" suggested potential for Communist penetration and subversion.[168] "Muscle gap" anxieties had coalesced to such an extent by 1960 that president-elect John Kennedy explicitly declared the nation's "growing softness" and "increasing lack of physical fitness" a "menace to our national security."[169] In many ways, muscle gap anxieties echoed the earlier masculinity crisis or "male panic" of the late nineteenth century, which had helped spur military interest in systematic physical training in the first place.

The 1950s also added a new fear of violent and out-of-control youth to other concerns about generational competence. This panic over juvenile delinquency had its roots in the World War II years. Massive disruptions to family life were among the consequences of calling millions of men to military service and of an unprecedented number of women entering the workforce. Many youths also entered the workforce at an early age, thereby earning a new degree of autonomy along with their wages. In the words of historian James Gilbert, "dislocation, disrupted families, and a spirit of abandon had lifted certain restraints from the behavior of young people."[170] Lessening restraints and increased autonomy potentially set the stage for crime, or at least immoral behavior and indiscipline. Fears of a coming crime wave, stoked by authorities ranging from the FBI to local parent-teacher associations and church groups in the 1940s, seemed to be confirmed by expert opinion and leading measures of crime statistics in the 1950s.[171] The degree of a juvenile delinquency wave's actual severity is open to interpretation and debate, but fear of delinquency in the public consciousness was real. An impetus for prehabilitation followed from that fear: beyond strengthening weak and effeminate youth, military service and systematic physical training could discipline wayward youth. Perhaps the most visible manifestation of the "individual reformation by way of military service" narrative was Elvis Presley's public conversion from "angry delinquent" to "patriotic young adult" during his time in uniform. In this narrative, physical fitness was a major component of the holistic approach that the Army claimed it applied and that it leveraged to help justify conscription.[172] Providing physical training to potential soldiers seemed to be a way to simultaneously improve the average conscript's quality and extend some social benefits of service to a wider swathe of American society. Some of these benefits related to physical health, but many derived from equating physical fitness with moral fitness.

Specific episodes punctuated general cultural anxieties about softness, inadequacy, delinquency, and lack of fitness to sustain federal interest in prehabilitation. For example, the Korean War once again set off hand-wringing and soul-searching about the state of the union's body politic. Of four million men examined for draft registration between 1948 and 1955, approximately 52 percent were rejected on the basis of physical or mental issues.[173] Those who donned Army fatigues scarcely seemed a match for their supposedly hardier forebears. Commanders in Korea bemoaned the poor condition of new troops arriving in theater.[174] Army commanders and national political leaders alike tended to attribute high rates of collaboration and death among the prisoner of war population, upward trends in courts martial, and an uptick in desertions to the soft new generation.[175] On the fields of friendlier strife, Soviet athletes performed well in the 1952 Helsinki Olympic Games, and then demolished the US teams at both the 1956 Winter and 1960 Summer Olympics.[176] Amid this, the highly publicized Kraus-Weber report that exploded into America's consciousness in 1955 seemed to lend scientific credence to existing beliefs about the nation's unfitness. Hans Kraus, a sports medicine professor, and Sonja Weber, a posture expert, tested American youth in the 1940s and 1950s using a six-event battery. Kraus and Weber compared the results to those of Austrian, Italian, and Swiss children and found a concerning gap. Across the board, Americans performed far worse than their European peers. Sixty percent of Americans failed at least one test, and 36 percent failed at least one strength test compared to a European failure rate of only about 1 percent.[177]

The Kraus-Weber report ultimately spurred a federal response. At a White House luncheon in the summer of 1955 attended by dozens of sports celebrities, the same man who prodded Roosevelt to action in 1940 resumed his efforts with Eisenhower. John Kelly brought Kraus and Weber before the luncheon's attendees, all of whom watched with mounting concern as the report's authors detailed their findings. Eisenhower was purportedly aghast. According to one reporter, the presentation convinced the president that the fitness problem was "even more alarming than he had imagined."[178] Eisenhower's mind supposedly went to his World War II experience, and specifically to his memory of draftee rejection rates.[179] For Eisenhower, youth fitness had become an issue of national security. The subsequent federal response developed between 1955 and 1956 through a series of conferences held at the nation's military academies, foregrounding the project's martial implications.[180] A consensus emerged from these meetings that the federal response had to avoid any whiff of totalitarianism.[181] This reflected a desire to maintain contrast with the Soviet Union's regimentation and to elide the taint of militarism.

Executive Order 10673 inaugurated this new prehabilitation effort, a Cabinet-level body titled the President's Council on Youth Fitness (PCYF), in July 1956. The PCYF did not intervene in America's schools, nor did it promulgate a compulsory program, directly sponsor activities, or fund research. Instead, it was essentially a "public relations firm for the notion of fitness." Shane MacCarthy, the PCYF's director, described the council as "a catalyst, a stimulator, a coordinator, a persuader, an urger, an idea-dropper, a direction-pointer."[182] The PCYF and its full-time staff of four partnered with media outlets, the Ad Council, voluntary organizations such as the Boy Scouts, and local community organizations such as schools and churches. Typical activities included publishing informational pamphlets, providing staff for television interviews, sponsoring annual Youth Fitness Weeks, and encouraging the adoption of fitness as a theme for state, local, and private organizations' events.[183] By leveraging its social and political capital, the PCYF strove to popularize physical activity, defined broadly and liberally, and to inform and arouse the American public to the issue of youth fitness.

The PCYF labeled the product it marketed "total fitness." Dr. G. Ott Romney, the council's deputy executive director, defined this concept for attendees at the 1958 USAIS physical fitness symposium as a combination of physical, mental, emotional, and social fitness. This model aligned remarkably well with the Army's own "total military fitness" concept.[184] But as a prehabilitation effort, the PCYF represented a new indirect approach despite the similarities in definitions of fitness. As Romney told the seminar's gathered officers, the PCYF was "not born to implement the Defense program," yet any improvement of youth fitness was "bound to improve the preparedness of youth for military service."[185] Improving preparedness did not require young males to don uniforms or sweat through the Army's specific exercise system. Instead, it encouraged activity, sport, and education to build a foundation that would prepare boys to "take basic training in stride" and to "accept the rigors [of service] with a grin instead of a whimper." According to Romney, the PCYF was not in the business of crafting protosoldiers, but at the same time it wanted to ensure that the military would not have to "cuddle and coddle carload lots of softies."[186] This approach, characterized by its advisory, noncompulsory, and civilian nature and its commitment to the general improvement of the population's health, proved more durable, widely influential, and popularly acceptable than earlier efforts. In fact, the PCYF is still active today as the President' Council on Sports, Fitness, and Nutrition.[187]

Between 1945 and 1957, the Army's physical culture remained consistent despite forecasted conditions on future battlefields that may have seemed to minimize the relevance of the individual soldier's fitness. New technologies might have modified the service's force structure and doctrine, but they did not generate commensurate change in the way the Army approached or valued exercise. Senior military leaders remained committed to fitness throughout. Indeed, they held to the trope of improving human resources to match or complement the capabilities of new military technologies. In the face of weapons that were able to level entire cities and whose yields were measured by the kilo- and megaton, the soldier needed to be able to "move farther, faster, oftener" than his predecessor while retaining "a reserve of strength from which to destroy or pursue enemy forces."[188] However, after 1945 a general lull set in at the lowest organizational levels during which recreational athletics reigned and the popular and official physical cultures did not align. The Korean War experience rekindled the Army's focus on physical training. That conflict demanded a high degree of fitness from front-line combatants and support troops alike. Furthermore, the Korean War pointed to psychological and ideological considerations in Cold War conflict that physical training might address.

After 1952, the Army's key physical culture producers and its senior leaders agreed that the existing culture and its expression in physical training doctrine were fundamentally sound. Insufficient command emphasis from inadequately educated officers had compromised the application of training since World War II, but the training system itself remained valid. The change that occurred within the culture between 1945 and 1957 was consequently minor. Producers of physical training doctrine consciously identified with the more scientific "new physical training concept" pioneered during World War II. Applying research methodology and empirical data, specialists sought to fine-tune the training system to improve specific performance characteristics effectively, efficiently, and safely. That system reflected a valuation of conditioning above all else. Though the official physical culture still accommodated beliefs about sculpting minds and spirits by way of exercise and sport, those outcomes remained ancillary to physical development, as they had since 1942. Additionally, the individual soldier's fitness continued accumulating attention within the official culture, but the most important individual remained the average man, not the elite athlete. With the growing focus on the individual also came an increased concern for health issues, especially weight control. For the first time, obesity came to be identified as a problem across the service, and one that physical training could help alleviate. Finally, the official physical culture remained centered on infantry combat, sustained especially by the Infantry School acquiring ownership of training research and doctrine. Publication of the field and technical manuals in 1957, coupled with the conscious decision to reinforce existing approaches and systems rather than change them, signified that the Army's official physical culture had reached a new level of maturation productive of stability, which it would maintain until 1980.

While the Army's physical culture did not change dramatically, the government's approach to prehabilitation did. Concerns about gaps between the quality of the United States' manpower and the demands of war, and now Cold War competition, endured. In addition to long-held anxieties about the deleterious effects of urbanization, industrialization, and mechanization, military and political leaders alike fretted about the impact of consumerism, abundance, juvenile delinquency, and the softening effects of new technologies on young male bodies. As the USAIS combat conditioning committee's chairman put it: "Ironically, the important breakthroughs which we have achieved in weapons and equipment, and which magnify our combat capabilities, also reduce our capabilities by contributing to the softening and deterioration of the soldier."[189] Between 1945 and 1957, evidence seemed to accumulate in support of these general worries. High draft rejection rates on physical grounds during World War II alarmed the nation. A lack of conditioning allegedly claimed lives in Korea and rendered servicemen susceptible to brainwashing. Critiques of mass-consumer society claimed that it induced numerous negative effects, ranging from physical, mental, and moral softness to widespread delinquency. The Kraus-Weber report also raised concerns about the physical "unfitness" of America's next generation of soldiers. The presumed physical unfitness of American youth fueled interest in prehabilitation to close the "muscle gap." Yet the approach to prehabilitation changed significantly during the 1940s and 1950s. The wartime Victory Corps and postwar Universal Military Training concept were designed to expose young men directly to the Army's physical culture. This approach generated resistance by spurring fears of militarism and totalitarianism. Eisenhower's President's Council on Youth Fitness sidestepped such fears by detaching fitness and military training, and by encouraging rather than mandating participation. Where the Army once took the lead in martial prehabilitation programs, it receded to the background in advisory state efforts. Preparation for military service still motivated federal prehabilitation efforts to a large degree through the 1950s, but broader and less explicitly martial health goals took priority. These made programs more publicly palatable, especially in the Cold War environment.

Mid-century prehabilitation programs hold many lessons for those seeking to address today's fears about the state of America's youth and its potential soldiery. First, Americans have proven consistently resistant to overtly martial initiatives. Though relatively more tolerant in times of emergency such as World War II, American society time and again displayed deep suspicion of compulsory, nationally organized, and regimented programs. Second, martial concerns offered persuasive arguments for the *need* of youth physical fitness, but prehabilitation programs oriented toward preparing youth for military service specifically have enjoyed only limited reach and lifespans. Finally, the most successful programs have leveraged what historian Rachel Moran calls "advisory state" methods to sell, counsel, and inform Americans on the how and why of physical fitness.[190] These programs did not just target future soldiers, and they didn't train youth directly for military service. Instead, they aimed to cultivate a broad awareness of and desire for healthy lifestyles and physical fitness in American society.

CONCLUSION
FASHIONING THAT "CERTAIN STRENGTH OF BODY AND SOUL," 1885–1957

In the summer of 2018, the US Army unveiled its first physical fitness test revamp since 1980—the Army Combat Fitness Test (ACFT). Comprising six events ostensibly correlated with common soldier tasks such as extracting casualties on a litter and throwing equipment over obstacles, the new age- and gender-neutral test was a major departure from its three-event predecessor, the Army Physical Fitness Test (APFT).[1] The ACFT epitomized a "generational, cultural change in fitness for the United States Army" and was to become the "cornerstone of individual soldier combat readiness," according to Maj. Gen. Malcolm Frost, who oversaw the test's final stages of development as the Center for Initial Military Training's commander.[2] The ACFT's introduction culminated more than six years of research, fueled largely by a drive across the Department of Defense to improve "lethality," and it bore significant implications for day-to-day training and service member promotions. For all the fanfare, critical reactions were also loud and widespread. Detractors argued that the test was problematic to administer, that it required too much specialized equipment, that its technicality made training for the test difficult, and that it would produce too many injuries.[3] Army leaders' responses framed the ACFT as a vehicle for ushering in a more holistic and combat-centered approach to fitness that would reduce injury rates, improve readiness, and save lives. "This fitness test is hard. No one should be under any illusions about it," then Army Chief of Staff Gen. Mark Milley stated, "but we really don't want to lose soldiers on the battlefield. We don't want young men and women to get killed in action because they weren't fit."[4]

Seen another way, the ACFT was an artifact representing the latest evolutions of the Army's official physical culture. Placing the test in historical context helps explain its character, the discourse around it, and the strong reactions the ACFT engendered from boosters and critics alike. Take the pivot to "combat" physical fitness, for instance. During the world wars and the Korean War, Army leaders felt compelled to reorient physical training toward practical preparation for combat. Given that the Army had been a force constantly at war for more than seventeen years at the time of the

ACFT's introduction, a similar turn from general to combat fitness could even be seen as overdue. Also, inasmuch as the ACFT represented a triumph of CrossFit principles over past fads such as the jogging craze of the mid-1970s and 1980s, the new test reflected the period's wider cultural influences.[5] Earlier configurations of the Army's physical culture had similarly reflected their popular fitness milieus. Rhythmic gymnastics and college athletics both influenced Army training in their times. Engaging with the physical culture underlying the ACFT can enhance the Army's efforts to enact real change. While most critiques of the ACFT to date seemed to be about the relative merits of push-ups, deadlifts, and other exercises, the issues actually went deeper. Just what does it mean to be fit? Fit for what? Who should be fit? How should fitness be measured? Who should decide? Answers to these questions have changed over time in response to imagined battlefields, actual wartime experiences, trends in civilian physical education, and popular fads. The responses embedded in the ACFT were just the most recent in a long history.

That history began more than a century ago. The nascent form of the Army's official physical culture emerged in a particular context at the turn of the twentieth century and was shaped by military demands, wider American culture, and the state of exercise science. It represented an intersection between popular and military cultures, just as it does now. Yet today's culture also reflects an additional influence—its own past. Understanding that chronicle of change over time is vital to understanding the culture today. Primary credit for its original formulation goes to Herman Koehler, father of both West Point's physical education program and systematic physical training in the US Army, who wrote at a time of great change in military science. A need seemed to exist at the dawn of the twentieth century to fit waning men for dispersed combat on emptying battlefields dominated by new technologies. Koehler aimed for goals beyond simple muscular and cardiovascular improvement. In war, he wrote, "physical fitness is the factor upon which, more than any other, the efficiency of a fighting machine depends." After fitness came "men, money, and materiel," but most importantly "morale" because it alone could "determine and bring out the full and true value of these . . . physical components."[6] Elaborating on this body-mind-soul synergy, Koehler contended that "mere physical endurance, hardihood and force, will accomplish but little as compared to physical fitness plus the development of those mental qualities that guide and control this force intelligently."[7]

Koehler's concept of war and the soldier's role in it harmonized then and now with deep-rooted cultural beliefs in the American military tradition that situate man as the "dominant instrument on the battlefield."[8] In this schema, improving the Army's manpower was and remains imperative for success in war. Koehler regarded physical training as a key tool for cultivating a superior soldiery, but not just because it could produce troops capable of marching further or lifting heavier loads. Rather, his mission in physical training was multifaceted and educative. This approach is the historical basis of the Army's official physical culture. Physical training was supposed to build bodies, shape minds, sculpt character, forge units, and make better citizens.

Over time, the Army's physical culture grew up and out from these roots while responding to a variety of stimuli that included its own inertia, military need, wider American culture, and the state of exercise science. For example, emphasis gradually shifted from manufacturing disciplined human machine cogs to fashioning individual warriors. Valuations of intangible character traits and quantifiable physiological performance measures similarly shifted over time from weighting the former to the latter. Likewise, the relative importance of combat-related functional fitness grew during wartime and when physical training policy came under the Infantry branch's control, but it generally flagged in peacetime. Projects of man-, soldier-, and citizen-making remained interrelated throughout, but their outward expressions in the form of prehabilitation programs morphed in response to resource constraints, popular acceptance, and expectations of a citizen's potential military service obligations. Three punctuated periods in the physical culture's evolution are evident between 1885 and 1957: Koehler's disciplinary era, the combat-readiness interregnum of 1917–1919, and the scientific measurement school's rise after 1942. All three eras shared a tension between tradition and innovation that reflects a paradox in military culture writ large. The core of that paradox derives from the need for conservative organizations to constantly adapt in order to maintain relevance and competitive advantage. Ultimately, the Army's physical culture proved sufficient for fitting men to modern war. However, the inertia it acquired, coupled with repeated failures to sustain evolutionary progress in peacetime, produced spasmodic change and forced those responsible for physical training during World War II and the Korean War to relearn old lessons.

Studying change in the Army's official physical culture over time also shows that its dominant definition of fitness has always been layered, constructed, changeable, and heavily influenced by American society.[9] Since cadets began sweating under Koehler's tutelage in 1885, more has been at stake in physical training than simply improving an individual's strength or endurance. Early on, fitness included elements such as symmetry and power, partly because muscle fiber was thought to be indicative of moral fiber and other qualities. Fit soldiers were masculine, disciplined, confident, selfless, and efficient parts in a larger machine who were also resistant to the pernicious effects of overcivilization in the modern world. During America's first great crusade in Europe between 1917 and 1918, fitness accumulated new meanings that reflected Progressives' worldviews and the demands of trench warfare. Later, scientific study yielded normalized measures of fitness in a physiological sense, yet the cultural definition of fitness retained immeasurable constituents such as teamwork, aggressiveness, confidence, a tough masculinity, and resistance to political subversion. Today, physical training remains a venue for the cultivation of mental toughness and a laboratory for character and leadership development. Notably, the dominant definition of fitness did not always correspond directly with the realities of combat. The ways in which cultural producers *imagined* combat and perceived the needs of the nation's young male population tended to be more influential. Fitness within the Army's official physical culture was always, and will likely continue to be, a malleable concept capable of sustaining many layers of meaning.

Part of the reason that fitness remains a malleable concept is that there is no objective, quantifiable standard of combat fitness. Indeed, such a standard may be impossible to define. None of the systems of exercise developed between 1885 and 1957 was premised on actual measures of soldiers' battle performance, or on remediating specific reasons for physical failures in combat. McCloy's and Esslinger's work during World War II came closest to delivering a quantifiable definition of fitness. But even that work proceeded from a generalized list of tasks thought to be necessary on the battlefield, such as jumping in and out of trenches or carrying heavy objects, and analysis of what could be expected of an average man in related and controlled tasks. Studies of combat motivation and soldier performance, and works of history in the face-of-battle vein, frequently highlight the intense physical demands of war and the interconnectedness of physical and mental stamina.[10] However, they are also consistently vague on the specific physical demands that soldiers face. Most scholarly studies and soldiers' recollections never get beyond meditations on the sheer exhaustion and fatigue native to battle. A precise, quantified definition of fitness may be an impossibility. Too many factors are at play in combat, and too little data collection is possible. Superior battlefield fitness is also a relative concept measurable only between combatants. The unquantifiability of fitness is significant to the Army's physical culture because it leaves much up to interpretation, values, beliefs, and reasoning by analogy. The application of science may yield practices that can render a body capable of lifting more weight or moving faster, but there is no comparable precision or certainty possible in making a person combat-ready.

Furthermore, though the Army's physical culture changed over time, it always existed at the intersection between soldier-, citizen-, and man-making projects. As a result, exercise was often a vehicle for moral, mental, and physical uplift. Fitness for combat alone was therefore never enough. This is still true today. Army leaders tend to assume that fit soldiers are good soldiers, and that characteristics conducive to superior conduct in battle can be revealed and refined through physical training and sport. The interaction of these three projects has also turned the Army's attention outward onto wider American society. Advocates of systematic training regularly promised that society would be enriched by men returning home who had been taught the value of fitness and ways of achieving it. But just returning healthy men was not enough. Men also needed to be made fit before entering the service so as to improve the overall quality of the nation's potential soldiery and the efficiency of basic military training. Between 1885 and 1957, every young man existed in a yet-to-be-mobilized reserve and in a social context where soldiering was crucial to citizenship and the masculine ideal, so it was only right to prehabilitate them for service. The urge to sculpt young Americans into better potential soldiers, better citizens, and better men became an enduring feature of the Army's official physical culture, informing the value of fitness within the Army and systems designed to achieve it. The American public's physical fitness, or more often the lack thereof, remains a national security concern today. If called upon to fight a war demanding mass mobilization, Americans would no doubt adapt. Yet that process of adaptation would not be easy, and the percentage of the population capable of shouldering the demands of combat training immediately is far smaller than it was in the early and mid-twentieth century.[11]

Beyond 1957, the Army's official physical culture continued evolving in response to familiar stimuli: military need, wider American culture, the state of exercise science, and the physical culture's own history. This is evident in the greater significance that running and exertion-recovery activities assumed within the Army's physical culture in the 1970s and 1980s. The move mirrored an aerobic exercise boom largely initiated by Dr. Kenneth Cooper's book *Aerobics*, published in 1968. Interpretations of wartime demands on humans held by the agencies most responsible for physical training doctrine and policy also influenced the culture's evolution. Wars featuring intensive ground combat, such as Korea and Vietnam, typically inclined the official physical culture toward individual combat readiness. In contrast, less demanding periods and a fascination with technology during the 1980s and 1990s inclined the Army's physical culture toward general, corporate health. In recent years, high-performance athlete training programs such as CrossFit and P90X exerted a powerful influence, due in part to combat operations in Iraq, Afghanistan, and elsewhere. Elite units such as the 75th Ranger Regiment, conceiving of fit soldiers as "combat tactical athletes," have been the vanguard in this movement.[12] Nevertheless, creating greater change across the entire Army requires action to change an ingrained *culture*. Implementing a new test is not enough. A broader and deeper effort to modify values, beliefs, assumptions, and standard day-to-day practices at the lowest organizational levels is necessary. It will also be challenging.

The Army's typical one-size-fits-all approach to fitness exemplifies the type of challenge the service faces in implementing change. According to official promotional and aspirational publications, today's soldier is supposed to be an elite warrior-athlete. For instance, the Army justified its "Soldier Athlete" initiative around 2010 on the premise that "our Soldiers must perform and excel at Soldiering at a professional level, just like any world-class athlete."[13] This elite warrior-athlete paradigm exists in tension with other factors. The Army is a massive organization that prefers applying singular standards and practices, which will by necessity be more productive of middling than elite outcomes. Also, since its inception the Army's physical culture has focused more on average unit performance and the ordinary soldier than on elite individuals. This ingrained tendency lives on. Most units still conduct mass physical training led by relatively junior and undertrained members. The onus for above-average performance rests on the individual soldier and requires him or her to invest personal time outside of the training day. Finally, the elite warrior-athlete paradigm centers on lethality in ground combat, but in truth this is only a requirement for a minority of the Army's population. Higher physical standards, especially those derived from an interpretation of ground combat's demands, preclude sizeable portions of the population from service, even if those precluded people have skills and aptitudes well suited to the highly technical demands of modern warfare.

High physical fitness standards are not undesirable or inappropriate, but the Army should diversify them or else face up to the challenges of enabling a large and varied population to meet them. Different performance benchmarks aligned with different types of duty positions, as proposed for the ACFT, are a step in the right direction. Yet the Army and its soldier population are more diverse than the ACFT's three degrees of performance. The Army Ground Forces learned a similar lesson during World War II, which led it to fashion a classification system that acknowledged many different categories of fitness. Ways should be found to retain service members whose contributions are not primarily physical, such as older soldiers and those working in highly technical fields. Additionally, producing truly elite warrior-athletes involves more than implementing new testing activities and standards. Deeper cultural change needs to occur at the company and battalion level. Physical training must move away from its focus on the mass, long valued for its supposed ability to instill discipline, and instead seek to maximize the capabilities of individual bodies. Old approaches will not work because they were designed to improve whole units and those units' weakest links. The scientific approach to physical training, pioneered during World War II and ascendant since, offers much promise, but units cannot sustain old practices and expect new results.

Changing the existing physical culture is no easy feat, but the culture's history suggests a possible approach. Historically, cultural change occurred most rapidly and was adopted most thoroughly during periods of expansion, such as during the world wars. Influxes of new leaders without entrenched values, assumptions, and approaches to physical training created windows of opportunity for implementing new ideas. Today, massive end-strength Army growth is theoretically possible, but highly unlikely. It should not be the basis of planning. Yet periods of rapid cultural change shared one more commonality—empowered experts who were also organizational outsiders. Herman Koehler, the original driving force behind a physical culture predicated on systematic training, arrived at West Point as a young, barely tested Turnverein teacher. He only earned an officer's commission after fourteen years of service. Joseph Raycroft and his hastily recruited team of civilian educators and coaches led a major reform of the

Army's physical culture during World War I. During World War II, Theodore Bank, Charles McCloy, and Arthur Esslinger dramatically altered the Army's official physical culture by ushering in a data-driven "new physical training concept" rooted in scientific research. In each case, unacculturated outsiders brought with them some of the latest ideas and practices from the world of physical education and were sanctioned by Army authorities to make changes. Similarly empowered outside experts could help realize change in today's Army. For example, performance coaches and nutritionists, uniformed or civilian, could plan programs full-time and tailor those programs to the needs of individual soldiers. Of course, making use of experts would require commanders to give up some authority and control. Experts would also be expensive, especially for such a large organization. However, if the Army truly seeks revolutionary change in physical fitness, then measures more drastic than introducing a new test will be necessary.

In implementing change, the Army should also address the gendered nature of its physical culture. A recurring urge to improve *men* has historically been a core component of the Army's physical culture. That urge creates a tendency to foster and reinforce traditional gender norms. Because cultural producers between the late nineteenth century and 1957 understood the task of building men and building soldiers to be one and the same, women had no place within the culture. Women's entry into the force in 1942 threatened the Army's man-building mission, even as the Army's physical culture appeared to threaten women's femininity in the eyes of many contemporary commentators. Thus, women required a different physical training system and culture, even though many men and women served in similar or even identical duty positions. Separate physical cultures, and the specific character of each, reinforced the notion that women were not real soldiers. Even when the Army's physical training system became gender-integrated and duty position–neutral in 1980, it set female performance standards for two of the three Army Physical Fitness Test events significantly lower than male standards.[14] Although designed to account for physiological differences between men and women, gender-based standards buttress conceptions of male superiority and arguments against gender-integrating combat arms units. If the Army wants to take gender integration seriously, then it must define fit *soldiers*, not fit men and women. The recently proposed gender-neutral test may help move the Army's physical culture in this direction. However, as some critics have observed, the ACFT is equal-opportunity, but statistically biased in ways that disadvantage women.[15] Consequences of a biased fitness test will manifest in the retention and promotion rates of female soldiers. Fortunately, testing standards and events can be modified to address this bias if the Army's leadership cares to do so. Precise measurements of what exactly combat demands of the human body cannot exist. Performance standards are thus by nature best guesses and generalized constructions, so they can be tailored and modified to ensure more statistically commensurate male and female outcomes without compromising their utility for assessing combat readiness.

Finally, this work offers important insights into relationships between citizen fitness and the Army's combat readiness. Poor national fitness negatively affects the military today as it did a century ago, but the problem has changed over time. Whereas the key concern between 1885 and 1957 was typically about quantity first and quality second, today the problem is chiefly one of quality. Between 1885 and 1957, the Army focused on conscription. Because young, male American citizens were also potential soldiers, they needed to be fit in order to enable the military's rapid expansion in time of war. High draft rejection rates during the world wars, along with narratives formulated to explain early Korean War failures and POW behavior, helped fuel the Army's conscription-related concerns. Practical mobilization issues regularly intersected with broader cultural anxieties about racial and masculine decline, and, especially during the Cold War, the nation's competitive edge relative to its adversaries. Army leaders and civilian policy-makers consequently gave increasing attention to the prehabilitation of American youth. Anxieties over national fitness have not disappeared. Commentators today still frame declining fitness as a national security concern. Approximately 71 percent of young people in the United States do not meet basic military entry standards.[16] However, the immediate problem for today's smaller, more selective, all-volunteer force is that poor national fitness denies the military access to a wide swathe of skilled citizens. From a purely military perspective, improving the nutrition, exercise, and general health habits of America's youth will produce more talented soldiers in addition to fitter soldiers. Exploring the history of prehabilitation in the first half of the twentieth century illuminates past approaches and suggests best practices. While this project offers no simple lessons or cookie-cutter solutions, historical awareness may help today's policy-makers approach issues with wisdom and sensitize them to possibilities, tendencies, and limitations.

A note of caution is necessary, however. Commentators and policy-makers must avoid the "youth these days" fallacy when discussing national fitness. This fallacy assumes that the current generation of young Americans is somehow innately weaker or less capable than earlier generations. It is worth remembering that elders of the men and women who won World War II doubted that the "Greatest Generation," as we know it today, was up to the task. In times of need, Americans have adapted and standards have adjusted to accommodate service by a larger percentage of the population. The US population is, in all likelihood, not in terminal decline. Assuming inherent generational softness obscures opportunities for intervention, systemic adjustment, and adaptation.

Writing in 1892, in the dawning years of the Army's physical culture rooted in systematic training, Capt. James Pilcher observed that the necessity for "individual action has again arisen." Pilcher posited a historical pendulum action. Where "individual strength and personal prowess" had been crucial characteristics for a warrior in the "days of Lysander and Scylla," gunpowder later "dethroned individuality in combat" and gave way to the methods of "hurling great masses of men against the enemy." Yet according to Pilcher, cutting-edge technological advances in his day denied soldiers "elbow-touch" encouragement and necessitated dispersion and individual action. "Duelling, although on a modified and vastly extended scale," he wrote, "has once more taken the chief place in the machinery of war." These new developments rendered the "culture of the soldier's physique . . . indispensable."[17] Pilcher, like all his peers who first advanced the cause of systematic training in the Army, believed he could enhance human performance to a degree never before known by applying science, rational exercise, and a modern, detailed knowledge of the body. Pilcher's generation inaugurated the Army's body-sculpting movement, which continues today. However, their efforts and the efforts of those who followed were influenced by more than a simple "detailed knowledge." Broad and shifting cultural, political, scientific, technological, social, and military contexts informed and constrained the imaginations of these advocates, as they still do now. War is an intensely physical activity. Participation in ground combat is perhaps man's supreme test of physical stamina, mental toughness, and character. Despite the promises of the most ardent technophiles, technology has not changed these fundamental facts. Nor is it likely to do so in the future. Where there is war, there will be a need for strong bodies to prosecute it. Even outside the demands of infantry combat, sufficiently strong bodies are necessary to endure the hardships and stresses intrinsic to war's nature. Much is bound up in those bodies—interleaved mental, spiritual, moral, and physical characteristics. How might the nation and its army best sculpt those bodies in pursuit of virtue, victory, and civic need? Answering this question will remain a process fraught by and freighted with layers of meaning that transcend the battlefield.

NOTES

INTRODUCTION: MODERN WAR, MODERN FITNESS

1. Ely J. Kahn, *Army Life* (Washington: Infantry Journal, 1943), 46.
2. Carl von Clausewitz, *On War*, trans. Michael Howard and Peter Paret, indexed ed. (Princeton: Princeton University Press, 1989), 101.
3. Harold M. Barrow and Janie P. Brown, *Man and Movement: Principles of Physical Education*, 4th ed. (Philadelphia: Lea & Febiger, 1988), 66–74.
4. Michael Anton Budd, *The Sculpture Machine: Physical Culture and Body Politics in the Age of Empire* (New York: New York University Press, 1997), x.
5. Barrow and Brown, *Man and Movement*, 83.
6. Kristin L. Hoganson, *Fighting for American Manhood: How Gender Politics Provoked the Spanish-American and Philippine-American Wars* (New Haven, CT: Yale University Press, 1998), 9–13.
7. John Keegan, *The Face of Battle* (New York: Penguin, 1978), 230.
8. Michael Howard, "Men against Fire: The Doctrine of the Offensive in 1914," in *Makers of Modern Strategy from Machiavelli to the Nuclear Age*, ed. Peter Paret (Princeton: Princeton University Press, 1986), 510–511.
9. Frederic N. Maude, *Notes on the Evolution of Infantry Tactics* (London: William Clowes and Sons, 1905), x.
10. Antulio J. Echevarria, "The 'Cult of the Offensive' Revisited: Confronting Technological Change before the Great War," *Journal of Strategic Studies* 25, no. 1 (2002): 209; Howard, "Men against Fire," 515–521.
11. Gail Bederman, *Manliness & Civilization: A Cultural History of Gender and Race in the United States, 1880–1917* (Chicago: University of Chicago Press, 1995), 4–5, 78–79, 92–93; Christopher E. Forth, *Masculinity in the Modern West: Gender, Civilization and the Body* (New York: Palgrave Macmillan, 2008), 142–145.
12. For a succinct summary of the "crisis in masculinity," and a critique of its classification as a "crisis," see Bederman, *Manliness & Civilization*, 11–15; for a deeper treatment of the crisis, see Forth, *Masculinity in the Modern West*; for more on the specific American context of the crisis, see John F. Kasson, *Houdini, Tarzan, and the Perfect Man: The White Male Body and the Challenge of Modernity in America* (New York: Hill and Wang, 2001), 10–11.
13. Wilhelm Balck, *Tactics*, trans. Walter Krueger, 4th ed., vol. 1 (Fort Leavenworth, KS: US Cavalry Association, 1911), 194.
14. Historians have thoroughly explored period beliefs in physical perfectibility,

but they have rarely applied this concept to military training. For some literature on perfectibility, see James C. Whorton, *Crusaders for Fitness: The History of American Health Reformers* (Princeton, NJ: Princeton University Press, 1982), 271–294; Joanna Bourke, *Dismembering the Male: Men's Bodies, Britain and the Great War* (Chicago: University of Chicago Press, 1996), 171–174, 209; Kasson, *Houdini, Tarzan, and the Perfect Man*, 7, 29, 49; Roberta J. Park, "Healthy, Moral, and Strong: Educational Views of Exercise and Athletics in Nineteenth-Century America," in *Fitness in American Culture: Images of Health, Sport, and the Body, 1830–1940*, ed. Kathryn Grover (Amherst: University of Massachusetts Press, 1989), 123, 46–58.

CHAPTER 1. BODIES AND BATTLEFIELDS: CONTEXTUALIZING MARTIAL FITNESS FOR MODERN WAR

1. Modern US Army physical training practices continue to evolve. The most recent doctrinal publication on physical training, Training Circular 3-22.20, dates to 2010. The current Army Physical Fitness Test (APFT) consisting of a two-mile run and two minutes each of push-ups and sit-ups dates to 1980. Testing only became mandatory in 1963. In late 2018, Army officials revealed a new six-event, age- and gender-neutral physical fitness test set to take effect in 2021.
2. War Department, *Manual of Physical Training for Use in the United States Army* (New York: Military Publishing, 1914), 3.
3. Hermann Hagedorn, *That Human Being, Leonard Wood* (New York: Harcourt, Brace, and Howe, 1920), 11.
4. War Department, *Manual of Physical Training for Use in the United States Army*, 3. The US Army's Army's implementation of systematic physical training had been haphazard and belated in comparison to European militaries and to wider American society. The US Military Academy, which was the US Army's torchbearer for physical training, introduced its first comprehensive program in 1859, but abandoned it during the Civil War. Physical training did not return in a systematic way until the late 1870s. Whitfield B. East, *A Historical Review and Analysis of Army Physical Readiness Training and Assessment* (Fort Leavenworth, KS: Combat Studies Institute Press, 2013), 28–31.
5. Kristin L. Hoganson, *Fighting for American Manhood: How Gender Politics Provoked the Spanish-American and Philippine-American Wars* (New Haven, CT: Yale University Press, 1998), 3.
6. E. Anthony Rotundo, "Body and Soul: Changing Ideals of American Middle-Class Manhood, 1770–1920," *Journal of Social History* 16, no. 4 (1983): 25–26.

7. E. Anthony Rotundo, *American Manhood: Transformations in Masculinity from the Revolution to the Modern Era* (New York: Basic, 1993), 248–250.
8. Frederick Jackson Turner, *The Frontier in American History* (New York: Henry Holt, 1920), 2–4; Michael S. Kimmel, *Manhood in America: A Cultural History*, 3rd ed. (New York: Oxford University Press, 2012), 87–89.
9. Kimmel, *Manhood in America*, 87.
10. Simultaneous threats came from working-class men and immigrants when political machines leveraged these populations' latent political power. See Gail Bederman, *Manliness & Civilization: A Cultural History of Gender and Race in the United States, 1880–1917* (Chicago: University of Chicago Press, 1995), 82–83.
11. Hoganson, *Fighting for American Manhood*, 109–116, 29–31.
12. Rotundo, "Body and Soul," 30.
13. G. Stanley Hall, "Feminization in School and Home," *World's Work* 16 (1908): 10238.
14. Bederman, *Manliness & Civilization*, 13; German military theorist Wilhelm Balck spoke directly to this point in blaming the day's "fast manner of living" for the Western soldier's decline. See Wilhelm Balck, *Tactics*, trans. Walter Krueger, 4th ed., vol. 1 (Fort Leavenworth, KS: U.S. Cavalry Association, 1911), 194.
15. Rotundo, *American Manhood*, 251–55; Bederman, *Manliness & Civilization*, 16–17.
16. Bederman, *Manliness & Civilization*, 77–84.
17. Rotundo, "Body and Soul," 29; Kimmel, *Manhood in America*, 119–20; Bederman, *Manliness & Civilization*, 18–19.
18. John F. Kasson, *Houdini, Tarzan, and the Perfect Man: The White Male Body and the Challenge of Modernity in America* (New York: Hill and Wang, 2001), 28–30.
19. Harvey Green, *Fit for America: Health, Fitness, Sport, and American Society* (New York: Pantheon, 1986), 137–39; "near epidemic" from Bederman, *Manliness & Civilization*, 85.
20. George M. Beard, *American Nervousness: Its Causes and Consequences* (New York: Putnam, 1881), 5–6.
21. Beard, viii.
22. Permutations of Beard's "American nervousness" and neurasthenia appeared in European societies also, especially France, Britain, and Germany. See Antulio J. Echevarria, "The 'Cult of the Offensive' Revisited: Confronting Technological Change before the Great War," *Journal of Strategic Studies* 25, no. 1 (2002): 205–207.

23. Beard, *American Nervousness,* vi; "brain workers" on ix.
24. Beard, 35.
25. Bederman, *Manliness & Civilization,* 84–88.
26. Beard, *American Nervousness,* ix.
27. For more on recapitulation, see Bederman, *Manliness & Civilization,* 88–101.
28. James C. Whorton, *Crusaders for Fitness: The History of American Health Reformers* (Princeton: Princeton University Press, 1982), 271–294; Joanna Bourke, *Dismembering the Male: Men's Bodies, Britain and the Great War* (Chicago: University of Chicago Press, 1996), 171–174; Kasson, *Houdini, Tarzan, and the Perfect Man,* 7, 29, 49; Roberta J. Park, "Healthy, Moral, and Strong: Educational Views of Exercise and Athletics in Nineteenth-Century America," in *Fitness in American Culture: Images of Health, Sport, and the Body, 1830–1940,* ed. Kathryn Grover (Amherst: University of Massachusetts Press, 1989), 123, 46–58.
29. Scholars often refer to this body of ideas as "Social Darwinism," though the term is problematic because of the diverse, often paradoxical conclusions biological thought produced in social sciences. For a brief but thorough exploration of the term, see Daniel Becquemont, "Social Darwinism: From Reality to Myth and from Myth to Reality," *Studies in History and Philosophy of Science* 42, no. 1 (2011): 12–19.
30. Hoganson, *Fighting for American Manhood,* 12–13; Carl N. Degler, *In Search of Human Nature: The Decline and Revival of Darwinism in American Social Thought* (New York: Oxford University Press, 1991), 14–15; Becquemont, "Social Darwinism," 16.
31. James J. Schneider, "The Theory of the Empty Battlefield," *Royal United Services Institute for Defence Studies Journal* 132, no. 3 (1987): 37.
32. Walter E. Kretchik, *U.S. Army Doctrine from the American Revolution to the War on Terror* (Lawrence: University Press of Kansas, 2011), 78–80.
33. James J. Schneider, "The Theory of the Empty Battlefield," *Royal United Services Institute for Defence Studies Journal* 132, no. 3 (1987): 37–38; Michael Howard, "Men against Fire: The Doctrine of the Offensive in 1914," in *Makers of Modern Strategy from Machiavelli to the Nuclear Age,* ed. Peter Paret (Princeton: Princeton University Press, 1986), 511; Kretchik, *U.S. Army Doctrine,* 66–86; Perry D. Jamieson, *Crossing the Deadly Ground: United States Army Tactics, 1865–1899* (Tuscaloosa: University of Alabama Press, 1994), 64–72.
34. Echevarria, "The 'Cult of the Offensive' Revisited," 202.
35. Kretchik, *U.S. Army Doctrine,* 66–72; Jamieson, *Crossing the Deadly Ground,* 64–72.
36. Kretchik, *U.S. Army Doctrine,* 84–86.

37. Azar Gat, *The Development of Military Thought: The Nineteenth Century* (Oxford: Clarendon, 1992), 138; Jamieson, *Crossing the Deadly Ground*, 75–86.
38. For an overivew and critique of the cult of the offensive's historiography, see Echevarria, "The 'Cult of the Offensive' Revisited," 199–201.
39. G. F. R. Henderson, *The Science of War: A Collection of Essays and Lectures, 1891–1903* (London: Longmans, Green, 1906), 159.
40. Henderson, 160.
41. Howard, "Men against Fire," 515.
42. Echevarria, "The 'Cult of the Offensive' Revisited," 200–201.
43. Charles Ardant du Picq, *Battle Studies: Ancient and Modern Battle*, trans. John N. Greely and Robert C. Cotton, 8th ed. (New York: Macmillan, 1921), 123.
44. Du Picq, 123–124.
45. Du Picq, 111.
46. Gat, *The Development of Military Thought*, 140.
47. Howard, "Men against Fire," 514–522.
48. Wilhelm Karl Friedrich Gustav von Sherff, *The New Tactics of Infantry*, trans. Lumley Graham (Leavenworth, KS: C. J. Smith, 1891), 17–18, 20–23.
49. US officers came to similar conclusions about the need for new tactics. The many manuals released between 1867 and the *Field Service Regulations* from 1914 attest to this doctrinal ferment. For more on US tactical development, which is closely related to European development, see Kretchik, *U.S. Army Doctrine*, 78–120 and Jamieson, *Crossing the Deadly Ground*, 92–112.
50. John A. English, *On Infantry*, rev. ed. (Westport, CT: Praeger, 1994), 4–5.
51. Henderson, *The Science of War*, 371.
52. Henderson, 373–374.
53. Howard, "Men against Fire," 517.
54. Kretchik, *U.S. Army Doctrine*, 114–115.
55. Echevarria, "The 'Cult of the Offensive' Revisited," 204–205.
56. The lessons derived from this interpretation most heavily influenced the tactical thought and practice of Western militaries in 1914. Studies of the Balkan Wars of 1912 and 1913 may have refuted some of these lessons, but World War I exploded before many militaries had time to process Balkan Wars experiences. English, *On Infantry*, 7.
57. Archibald F. Becke, *An Introduction to the History of Tactics, 1740–1905* (London: Hugh Rees, 1909), 95.
58. Frederic N. Maude, *Notes on the Evolution of Infantry Tactics* (London: William Clowes and Sons, 1905), 146.
59. Becke, *An Introduction to the History of Tactics, 1740–1905*, 65.
60. For a concise statement of the "cult of the offensive" argument and a guide to

further reading, see Stephen Van Evera, "The Cult of the Offensive and the Origins of the First World War," *International Security* 9, no. 1 (1984).

61. Howard, "Men against Fire," 510–511; Echevarria, "The 'Cult of the Offensive' Revisited," 199–202; "compelling rationale" on 201.
62. Quoted in Howard, "Men against Fire," 520.
63. Echevarria, "The 'Cult of the Offensive' Revisited," 208–209.
64. Balck, *Tactics*, 1:194.
65. Balck, 1:194–195.
66. Brian McAllister Linn, *Echo of Battle: The Army's Way of War* (Cambridge, MA: Harvard University Press, 2007), 110–111.
67. Muscular Christianity originated in England in the first half of the nineteenth century and migrated to America, chiefly the northeast, beginning in the 1850s. Harvey Green, "Introduction," in *Fitness in American Culture: Images of Health, Sport, and the Body, 1830–1940*, ed. Kathryn Grover (Amherst: University of Massachusetts Press, 1989); Whorton, *Crusaders for Fitness*, 271. For a thorough analysis of the movement, see Clifford Putney, *Muscular Christianity: Manhood and Sports in Protestant America, 1880–1920* (Cambridge, MA: Harvard University Press, 2001).
68. Green, *Fit for America*, 195–197; T. J. Jackson Lears, "American Advertising and the Reconstruction of the Body, 1880–1930," in Grover, *Fitness in American Culture*.
69. Macfadden and his magazine are the subject of many studies. See, for example, Mark Adams, *Mr. America: How Muscular Millionaire Bernarr Macfadden Transformed the Nation through Sex, Salad, and the Ultimate Starvation Diet* (New York: Harper, 2009); Lisa Robin Grunberger, *Bernarr Macfadden's "Physical Culture": Muscles, Morals, and the Millennium* (PhD diss., University of Chicago, 1997); Robert Ernst, *Weakness Is a Crime: The Life of Bernarr Macfadden* (Garden City, NY: Syracuse University Press, 1991); William R. Hunt, *Body Love: The Amazing Career of Bernarr Macfadden* (Bowling Green, OH: Bowling Green State University Popular Press, 1989).
70. Gertrud Pfister, "The Role of German Turners in American Physical Education," *International Journal of the History of Sport* 26, no. 13 (October 2009): 1910.
71. Green, *Fit for America*, 181–182.
72. Edward Mussey Hartwell, *Physical Training Treated from American and European Points of View* (Boston: G. H. Ellis, 1890), 8.
73. Frederic L. Paxson, "The Rise of Sport," *Mississippi Valley Historical Review* 4, no. 2 (1917): 145.
74. Donald J. Mrozek, *Sport and American Mentality, 1880–1910* (Knoxville: University of Tennessee Press, 1983), 28–31.

75. Steven Pope, *Patriotic Games: Sporting Traditions in the American Imagination, 1876–1926* (New York: Oxford University Press, 1997), 3–6.
76. For extended treatments of this point, see Wanda Ellen Wakefield, *Playing to Win: Sports and the American Military, 1898–1945* (Albany: State University of New York Press, 1997); Steven Pope, "An Army of Athletes: Playing Fields, Battlefields, and the American Military Sporting Experience, 1890–1920," *Journal of Military History* 59, no. 3 (1995).
77. The Master of the Sword was (and remains) responsible for the physical development of cadets. Calls for physical training in the Army predated Koehler's appointment, but Koehler was deeply influential in securing official sanction for standardized, systematic physical training.
78. James Huff McCurdy, *The Objectives of the American Physical Education Association* (Springfield, MA: American Physical Education Association, 1927), 1–2.
79. Roberta J. Park, "Physiologists, Physicians, and Physical Educators: Nineteenth-Century Biology and Exercise, *Hygienic* and *Educative*," in *Sport and Exercise Science: Essays in the History of Sports Medicine*, ed. Jack W. Berryman and Roberta J. Park (Urbana: University of Illinois Press, 1992), 138.
80. Isabel C. Barrows, ed., *Physical Training: A Full Report of the Papers and Discussions of the Conference Held in Boston in November, 1889* (Boston: Press of George H. Ellis, 1890), 1–2.
81. Park, "Physiologists, Physicians, and Physical Educators," 138–139.
82. Fred Eugene Leonard, *Pioneers of Modern Physical Training* (New York: Association Press, 1919), 147–155.
83. Edward Mussey Hartwell, "The Nature of Physical Training, and the Best Means of Securing Its Ends," in *Physical Training: A Full Report of the Papers and Discussions of the Conference Held in Boston in November, 1889*, ed. Isabel C. Barrows (Boston: Press of George H. Ellis, 1890), 5.
84. Hartwell, 8–17.
85. Hartwell, 20.
86. Jakob Bolin, *What Is Gymnastics?* (New York: Willett Press, 1902), 3.
87. Park, "Physiologists, Physicians, and Physical Educators," 166–168.

CHAPTER 2. ORIGINS OF A US ARMY PHYSICAL CULTURE, 1885–1916

1. Charles R. Greenleaf, "Physical Training in the U.S. Army," in *Proceedings of the American Association for the Advancement of Physical Education at Its Sixth Annual Meeting* (Ithaca, NY: Andrus & Church, 1891), 58–59.
2. Greenleaf, 59.
3. T. Gentz, "Gymnastics as a Branch of Military Education," *Army and Navy Journal* 9, no. 35 (1872): 562.

4. Gentz, 593.
5. James E. Pilcher, "The Building of the Soldier," *United Service* 7, no. 4 (1892): 336.
6. The French gymnastic school accepted one sergeant or corporal from every regiment and independent battalion for a six-month program. Graduates returned to their units as trainers, and the best remained at the school for another six months as assistant instructors. The course included training in "gymnastics, scaling walls, swimming, fencing with the bayonet, singing, dancing, reading, writing," and more. McClellan reported that the "efficiency of the French infantry is in no small degree attributable to the great attention paid to these points throughout the army." George B. McClellan, *Report of the Secretary of War Communicating the Report of Captain George B. McClellan, One of the Officers Sent to the Seat of War in Europe in 1855 and 1856* (Washington: A.O.P. Nicholson, Printer, 1857), 44.
7. Greenleaf, "Physical Training in the U.S. Army," 60.
8. Edward Mussey Hartwell, "Physical Training in American Colleges and Universities," in *Circulars of Information of the Bureau of Education* (Washington, DC: Bureau of Education, 1886), 180; more on Hartwell's analysis of gymnastics training in European militaries can be found in his comments on Lieutenant Colonel Greenleaf's presentation to the AAAPE in 1891, see Greenleaf, "Physical Training in the U.S. Army," 77–80.
9. Greenleaf, "Physical Training in the U.S. Army," 59.
10. Pilcher, "The Building of the Soldier," 323. American experience in Cuba and the Philippines between 1898 and 1902 tended to reinforce these earlier assessments. For instance, Brig. Gen. W. H. Carter claimed in 1905 that American success in the Spanish-American War derived largely from a training system that "aimed to secure its results in war by putting every man on the firing line in physical condition to run from cover to cover without becoming so winded as to be unable to shoot straight." See W. H. Carter, "A Meet in the Philippines: A Rational Plan of Athletic Training," *Journal of the Military Service Institution of the United States* 36, no. 135 (1905): 455–456.
11. Bowers Davis, "A System for Army Athletics," *Infantry Journal* 3, no. 2 (1906): 83.
12. John Stewart Kulp, "What to Avoid in Army Athletics," in *Proceedings of the Seventh Annual Meeting of the Association of Military Surgeons of the United States*, ed. James E. Pilcher (Columbus: Berlin Publishing, 1897), 314.
13. Edmund Butts, "Athletic Training," *Infantry Journal* 2, no. 1 (1905): 18.
14. War Department, *Manual of Physical Training for Use in the United States Army* (New York: Military Publishing, 1914), 3.
15. Frank S. Besson, "Physical Training in the Army," *Journal of the Military Ser-*

vice Institution of the United States 55 (1914): 39–40; criticisms of the Army's proliferation of manuals, circulars, and orders on physical training were not new, nor were complaints that this proliferation prevented systematic training. For instance, see Guy G. Palmer, "Physical Culture and Training in the Army," *Journal of the United States Infantry Association* 2, no. 4 (1906): 126.

16. Besson, "Physical Training in the Army," 42.
17. The two other board members were Lt. Col. Fred Sladen and 1st Lt. Philip Mathews. The former was West Point's commandant of cadets and Koehler's superior in the Department of Tactics. Sladen likely provided supervision and the weight of his rank and position. Mathews was an officer in the Department of Tactics and Koehler's assistant instructor of gymnastics. Besson, 42; *Official Register of the Officers and Cadets United States Military Academy* (West Point, NY: United States Military Academy Printing Office, 1913), 7.
18. Michael J. Reagor, "Herman J. Koehler: The Father of West Point Physical Education," *Assembly* 51, no. 3 (1993).
19. Robert Degen, "The Evolution of Physical Education at the United States Military Academy" (master's thesis, University of Wisconsin, 1966), 46–49; Herman J. Koehler, "The Physical Training of Cadets, 1802–1902," in *The Centennial of the United States Military Academy at West Point, New York, 1802–1902* (Washington, DC: Government Printing Office, 1904), 897–898.
20. *Annual Report of the Board of Visitors to the United States Military Academy for the Year 1881* (Washington, DC: Government Printing Office, 1881), 7.
21. For a complete overview of Farrow's system, see Edward Samuel Farrow, *A Military System of Gymnastic Exercises and a System of Swimming* (New York: Metropolitan, 1881). Farrow's system descended directly from Archibald MacLaren's *A System of Physical Education* (1869).
22. Koehler, "The Physical Training of Cadets," 898–899.
23. Whitfield B. East, *A Historical Review and Analysis of Army Physical Readiness Training and Assessment* (Fort Leavenworth, KS: Combat Studies Institute Press, 2013), 31.
24. The Milwaukee Normal School was one of the nation's premier schools for physical educators.
25. Brosius came to the search committee's notice for two reasons. First, his 1880 team's success at the Fifth German Turner Festival in Frankfurt won wide recognition in Turner circles and in American newspapers. Second, one of his former students, a Captain Reed, was involved in the search. Reed was an advocate of applying the "Milwaukee idea of physical exercises" at West Point. George Brosius, *Fifty Years Devoted to the Cause of Physical Culture, 1864–1914* (Milwaukee, WI: Germania, 1914), 89–90.

26. Lance Betros, *Carved from Granite: West Point since 1902* (College Station: Texas A & M University Press, 2012), 164–166.
27. Elliott C. Cutler, "Lt. Col. Herman J. Koehler, Master of the Sword: An Account of His Service and Influence," *Assembly* 39, no. 3 (1980): 20.
28. Koehler, "The Physical Training of Cadets," 899.
29. Koehler, 900.
30. Koehler, 902, 904.
31. *Report of the Board of Visitors to the United States Military Academy for the Year 1889* (Washington, DC: Government Printing Office, 1889), 38–39.
32. The manual of 1892 resulted from a suggestion by the West Point superintendent, Col. John Wilson, to Koehler that he publish his system for use in the wider Army. The Army's adjutant-general reviewed the manual and the secretary of war urged calisthenic instruction of enlisted soldiers to conform to Koehler's system. However, little seems to have come of this urging, given continued complaints about a lack of system two decades later. Herman J. Koehler, *Manual of Calisthenic Exercises* (Washington, DC: Government Printing Office, 1892), v.
33. Degen, "The Evolution of Physical Education," 63–68.
34. Degen, 64–65.
35. Fred Eugene Leonard, *A Guide to the History of Physical Education*, ed. George Baird Affleck, 3rd ed. (Philadelphia, PA: Lea & Febiger, 1947), 86–87.
36. Gertrud Pfister, "The Role of German Turners in American Physical Education," *International Journal of the History of Sport* 26, no. 13 (2009): 1896; Deobald B. Van Dalen and Bruce L. Bennett, *A World History of Physical Education: Cultural, Philosophical, Comparative*, 2nd ed. (Englewood Cliffs, NJ: Prentice Hall, 1971), 96, 399.
37. At least five thousand Turners served in the Union Army, which represented more than 50 percent of the total Turners in America at the time. Leonard, *A Guide to the History of Education*, 298.
38. Pfister, "The Role of German Turners," 1908–1916.
39. Pfister, 1902.
40. Paula D. Welch, *History of American Physical Education and Sport*, 3rd ed. (Springfield, IL: Charles C. Thomas, 2004), 111; Van Dalen and Bennett, *A World History of Physical Education*, 425.
41. The manual listed ten categories: setting-up exercises (calisthenics), marching and running, work with dumbbells and other implements, climbing, jumping, apparatus work, gymnastic contests, athletics (track-and-field), swimming, and boxing and wrestling. War Department, *Manual of Physical Training*, 6.
42. Cutler, "Lt. Col. Herman J. Koehler," 21.

43. Herman Koehler Biographical Sketch; 201 File, Headquarters, USMA, February 17, 1919, United States Military Academy Special Collections.
44. Herman J. Koehler, "Physical Training in the Army," *Infantry Journal* 1, no. 1 (1904): 11–13; Greenleaf, "Physical Training in the U.S. Army," 64–66.
45. Palmer, "Physical Culture and Training in the Army," 119–120. Gym construction boomed in the 1890s, but it began a few years earlier. For instance, Maj. Gen. Nelson Miles wrote enthusiastically about a new gym at Vancouver Barracks (Washington Territory) in 1884. Greenleaf, "Physical Training in the U.S. Army," 65.
46. Congress appropriated funds for construction of these gymnasia in June 1890 and also authorized construction of similar buildings at other posts as deemed necessary by the secretary of war. Greenleaf, 67.
47. A. B. Donworth, "Gymnasium Training in the Army," *Journal of the Military Service Institution of the United States* 21 (1897): 509–512; for pictures and diagrams of an sample gym, see *Photographs of Gymnastic Apparatus in United States Army Post Plattsburg, N.Y.: Arranged to List and Plans of Lieut. Herman J. Koehler, U.S.A.* (Providence, RI: Narragansett Machine, 1903). Book is available in the United States Military Academy library.
48. Koehler, "Physical Training in the Army," 10; Herschel Tupes, "Annual Athletic and Gymnastic Tests for the Army," *Infantry Journal* 2, no. 2 (1905): 103.
49. Herman J. Koehler, *Manual of Gymnastic Exercises: Prepared for Use in Service Gymnasiums* (Washington, DC: Government Printing Office, 1904), 17.
50. Edmund L. Butts, "Physical Training of the American Soldier," *Journal of the Military Service Institution of the United States* 61, no. 75 (1895): 499.
51. Butts, 500–501.
52. Edmund L. Butts, "Soldierly Bearing, Health and Athletics," *Outing*, March 1904, 707.
53. Butts, "Physical Training of the American Soldier," 506.
54. Butts, 506–509.
55. Butts, "Soldierly Bearing, Health and Athletics," 707.
56. *Manual of Physical Drill, United States Army* (New York: D. Appleton, 1900), iii.
57. *Manual of Physical Drill*, iii.
58. *Manual of Physical Drill*, 1.
59. *Manual of Physical Drill*, 3–4.
60. Butts, "Physical Training of the American Soldier," 505.
61. Robert Smart, "The Physical Development of the Recruit," in *Proceedings of the Association of Military Surgeons of the United States at Its Tenth Annual Meeting* (Carlisle: Association of Military Surgeons, 1901), 572–573.
62. Smart, 575.

63. Koehler, "Physical Training in the Army," 8.
64. Koehler, 10.
65. Robert L. Bullard and H. S. Hawkins, "Athletics in the Army," *Journal of the Military Service Institution of the United States* 37 (1905): 400.
66. Herman J. Koehler, "General Remarks on Physical Training in the Service," *Infantry Journal* 3, no. 4 (1907): 103.
67. Koehler, 103.
68. The Army Gymnastic Staff was renamed the Army Physical Training Staff in 1918, was made a corps in 1940, and is known today as the Royal Army Physical Training Corps. For more on this center's development and structure, see James D. Campbell, *"The Army Isn't All Work": Physical Culture in the Evolution of the British Army, 1860–1920* (Burlington, VT: Ashgate, 2012).
69. Greenleaf, "Physical Training in the U.S. Army," 74.
70. Greenleaf, 75. Medical officers, citing possession of expert knowledge, typically argued for other medical officers to take charge of physical training. For other examples, see Pilcher, "The Building of the Soldier," 334–335; Smart, "The Physical Development of the Recruit," 575.
71. Koehler, *Manual of Calisthenic Exercises*, v; Brigadier General Albert L. Mills, August 6, 1906, Herman Koehler Vertical File, United States Military Academy Special Collections.
72. Palmer, "Physical Culture and Training in the Army," 121.
73. "Showing Off His Stamina, Gen. Miles Making Ninety-Mile Horseback Ride," *Los Angeles Times*, July 15, 1903, 11.
74. Michael D. Krause, "History of U.S. Army Soldier Physical Fitness," in *National Conference on Military Physical Fitness: Proceedings Report*, ed. Lois A. Hale (Washington, DC: US Department of Health and Human Services in cooperation with the National Defense University, 1990), 21.
75. East, *A Historical Review and Analysis*, 42.
76. Krause, "History of U.S. Army Soldier Physical Fitness," 21.
77. *General Order, No. 44* (Washington: War Department, March 1, 1906), 1–2.
78. East, *A Historical Review and Analysis*, 43.
79. "Roosevelt Led 60 on a Bully Tramp," *New York Times*, November 8, 1908.
80. East, *A Historical Review and Analysis*, 43.
81. Edward M. Coffman, *The Regulars: The American Army, 1898–1941* (Cambridge, MA: Belknap Press of Harvard University Press, 2004), 87–88.
82. War Department, *Manual of Physical Training*, 5–6.
83. War Department, 6.
84. War Department, 6.
85. Roberta J. Park, "Physiologists, Physicians, and Physical Educators: Nineteenth-

Century Biology and Exercise, *Hygienic* and *Educative*," in *Sport and Exercise Science: Essays in the History of Sports Medicine*, ed. Jack W. Berryman and Roberta J. Park (Urbana: University of Illinois Press, 1992), 137–142.

86. War Department, *Manual of Physical Training*, 14.
87. War Department, 14–15.
88. War Department, 12.
89. War Department, 12.
90. War Department, 3.
91. War Department, 193–196.
92. War Department, 10.
93. War Department, 3.
94. Herman J. Koehler, "Letter from Captain Herman J. Koehler," *American Physical Education Review* 21, no. 3 (1916): 149.
95. War Department, *Manual of Physical Training*, 6. Variations on the confidence theme can be found in Edmund L. Butts, "Military Athletics," *Harper's Weekly*, no. 41 (January 9, 1897): 41; Merch B. Stewart, *The Physical Development of the Infantry Soldier* (Menasha: George Banta, 1913), 7; Edward L. King, "Athletics for the Physical Betterment of the Enlisted Men in the Army," *Outing*, January 1902, 432.
96. Edmund L. Butts, "Soldierly Bearing, Health and Athletics," 707.
97. Koehler, "Letter from Captain Herman J. Koehler," 149.
98. Koehler, 151.
99. G. Stanley Hall, "Some Relations between Physical and Mental Training," in *Report of the Ninth Annual Meeting of the American Association for the Advancement of Physical Education* (New Haven, CT: Press of Clarence H. Ryder, 1894), 31.
100. Draft of *Manual of Physical Training*, 2, Herman Koehler Vertical File, United States Military Academy Special Collections.
101. James E. Pilcher, "The Place of Physical Training in the Military Service," in *The Proceedings of the Fourth Annual Meeting of the Association of Military Surgeons of the United States* (St. Louis: Suxton & Skinner Stationery, 1894), 178.
102. Donworth, "Gymnasium Training in the Army," 513.
103. Park, "Physiologists, Physicians, and Physical Educators," 139, 144–146, 155.
104. Koehler, "Physical Training in the Army," 10.
105. L. S. Upton, "Physical Training in the Army," *Infantry Journal* 2, no. 2 (1905): 110.
106. Butts, "Physical Training of the American Soldier," 502.
107. War Department, *Manual of Physical Training*, 13.
108. For examples, see Koehler, *Manual of Calisthenic Exercises*, 2; Koehler, "General

Remarks on Physical Training in the Service," 121; Edmund L. Butts, *Manual of Physical Drill, United States Army* (New York: D. Appleton, 1900), 2; Enoch B. Garey, *Manual of Physical Drill* (Kansas City: Franklin Hudson, 1911), 54.

109. Pilcher, "The Building of the Soldier," 334–335.
110. Koehler, *Manual of Gymnastic Exercises*, 9.
111. Koehler, "Physical Training in the Army," 11–12.
112. Butts, "Physical Training of the American Soldier," 512.
113. Palmer, "Physical Culture and Training in the Army," 121.
114. Henry S. Kilbourne, "The Physical Proportions of the American Soldier," in *Proceedings of the Seventh Annual Meeting of the Association of Military Surgeons of the United States*, ed. James E. Pilcher (Columbus: Berlin, 1897), 332, quote on 39.
115. Draft of *Manual of Physical Training*, 2–4.
116. Stewart, *The Physical Development of the Infantry Soldier*, 2–4.
117. Jeffery Allen Charlston, "Disorganized and Quasi-Official but Eventually Successful: Sport in the U.S. Military, 1814–1914," *International Journal of the History of Sport* 19, no. 4 (2002): 76–78.
118. Steven Pope, "An Army of Athletes: Playing Fields, Battlefields, and the American Military Sporting Experience, 1890–1920," *Journal of Military History* 59, no. 3 (1995): 438–441.
119. On synergy, see Charlston, "Disorganized and Quasi-Official," 76.
120. Henry G. Beyer, "Military Physical Training," in Pilcher, *Proceedings of the Seventh Annual Meeting of the Association of Military Surgeons of the United States*, 266.
121. Bullard and Hawkins, "Athletics in the Army," 405. In a response to this set of articles, Lt. Col. A. C. Sharpe characterized field days as the "most irrational feature of our garrison life." A. C. Sharpe, "Comment & Criticism: Athletics in the Army," *Journal of the Military Service Institution of the United States* 38, no. 141 (1906): 538.
122. Bullard and Hawkins, "Athletics in the Army," 402.
123. Butts, "Physical Training of the American Soldier," 707.
124. Butts never listed a program of events, but for an example of one that meets Butts's criteria and intent, see Davis, "A System for Army Athletics," 79–80.
125. Butts, "Physical Training of the American Soldier," 511.
126. Also, Butts did not author the chapter on track-and-field competition. Instead, he borrowed the material from a book titled "Track Athletic in Detail." Butts, *Manual of Physical Drill*, iii, 136.
127. William H. Edwards, *Football Days: Memories of the Game and of the Men Behind the Ball* (New York: Moffat, Yard, 1916), 214–215.
128. Koehler, "Physical Training in the Army," 2.

129. Koehler, "General Remarks on Physical Training in the Service," 103–104, 15.

130. Herman Koehler, *The Theory and Practice of Athletics at the Military Academy* (West Point, NY: Military Academy Printing Office, 1909), 2.

131. Koehler, "Physical Training in the Army," 9.

132. The Army Athletic Association, renamed in 1903, was originally known as the Army Officers Athletic Association.

133. Betros, *Carved from Granite*, 168–171.

134. Roberta J. Park, "Healthy, Moral, and Strong: Educational Views of Exercise and Athletics in Nineteenth-Century America," in *Fitness in American Culture: Images of Health, Sport, and the Body, 1830–1940*, ed. Kathryn Grover (Amherst: University of Massachusetts Press, 1989) 138–143.

135. For a concise statement of this position, see Edward Mussey Hartwell, "The Nature of Physical Training, and the Best Means of Securing Its Ends," in *Physical Training: A Full Report of the Papers and Discussions of the Conference Held in Boston in November, 1889*, ed. Isabel C. Barrows (Boston: Press of George H. Ellis, 1890), 5–22, 20.

136. Park, "Healthy, Moral, and Strong," 167–171.

CHAPTER 3. THE US ARMY'S BATTLE OF THE SYSTEMS, 1914–1920

1. Antulio J. Echevarria, "The 'Cult of the Offensive' Revisited: Confronting Technological Change before the Great War," *Journal of Strategic Studies* 25, no. 1 (2002): 199–202.

2. Luther H. Gulick, "Physical Fitness in the Fighting Armies," *American Physical Education Review* 23, no. 6 (1918): 341–350.

3. Jennifer D. Keene, *Doughboys, the Great War, and the Remaking of America* (Baltimore: Johns Hopkins University Press, 2001), 9.

4. Herman J. Koehler, *Manual of Gymnastic Exercises: Prepared for Use in Service Gymnasiums* (Washington, DC: Government Printing Office, 1904), 9.

5. George J. Fisher, "Physical Training in the Army," *American Physical Education Review* 23, no. 2 (1918): 65.

6. Keene, *Doughboys*, 24–25.

7. James Mennell, "The Service Football Program of World War I: Its Impact on the Popularity of the Game," *Journal of Sport History* 16, no. 3 (1989), 251–252.

8. For the CTCA's portrayal of its task, purpose, and method, see Edward Frank Allen, *Keeping Our Fighters Fit for War and After* (New York: Century, 1918), 3–8, quotation on 16; War Department, *Commission on Training Camp Activities* (Washington, DC: Government Printing Office, 1917), 3–5; Raymond B. Fosdick, "The Commission on Training Camp Activities," *Proceedings of the Academy of Political Science in the City of New York* 7, no. 4 (1918): 163–170.

9. Allen, *Keeping Our Fighters Fit*, preface.
10. Nancy K. Bristow, *Making Men Moral: Social Engineering during the Great War* (New York: New York University Press, 1996), 1–8; War Department, *Commission on Training Camp Activities*, 3–6; Fosdick, "Commission," 819; on the Progressive-era cultural debate about the identity of American soldiers as either innocent boys or adult men and the moral implications of that identity, see Anni Baker, "The Abolition of the U.S. Army Canteen, 1898–1914," *Journal of Military History* 80, no. 3 (2016).
11. Bristow, *Making Men Moral*, 11.
12. Allen, *Keeping Our Fighters Fit*, preface.
13. Bristow, *Making Men Moral*, 4–7.
14. Allen, *Keeping Our Fighters Fit*, 3–6.
15. Bristow, *Making Men Moral*, 38–40.
16. Allen, *Keeping Our Fighters Fit*, 40.
17. Noted football coach Walter Camp headed the Athletic Division in the Navy's CTCA. Camp created and promoted the now-famous "Daily Dozen" exercise program. Although the Daily Dozen became extremely popular and appeared occasionally in the physical training practices of some Army units, it was never part of the Army's official physical culture.
18. Quotation in Joseph E. Raycroft, "Safeguarding the Health of College Students," *Science* 39, no. 1011 (1914): 709, 711; Curriculum Vitae: Joseph Edward Raycroft, 1948, Series 1, Biographical, Box 2, Joseph Edward Raycroft Papers (JERP), Department of Rare Books and Special Collections, Princeton University Library (PUL); Joseph E. Raycroft, "The Educational Value of Athletics in Schools and Colleges," *School and Society* 3, no. 61 (1915): 295–296; Joseph E. Raycroft, "Training Camp Activities," *American Physical Education Review* 23, no. 3 (1918): 143.
19. "Proceedings of the Society of Directors of Physical Education in Colleges," *American Physical Education Review* 22, no. 4 (1917): 190–192.
20. Joseph E. Raycroft, Memorandum Concerning Physical Training in the New Army, May 1917, Box 4, JERP, PUL.
21. For a brief overview of the YMCA's involvement in military athletics, see Steven Pope, "An Army of Athletes: Playing Fields, Battlefields, and the American Military Sporting Experience, 1890–1920," *Journal of Military History* 59, no. 3 (1995): 442–444.
22. Joseph E. Raycroft, Memorandum Concerning Physical Training in the New Army, May 1917, Box 4, JERP, PUL.
23. Raycroft, Memorandum, May 1917, Box 4, JERP, PUL.
24. Draft of Efficiency in Army Physical Training, Presented to the Athletic Re-

search Society, Joseph E. Raycroft, pg. 2, 1920, Series 3, Physical Education During Wartime, 1917–1944, Box 4, JERP, PUL.

25. Joseph E. Raycroft, Memorandum Concerning Physical Training in the New Army, May 1917, Box 4, JERP, PUL.

26. Joseph Raycroft to Raymond Fosdick, 14 June 1917; Fosdick No. 1, box 25; Records of the War Department General & Special Staffs, Commission on Training Camp Activities, Correspondence of the Athletic Division, 1917–1919, Record Group (RG) 165, National Archives at College Park, MD (NACP).

27. Joseph E. Raycroft, Memorandum Concerning Physical Training in the New Army, May 1917, Box 4, JERP, PUL.

28. Joseph E. Raycroft, Memorandum Outlining the Various Steps Taken in the Development of a Program of Physical Training, Boxing, Bayonet Fighting, Athletics, Etc., as a Part of the Training Program of a Soldier, 1917–1920, pg. 3, 1941, Box 4, JERP, PUL; for a description of the Canadian physical training system and its use of boxing in bayonet training, see Percy Hobbs, "Bayonet Fighting and Physical Training," *Infantry Journal* 14, no. 2 (1917).

29. Studies of foreign practices generated much literature in the United States. For a sample, see Fisher, "Physical Training in the Army," 69; "Military Training in Foreign Countries," *American Physical Education Review* 22, no. 8 (1917); Army War College, *Notes on Bayonet Training Compiled from Foreign Reports* (Washington, DC: Government Printing Office, 1917); Marc Bellin du Coteau, "The Physical Education of the Fighting Man: Method in Use in the National Military School of St. Cyr, France," *American Physical Education Review* 22, no. 9 (1917); Raycroft, "Training Camp Activities," 145.

30. House of Representatives Select Committee on Expenditures in the War Department, *War Expenditures: Hearings before the Select Committee on Expenditures in the War Department* (Washington, DC: Government Printing Office, 1919), 157.

31. James D. Campbell, *"The Army Isn't All Work": Physical Culture in the Evolution of the British Army, 1860–1920* (Burlington, VT: Ashgate, 2012), 63–64, 70–71, 112.

32. Select Committee on Expenditures in the War Department, *War Expenditures,* 157.

33. Select Committee on Expenditures in the War Department, 157; Herbert Reed, "'Not a Minute' Koehler Takes the Team," *Independent,* July 14, 1917.

34. Issued in May 1917, this publication was a stripped-down version of the *Manual of Physical Training* of 1914. Koehler's disciplinary drill formed this document's core. Most elements of the manual of 1914 that required additional equipment or apparatus were removed, as were the sections dealing with athletics.

35. Select Committee on Expenditures in the War Department, *War Expenditures*, 157.
36. Joseph E. Raycroft, Memorandum Outlining the Various Steps Taken in the Development of a Program of Physical Training, Boxing, Bayonet Fighting, Athletics, Etc., as a Part of the Training Program of a Soldier, 1917–1920, pg. 2, 1941, Box 4, JERP, PUL.
37. Raycroft, 5; Letter, Major General J. Franklin Bell to Colonel Traub, 12 July 1917, Series 3, Physical Education during Wartime, 1917–1944, Box 4, JERP, PUL; Letter, Joseph Raycroft to Col. Samuel W. Miller, 29 June 1917, Series 3: Physical Education During Wartime, 1917–1944, Box 4, JERP, PUL.
38. Meeting of War Department Commission on Training Camp Activities Report, 21 November 1917; Fosdick Letters No. 1; Commission on Training Camp Activities, Correspondence of the Athletic Division, 1917–1919, box 25; RG 165, NACP.
39. Joseph E. Raycroft, Memorandum Outlining the Various Steps Taken in the Development of a Program of Physical Training, Boxing, Bayonet Fighting, Athletics, Etc., as a Part of the Training Program of a Soldier, 1917–1920, pg. 5–6, 1941, Box 4, JERP, PUL.
40. Raycroft, 7.
41. Letter, Joseph Raycroft to James A. Babbitt, 9 December 1942, Series 1, Personal Correspondence—Professional Career, Box 1, JERP, PUL.
42. Keene, *Doughboys*, 41.
43. Report of Fred W. Marvel, (Temporary) Inspector of Athletics, to Joseph E. Raycroft, MD, 1918, Series 3, Box 4, JERP, PUL.
44. Fisher, "Physical Training in the Army," 66.
45. Raycroft's association with President Wilson (both were Princeton men) probably helped too. Letter, John L. Griffith to George A. Barton, 19 April 1944, Series 1, Personal Correspondence—Professional Career, Box 1, JERP, PUL.
46. Letter, Newton Baker to Raymond Fosdick, 21 June 1917, Series 3, Box 4, JERP, PUL.
47. Thomas Browne to Joseph Raycroft, 16 June 1918; Commission on Training Camp Activities, Correspondence of the Athletic Division, 1917–1919, box 8; RG 165, NACP.
48. Letter, Joseph Raycroft to Raymond Fosdick, 26 May 1917, Series 3, Physical Education during Wartime, 1917–1944, Box 4, JERP, PUL.
49. Raymond Fosdick to Joseph Raycroft, 14 December 1917; Fosdick Letters No. 1; Commission on Training Camp Activities, Correspondence of the Athletic Division, 1917–1919, box 25; RG 165, NACP.
50. John Biddle, Memorandum for the Adjutant General of the Army, Subject:

Commission for Athletic Directors, 26 January 1918, Series 3, Physical Education During Wartime, 1917–1944, Box 4, JERP, PUL.

51. Joseph Raycroft to J. S. Tichenor, undated; folder 45; Commission on Training Camp Activities, Correspondence of the Athletic Division, 1917–1919, box 35; RG 165, NACP.
52. Memorandum Regarding the Relationship in Camps That Should Exist between YMCA Directors and War Department Athletic Directors, 18 January 1918; folder 45; Commission on Training Camp Activities, Correspondence of the Athletic Division, 1917–1919, box 35; RG 165, NACP.
53. Report of Fred W. Marvel, (Temporary) Inspector of Athletics, to Joseph E. Raycroft, MD, 1918, pg. 8, Series 3, Box 4, JERP, PUL.
54. Joseph E. Raycroft, Suggestions for Colleges from the Army Experience in Physical Training, pg. 14, December 1918, Series 3, Physical Education during Wartime, 1917–1944, Box 4, JERP, PUL.
55. Fisher, "Physical Training in the Army," 66; for an example of sharing diverse experiences, see "Extracts from Occasional Letters from Physical Directors in Army Camps to Dr. George J. Fisher, Director, War Work Council, Young Men's Christian Association," *American Physical Education Review* 22, no. 9 (1917): 558–566.
56. Draft of History of War Department Commission on Training Camp Activities Athletic Division, April 1917—January 1919, pg. 17, Series 3, Physical Education during Wartime, 1917–1944, Box 4, JERP, PUL; Draft of Efficiency in Army Physical Training, Presented to the Athletic Research Society, pg. 3, 1920, Series 3, Physical Education during Wartime, 1917–1944, Box 4, JERP, PUL.
57. Joseph E. Raycroft, Memorandum Outlining the Various Steps Taken in the Development of a Program of Physical Training, Boxing, Bayonet Fighting, Athletics, Etc., as a Part of the Training Program of a Soldier, 1917–1920, pg. 10–11, 1941, Box 4, JERP, PUL.
58. Report of Fred W. Marvel, (Temporary) Inspector of Athletics, to Joseph E. Raycroft, MD, 1918, pg. 4, Series 3, Box 4, JERP, PUL; Fisher, 69.
59. Joseph E. Raycroft, Memorandum Outlining the Various Steps Taken in the Development of a Program of Physical Training, Boxing, Bayonet Fighting, Athletics, Etc., as a Part of the Training Program of a Soldier, 1917–1920, pg. 11–13, 1941, Box 4, JERP, PUL.; Raycroft, "Training Camp Activities," 147.
60. War Plans Division, *Training Circular No. 19: Organization of Physical and Bayonet Training* (Washington, DC: War Department, 1918), 8.
61. Raycroft claimed that such schools had trained "tens of thousands" of commissioned and noncommissioned officers in his system by November 1918. Draft

of Efficiency in Army Physical Training, Presented to the Athletic Research Society, pg. 3, 1920, Series 3, Physical Education during Wartime, 1917–1944, Box 4, JERP, PUL.

62. Joseph E. Raycroft, Memorandum Outlining the Various Steps Taken in the Development of a Program of Physical Training, Boxing, Bayonet Fighting, Athletics, Etc., as a Part of the Training Program of a Soldier, 1917–1920, pg. 14, 1941, Box 4, JERP, PUL.
63. Raycroft, 14–15.
64. Joseph E. Raycroft, Suggestions for Colleges from the Army Experience in Physical Training, pg. 4, December 1918, Series 3, Physical Education during Wartime, 1917–1944, Box 4, JERP, PUL.
65. Joseph Raycroft to Johnny Griffiths, 14 December 1918, Commission on Training Camp Activities, Correspondence of the Athletic Division, 1917–1919, box 1; RG 165, NACP.
66. "Physical and Bayonet Training (Editorial)," *Infantry Journal* 16, no. 6 (1919): 515; Whitfield B. East, *A Historical Review and Analysis of Army Physical Readiness Training and Assessment* (Fort Leavenworth, KS: Combat Studies Institute Press, 2013), 70.
67. Memorandum, Joseph Raycroft to Captain Brosius, George V. Blake, and Lt. Brook Leman, 30 August 1919, Series 3, Physical Education During Wartime, 1917–1944, Box 4, JERP, PUL.
68. Notably, one of the first three instructors assigned was Koehler's cousin, Capt. Carl Brosius. Joseph E. Raycroft, *Mass Physical Training for Use in the Army and the Reserve Officers' Training Corps* (Washington, DC: United States Infantry Association, 1920), ix; for a full instructor roster, see J. C. Drain, "New Physical and Bayonet Training Course," *Infantry Journal* 16, no. 6 (1919): 475.
69. "Physical and Bayonet Training (Editorial)," 515–516.
70. War Department, *Commission on Training Camp Activities* (1917), 3–4.
71. Raycroft, *Mass Physical Training*, vi, viii.
72. War Plans Division, *Training Circular No. 19*, 8.
73. Joseph E. Raycroft, Draft of Efficiency in Army Physical Training, Presented to the Athletic Research Society, pg. 1, 1920, Series 3, Physical Education during Wartime, 1917–1944, Box 4, JERP, PUL.
74. Joseph E. Raycroft, Suggestions for Colleges from the Army Experience in Physical Training, pg. 8, December 1918, Series 3, Physical Education during Wartime, 1917–1944, Box 4, JERP, PUL.
75. Joseph E. Raycroft, Draft of Efficiency in Army Physical Training, Presented to the Athletic Research Society, pg. 23–25, 1920, Series 3, Physical Education during Wartime, 1917–1944, Box 4, JERP, PUL. In examining Raycroft's and

the CTCA's files, I have found no evidence for a comprehensive effort to quantify and measure physiological performance requirements in the US Army prior to 1942. More research may yet bring such data to light.

76. Raycroft, *Mass Physical Training*, 1–2.
77. Raycroft, "Training Camp Activities," 144–145.
78. Joseph E. Raycroft, Draft of Efficiency in Army Physical Training, Presented to the Athletic Research Society, pg. 2, 1920, Series 3, Physical Education during Wartime, 1917–1944, Box 4, JERP, PUL.
79. Joseph E. Raycroft, Suggestions for Colleges from the Army Experience in Physical Training, pg. 2, December 1918, Series 3, Physical Education during Wartime, 1917–1944, Box 4, JERP, PUL.
80. Hilton Howell Railey, "Your Boy in Camp," *Independent*, August 11, 1917.
81. Raycroft, "Training Camp Activities," 144.
82. Allen, *Keeping Our Fighters Fit*, 42.
83. Letter, Joseph Raycroft to John G. Hibben, 13 November 1919, Series 3, Physical Education during Wartime, 1917–1944, Box 4, JERP, PUL.
84. Raycroft, *Mass Physical Training*, iii–iv.
85. Raycroft, iv.
86. Raycroft, 4.
87. Thomas Browne to Joseph Raycroft, 19 May 1918; Commission on Training Camp Activities, Correspondence of the Athletic Division, 1917–1919, box 8; RG 165, NACP.
88. Raycroft, *Mass Physical Training*, vii.
89. Joseph E. Raycroft, Suggestions for Colleges from the Army Experience in Physical Training, pg. 9, December 1918, Series 3, Physical Education during Wartime, 1917–1944, Box 4, JERP, PUL.
90. Raycroft, *Mass Physical Training*, 45.
91. Raycroft, vii, quotation on 40.
92. Raycroft, 34.
93. Raycroft, vii–viii.
94. War Department, *Manual of Physical Training for Use in the United States Army* (New York: Military Publishing, 1914), 9.
95. Raycroft, *Mass Physical Training*, 71.
96. Raycroft, viii.
97. Raycroft, 110.
98. High valuation of the bayonet was not a feature exclusive to US military culture. Practically all Western-style armies embraced the bayonet before World War I. As historian Hew Strachan has observed, the bayonet was representative of an acknowledgment that morale was of "increasing and legitimate

importance" on modern battlefields. According to Strachan, technology "did not remove the need for men to cope, but increasing the pressures loaded on them, intensified the search for palliatives." Bayonet training cultivated an aggressive spirit and the individual soldier's confidence, and was therefore useful to improving an organization's moral forces. Hew Strachan, "Training, Morale and Modern War," *Journal of Contemporary History* 41, no. 2 (2006): 218.

99. Raycroft, *Mass Physical Training*, 3.
100. Quotation on War Department, *Commission on Training Camp Activities* (1917), 13; see also Raycroft, *Mass Physical Training*, 84; Joseph E. Raycroft, Memorandum Outlining the Various Steps Taken in the Development of a Program of Physical Training, Boxing, Bayonet Fighting, Athletics, Etc., as a Part of the Training Program of a Soldier, 1917–1920, pg. 7, 1941, Box 4, JERP, PUL.
101. Allen, *Keeping Our Fighters Fit*, 55–56.
102. Raycroft, "Training Camp Activities," 146.
103. "Defence Opposed in Boxing Rules for Army Camps," *New York Tribune*, June 23, 1918; War Department Commission on Training Camp Activities, *Rules for Boxing* (Washington, DC: Government Printing Office, 1918).
104. War Department, *Commission on Training Camp Activities* (1917), 13.
105. Hiram A. Jones, "The Revised Preparedness Bill: The Status of the Physical Preparedness Legislation," *Journal of Health and Physical Education* 12, no. 2 (1941).
106. War Department, *Outline of Plan for Military Training in Public Schools of the United States* (Washington, DC: Government Printing Office, 1916), 1.
107. War Department, *Outline of Plan*, 1.
108. Joseph E. Raycroft, Memorandum Outlining the Various Steps Taken in the Development of a Program of Physical Training, Boxing, Bayonet Fighting, Athletics, Etc., as a Part of the Training Program of a Soldier, 1917–1920, pgs. 7–8, 1941, Box 4, JERP, PUL.
109. Raycroft, 8.
110. J. V. Fitzgerald, "See a Revival of Boxing as Army Takes up Sport," *Washington Post*, November 5, 1917.
111. Quotation in Allen, *Keeping Our Fighters Fit*, 53–54.
112. Allen, 57–58.
113. War Department, *Commission on Training Camp Activities* (1917), 12.
114. Pope, "An Army of Athletes," 436–40; Wanda Ellen Wakefield, *Playing to Win: Sports and the American Military, 1898–1945* (Albany: State University of New York Press, 1997), 6–9; Mrozek, *Sport and American Mentality*, 51–59.

115. War Department, *Manual of Physical Training for Use in the United States Army*, 309.
116. War Department, 309.
117. War Department, 309–13; Herman J. Koehler, "General Remarks on Physical Training in the Service," *Infantry Journal* 3, no. 4 (1907): 103–104.
118. Drain, "New Phyiscal and Bayonet Training Course," 475.
119. Quotation in Raycroft, "Training Camp Activities," 143; see also "Raycroft Tells of Sports in the Army," *Sporting Goods Dealer*, 1918.
120. Raycroft, *Mass Physical Training*, viii; Joseph E. Raycroft, Memorandum Outlining the Various Steps Taken in the Development of a Program of Physical Training, Boxing, Bayonet Fighting, Athletics, Etc., as a Part of the Training Program of a Soldier, 1917–1920, pg. 6, 1941, Box 4, JERP, PUL.
121. Allen, *Keeping Our Fighters Fit*, 52–53.
122. Allen, 47–48.
123. Koehler, "General Remarks on Physical Training in the Service," 103–105.
124. Joseph E. Raycroft, Suggestions for Colleges from the Army Experience in Physical Training, pgs. 8–10, December 1918, Series 3, Physical Education during Wartime, 1917–1944, Box 4, JERP, PUL.
125. Raycroft, 11; Raycroft, "Training Camp Activities," 147.
126. Raycroft, *Mass Physical Training*, viii.
127. Obstacle courses were a new feature in US Army physical training. The idea for them had largely been borrowed from contemporary British training practices intended to deliver realistic combat training.
128. Raycroft, *Mass Physical Training*, 142–148.
129. Koehler had used an intensive program body and performance measurements of his own creation at West Point since the mid-1880s. In 1906 President Theodore Roosevelt mandated a three-day, ninety-mile horseback-riding test for all field-grade officers. East, *A Historical Review*, 42–43; the riding test fell into disuse just prior to World War I and the Army discarded it formally after the war. "Physical Fitness," *Military Engineer* 14, no. 75 (1922): 163.
130. Joseph E. Raycroft, Draft of Efficiency in Army Physical Training, Presented to the Athletic Research Society, pg. 4, 1920, Series 3, Physical Education during Wartime, 1917–1944, Box 4, JERP, PUL.
131. War Plans Division, *Training Circular No. 19*, 7.
132. Raymond B. Fosdick, Memorandum Concerning Suggestions for Demobilizing the Work of the Commission on Training Camp Activities, 25 November 1918, Series 3, Physical Education during Wartime, 1917–1944, Box 4, JERP, PUL.

133. Joseph E. Raycroft, Memorandum Outlining the Various Steps Taken in the Development of a Program of Physical Training, Boxing, Bayonet Fighting, Athletics, Etc., as a Part of the Training Program of a Soldier, 1917–1920, pgs. 18–19, 1941, Box 4, JERP, PUL.
134. Raycroft.
135. William H. Waldron, *Army Physical Training* (New York: H. Holt, 1919), iii.

CHAPTER 4. REVERSION, DISAGGREGATION, AND "PREHABILITATION," 1919–1940

1. F. J. Morrow, "Military Preparedness," *American Physical Education Review* 24, no. 5 (1919): 280.
2. Morrow, 280.
3. A. D. Browne, "Physical Education in the Light of the Present National Situation," *American Physical Education Review* 24, no. 2 (1919): 74.
4. Joseph E. Raycroft, *Mass Physical Training for Use in the Army and the Reserve Officers' Training Corps* (Washington, DC: United States Infantry Association, 1920), ix; full instructor roster in J. C. Drain, "New Physical and Bayonet Training Course," *Infantry Journal* 16, no. 6 (1919): 475.
5. Joseph E. Raycroft, Memorandum Outlining the Various Steps Taken in the Development of a Program of Physical Training, Boxing, Bayonet Fighting, Athletics, Etc., as a Part of the Training Program of a Soldier, 1917–1920, pp. 18–19, box 4, folder 8, Joseph Edward Raycroft Papers (JERP), Department of Rare Books and Special Collections, Princeton University Library (PUL).
6. The service schools represented the Infantry, Cavalry, Field Artillery, Coast Artillery, and Engineer branches.
7. Memorandum from Maj. Gen. Charles S. Farnsworth to the Chief of the Training and Instruction Branch, General Staff, 25 September 1919, Box 4, JERP, PUL.
8. Letter, Joseph Raycroft to John G. Hibben, 13 November 1919, Series 3, Physical Education during Wartime, 1917–1944, Box 4, JERP, PUL.
9. Drain, "New Physical and Bayonet Training Course," 474.
10. Drain, 475–476.
11. Drain, 484.
12. "Physical and Bayonet Training (Editorial)," *Infantry Journal* 16, no. 6 (1919): 515–516.
13. Office of the Chief of Staff, Resume of Important Papers in the Day's Work, January 23, 1920, Box 4, JERP, PUL.
14. Whitfield B. East, *A Historical Review and Analysis of Army Physical Readiness*

Training and Assessment (Ft. Leavenworth, KS: Combat Studies Institute Press, 2013), 199.

15. Joseph E. Raycroft, Memorandum Outlining the Various Steps Taken in the Development of a Program of Physical Training, Boxing, Bayonet Fighting, Athletics, Etc., as a Part of the Training Program of a Soldier, 1917–1920, pp. 18–19, box 4, folder 8, JERP, PUL.
16. Drain, "New Physical and Bayonet Training Course," 475.
17. Letter, Major General Charles Farnsworth to Joseph Raycroft, 5 March 1920, Box 4, JERP, PUL.
18. Series of correspondence between Farnsworth, Raycroft, and later CPT Braun between MAR 1920 and SEP 1923, Box 4, Series 3, JERP, PUL.
19. A. W. Bjornstad, "Athletic Policy of Infantry School," *Infantry Journal* 26, no. 1 (1925): 44.
20. G. J. Braun, "Physical Training at Infantry School," *Infantry Journal* 25, no. 2 (1924): 149.
21. On the haphazard development of military sport, see Jeffery Allen Charlston, "Disorganized and Quasi-Official but Eventually Successful: Sport in the U.S. Military, 1814–1914," *International Journal of the History of Sport* 19, no. 4 (2002): 70–88, quotation at 70–71.
22. Raycroft, *Mass Physical Training*, iii–iv.
23. East, *A Historical Review*, 70. Stewart served as superintendent between 1926 and 1927. Though he departed the office before *TR 115-5* was published, Stewart had supervised the regulations' development during his tenure.
24. Merch B. Stewart, *The Physical Development of the Infantry Soldier* (Menasha, WI: George Banta, 1913), 2.
25. Stewart, 4.
26. Merch B. Stewart, "A Thirty-Minute Talk: Military Discipline," *Infantry Journal* 16, no. 6 (1919): 492.
27. Stewart, *Physical Development*, 6–7.
28. These included setting-up exercises, gymnastics, calisthenics, rifle drills, and limited use of games as a supplement to make drill more interesting. Stewart, *Physical Development*, 24–27.
29. War Department, *Training Regulations No. 115-5: Physical Training* (Washington, DC: Government Printing Office, 1928), 1–2.
30. War Department, 2.
31. *Training Regulations 115-5* was divided into two parts. The first and most commonly used part represented a basic program that units could implement anywhere, even without additional equipment. Activities covered included

setting-up drills, marching, running, and group games. The second part was designed for use by trained instructors with access to equipment and included activities such as rifle and dumbbell exercises, and gymnastic drills requiring an apparatus.

32. War Department, *Training Regulations No. 115-5: Physical Training*, 3.
33. War Department, 49.
34. War Department, 49.
35. War Department, 50.
36. War Department, 56.
37. War Department, 55–56.
38. Raycroft, *Mass Physical Training*, 149.
39. War Department, *Training Regulations No. 115-5: Physical Training*, 3; War Department, *Manual of Physical Training for Use in the United States Army* (New York: Military Publishing, 1914), 310–311.
40. Herman J. Koehler, *Koehler's West Point Manual of Disciplinary Physical Training* (New York: E. P. Dutton, 1919).
41. War Department, *Basic Field Manual*, vol. 1, chap. 4, *Physical Training* (Washington, DC: Government Printing Office, 1936).
42. War Department, *Field Manual 21-20: Basic Field Manual—Physical Training* (Washington, DC: Government Printing Office, 1941), 2.
43. Steven Pope, "An Army of Athletes: Playing Fields, Battlefields, and the American Military Sporting Experience, 1890–1920," *Journal of Military History* 59, no. 3 (1995): 453.
44. This represented a notable break from the debates over the faddishness of sport and physical training in the Army that had been active less than they had been two decades earlier. R. H. Allen, "Athletics and the Infantry Spirit," *Infantry Journal* 28, no. 1 (1926): 24.
45. Allen, "Athletics and the Infantry Spirit," 26.
46. Wanda Ellen Wakefield, *Playing to Win: Sports and the American Military, 1898–1945* (Albany: State University of New York Press, 1997), 62.
47. Quotation in Wakefield, 63.
48. Wakefield, 62–78.
49. United States Military Academy, *Annual Report of the Superintendent* (West Point, NY: United States Military Academy Press, 1922), 10.
50. Herman J. Koehler, "Competitive Athletics at the United States Military Academy," *Pointer* (September 29, 1923): 11.
51. Allen, "Athletics and the Infantry Spirit," 24.
52. War Department, *Army Regulations No. 850–120: Athletics* (Washington: War Department, 1928).

53. Wakefield, *Playing to Win*, 54.

54. Allen, "Athletics and the Infantry Spirit," 24.

55. For the full analysis, see Albert G. Love and Charles B. Davenport, *Defects Found in Drafted Men* (Washington, DC: Government Printing Office, 1920); for a summary of key findings, see Albert G. Love and Charles B. Davenport, "Defects Found in Drafted Men," *Scientific Monthly* 10, no. 1 (1920): 5–25; Albert G. Love and Charles B. Davenport, "Defects Found in Drafted Men, II," *Scientific Monthly* 10, no. 2 (1920): 125–141.

56. Love and Davenport, "Defects Found in Drafted Men," 7.

57. Defects rendering men unsuitable for service were included in categories Vg, which were rejected by local draft boards, and D. Men sufficiently fit for immediate service fell in category A, while men eligible for service after remedial action fell in category B. Category C included men who were only deemed capable of limited military service, such as in clerical positions. Love and Davenport, 8–10.

58. Love and Davenport, 11.

59. Paula D. Welch, *History of American Physical Education and Sport*, 3rd ed. (Springfield, IL: Charles C. Thomas, 2004), 172.

60. Walter Camp, *Keeping Fit All the Way: How to Obtain and Maintain Health, Strength, and Efficiency* (New York: Harper, 1919), chap. 7, kindle.

61. Willard S. Small, "The Nation's Need of Physical Education," *American Journal of Public Health* 8, no. 11 (1918): 830.

62. Thomas A. Storey, "War-Time Revelations in Physical Education," *American Physical Education Review* 25, no. 2 (1920): 47.

63. Storey, 47.

64. John Sundwall, "Health Education and Activities in Colleges and Universities," *American Physical Education Review* 26, no. 4 (1921): 164.

65. Sundwall, 165.

66. Dudley A. Sargent, "Taking Account of Stock," *American Physical Education Review* 27, no. 2 (1922): 49–50.

67. George J. Fisher, "Points of Emphasis in a Post-War Program of Physical Training," *American Physical Education Review* 24, no. 3 (1919): 126.

68. F. W. Maroney, "Physical Education Looks Ahead," *Journal of Health and Physical Education* 5, no. 8 (1933): 4.

69. Marilyn J. Gibbs and Claudius W. Griffin, "Physical Fitness," in *Handbook of American Popular Culture*, ed. M. Thomas Inge (New York: Greenwood, 1989), 931; Maroney, "Physical Education Looks Ahead," 4.

70. James Huff McCurdy, "Physical Efficiency as a National Asset," *American Physical Education Review* 25, no. 3 (1920): 101.

71. McCurdy, 101.
72. Fisher, "Points of Emphasis," 126.
73. "The Army Builds Men," *Infantry Journal* 18, no. 1 (1921): 80–81.
74. Deobald B. Van Dalen and Bruce L. Bennett, *A World History of Physical Education: Cultural, Philosophical, Comparative,* 2nd ed. (Englewood Cliffs, NJ: Prentice Hall, 1971), 468.
75. Van Dalen and Bennett, 460–461.
76. Van Dalen and Bennett, 461.
77. McCurdy, "Physical Efficiency," 105.
78. This was a joint statement also approved by the Navy Department, US Civil Service Commission, Department of the Interior, and the Commissioner of Education. "The Need in the Army and Navy," *American Physical Education Review* 23, no. 4 (1918): 251.
79. Morrow, "Military Preparedness," 280–281.
80. Early advocates of systematic physical training had long urged this line of thinking within the Army. For instance, Koehler wrote in vehement opposition to the use of military drill in schools as early as 1896. Herman J. Koehler, "Military Drill Vs. Gymnastics," *Mind and Body* 3, no. 28 (1896): 79–80.
81. Joseph E. Raycroft, Suggestions for Colleges from the Army Experience in Physical Training, 26 December 1918, Box 4, JERP, PUL.
82. Raycroft, 8.
83. Raycroft, 10–11.
84. Raycroft, 11–14; the popularity of intercollegiate athletics, which was already growing rapidly, exploded after World War I. For more, see Van Dalen and Bennett, *A World History of Physical Education,* 430, 45–53.
85. Van Dalen and Bennett, *A World History of Physical Education,* 431–432.
86. James Edward Rogers, "Trends in Physical Education," *Journal of Health and Physical Education* 2, no. 8 (1931): 19, 47.
87. This reflected traditional conceptions of citizenship that closely associated citizenship with military duty. Mass armies reinforced and amplified this connection. Derek Heater, *A Brief History of Citizenship* (Edinburgh: Edinburgh University Press, 2004), 4–5; Keith Faulks, *Citizenship* (New York: Routledge, 2000), 169.
88. Morrow, "Military Preparedness," 280; Storey, "War-Time Revelations," 47, 51; Sundwall, "Health Education," 104; McCurdy, "Physical Efficiency," 101–105; Welch, *History of American Education and Sport,* 172–173.
89. Morrow, "Military Preparedness," 280.
90. Thomas D. Wood, "Schools Hold Health Key for All Future Citizens," *Journal of Health and Physical Education* 1, no. 3 (1930): 3.

91. Quotation in R. J. Francis, "Toward a Philosophy of Physical Education," *Journal of Health and Physical Education* 10, no. 4 (1939): 216–217. Interest in European physical education systems ran high in the 1930s, especially as they related to nationalist efforts to mold young citizens: see Charles Edward Merriam, *The Making of Citizens: A Comparative Study of Methods of Civic Training* (Chicago: University of Chicago Press, 1931), 328–329; Maroney, "Physical Education Looks Ahead," 45; Van Dalen and Bennett, *A World History of Physical Education*, 479.
92. P. S. Bond et al., *The Red, White and Blue Manual: A Text Book for the Citizens' Military Training Camp*, vol. 1, Red Course (Baltimore: Johns Hopkins Press, 1921), 1.
93. Very little scholarship exists on the CMTC. For one of the only manuscripts on the subject, see Donald M. Kington, *Forgotten Summers: The Story of the Citizens' Military Training Camps, 1921–1940* (San Francisco: Two Decades, 1995), 1–5.
94. Generally speaking, each camp was aligned with an Army Corps Area. The initial camps were held at Camp Devens, Fort Snelling, Plattsburg, the Presidio, Camp Lewis, Camp Meade, Camp Jackson, Camp Knox, Camp Grant, Camp Pike, Fort Logan, and Camp Travis. Kington, *Forgotten Summers*, 14–16.
95. Kington, 107.
96. On the campaign for universal compulsory military training, see John Garry Clifford, *The Citizen Soldiers: The Plattsburg Training Camp Movement, 1913–1920* (Lexington: University Press of Kentucky, 1972), 193.
97. George Wheeler Hinman, "Citizens Military Training Camps," *Infantry Journal* 18, no. 6 (1921): 579–83, quotation on 581.
98. Hinman, 581.
99. Bond et al., *The Red, White and Blue Manual*, 1–2.
100. Bond et al., 2.
101. P. S. Bond, *Your Boy & the Other in Universal Training: The Nation's School for Citizenship* (Washington, DC: Press of the Military Engineer, 1920), 92.
102. Love and Davenport, "Defects Found in Drafted Men," 7–8.
103. About 218 of every one thousand men examined revealed defects in this category. Of these, about ninety involved deformed or injured appendages, or hernias. Love and Davenport, 8.
104. Bond, *Your Boy*, 100–101; the emphasis on health education was also in keeping with trends in civilian physical education. See Rogers, "Trends in Physical Education," 18–19, 47.
105. Bond et al., *The Red, White and Blue Manual*, 4–5.
106. Bond et al., 1.

107. For the series of exercises used by the CMTC, see Bond et al., 1–22; among the existing manuals, the CMTC's routine most closely resembled that found in War Department, *Special Regulations, No. 23: Field Physical Training of the Soldier* (Washington, DC: Government Printing Office, 1917); Raycroft's manual also included a similar system, though it was borrowed from Koehler's earlier work. See Raycroft, *Mass Physical Training,* 8–33.
108. H. W. Fleet, "Citizens' Military Training Camps," *Infantry Journal* 32, no. 5 (1928): 497–498.
109. Bond et al., *The Red, White and Blue Manual,* 2.
110. Bond, *Your Boy,* 26.
111. Bond et al., *The Red, White and Blue Manual,* 22.
112. Wakefield, *Playing to Win,* 78.
113. Fleet, "Citizens' Military Training Camps," 498.
114. Kington, *Forgotten Summers,* 115–117.
115. Bond et al., *The Red, White and Blue Manual,* part 8, 1.
116. For several years, Babe Ruth even contributed autographed balls and bats to the best player at each camp. Kington, *Forgotten Summers,* 115–117.
117. Bond et al., *The Red, White and Blue Manual,* part 8, 1.
118. Fleet, "Citizens' Military Training Camps," 499.
119. Bond, *Your Boy,* 97.
120. Christina S. Jarvis, *The Male Body at War: American Masculinity during World War II* (DeKalb: Northern Illinois University Press, 2004), 19.
121. James J. McEntee, *Now They Are Men: The Story of the CCC* (Washington, DC: National Home Library Foundation, 1940), 1–7.
122. Jarvis, *The Male Body at War,* 20.
123. A typical camp leadership cadre included two Regular Army officers, one acting as commander and the other as a deputy, plus two noncommissioned officers and four or five enlisted men. Charles E. Heller, "The U.S. Army, the Civilian Conservation Corps, and Leadership for World War II, 1933–1942," *Armed Forces & Society* 36, no. 3 (2010): 442–444.
124. Heller, 444.
125. Jarvis, *The Male Body at War,* 21.
126. McEntee, *Now They Are Men,* 18.
127. Jarvis, *The Male Body at War,* 23; McEntee, *Now They Are Men,* 60–61.
128. McEntee, *Now They Are Men,* 58.
129. McEntee, 27.
130. McEntee, 37.
131. For more on the daily life of a CCC enrollee, see John A. Salmond, *The Civilian*

Conservation Corps, 1933–1942: A New Deal Case Study (Durham, NC: Duke University Press, 1967), 135–144.

132. The article's purpose appears to have been to reassure officers about the quality of the new draftees, but the authors had to acknowledge lower standards in doing so. Lewis B. Hershey and Thomas M. Watlington, "The Man Selected for Service," *Infantry Journal* 47, no. 6 (1940): 533.

CHAPTER 5. PHYSICAL CULTURES FOR TOTAL WAR, 1936–1946

1. "Kelly Says Nation Must Toughen Up," *New York Times*, November 6, 1942.
2. "Kelly Says Nation Must Toughen Up."
3. Peter R. Mansoor, *The GI Offensive in Europe: The Triumph of American Infantry Divisions, 1941–1945* (Lawrence: University Press of Kansas, 2002), 2. This argument is a historiographical reaction to arguments made by John Ellis and others that Allied superiority in terms of manpower, materiel, and production alone determined victory. See also Richard Overy, *Why the Allies Won* (New York: W. W. Norton, 1997); Williamson Murray and Allan R. Millett, *A War to Be Won: Fighting the Second World War* (Cambridge, MA: Harvard University Press, 2000).
4. "President Asks Fitness Training, Picks John B. Kelly, Olympic Sculler, to Devise 'Physical Preparedness' Program for Nation's Manhood," *New York Times*, September 13, 1940.
5. William B. Foster et al., *Physical Standards in World War II* (Washington, DC: Office of the Surgeon General, Department of the Army, 1967), 2.
6. In late December 1941, new regulations made local induction procedures more uniform. Local boards began using DSS Form 220, a "List of Defects," in lieu of the MR 1–9 standards. Local boards made determinations just on "easily detectable defects disqualifying for general service" and Army reception centers conducted more detailed examinations involving physical profiling, blood typing, and immunizations. Foster et al., 11–14.
7. Foster et al., 16.
8. Leonard G. Rowntree, "National Program for Physical Fitness," *Journal of American Medical Association* 125, no. 12 (1944): 821; Hiram A. Jones, "Report on National Fitness: A Program through Schools and Colleges," *Journal of Health and Physical Education* 13, no. 3 (1942): 133.
9. G. St. J. Perrott, "Selective Service Rejection Statistics and Some of Their Implications," *American Journal of Public Health* 36 (April 1946): 336.
10. Michael M. Davis, "How Healthy Are We?," *New York Times*, February 22, 1942.

11. "Urges Rebuilding of Rejected Men: Rehabilitation Board Presses Plan for U.S. Financing of Voluntary Health Plan," *New York Times*, August 16, 1941.
12. Luther Huston, "Draft System Assays Man Power: Quantity and Quality of Human Material Is Measured," *New York Times*, April 20, 1941.
13. "Health of the Youth of the Nation (Editorial)," *Journal of American Medical Association* 114, no. 5 (1940): 414–415; "U.S. Army Standards Put above Reich's," *New York Times*, November 16, 1941.
14. John H. Shaw, "American Physical Fitness," *Phi Delta Kappan* 24, no. 7 (1942): 285; "The Nation's Health," *New York Times*, October 12, 1941; for a general treatment of the public discourse, see Christina S. Jarvis, *The Male Body at War: American Masculinity during World War II* (DeKalb: Northern Illinois University Press, 2004), 60–62; on the response of physical educators to accusations of prewar failures on behalf of schools to address remedial defects, see Deobald B. Van Dalen and Bruce L. Bennett, *A World History of Physical Education: Cultural, Philosophical, Comparative*, 2nd ed. (Englewood Cliffs, NJ: Prentice Hall, 1971), 484–485.
15. Davis, "How Healthy Are We?"
16. Foster et al., *Physical Standards in World War II*, 19–20.
17. Davis, "How Healthy Are We?"
18. The six elements included general stamina, upper extremities, lower extremities, hearing, vision, and emotional stability. Physical ratings appeared as a six-digit code. The highest physical grade was a 111111. A man whose hearing qualified him only for limited service but was otherwise healthy received a rating of 111311. Robert R. Palmer, "Manpower for the Army: How the Physical Profile System Affected the Infantry," *Infantry Journal* 41, no. 6 (1947): 38–45.
19. Robert R. Palmer, I. Wiley Bell, and William R. Keast, *The Army Ground Forces: The Procurement and Training of Ground Combat Troops* (Washington, DC: Center of Military History, 1991), 66–69.
20. "Army to Build up Health of 200,000 Dropped in Draft," *New York Times*, October 11, 1941. The rehabilitation policy had a precedent in registrants with correctable defects being rejected for service in 1917–1918 being classified as "remediable." Foster et al., *Physical Standards in World War II*, 17–19.
21. William L. Hughes, "The Civilian Defense Physical Fitness Program," *Journal of Health and Physical Education* 13, no. 2 (1942): 71.
22. Hughes, 73; "National Physical Fitness Program: A Statement by the Board of Directors," *Journal of Health and Physical Education* 12, no. 10 (1941): 548.
23. Executive Office of the Committee on Physical Fitness, "Civilian Physical Fitness," *Journal of Health and Physical Education* 14 (1943): 518.
24. Jarvis, *The Male Body at War*, 66–69; Whitfield B. East, *A Historical Review and*

Analysis of Army Physical Readiness Training and Assessment (Fort Leavenworth, KS: Combat Studies Institute Press, 2013), 80, 97.

25. Rowntree, "National Program for Physical Fitness," 822–823.
26. Shaw, "American Physical Fitness," 285.
27. Rowntree, "National Program for Physical Fitness," 825.
28. Theodore P. Bank, "The Army Physical Conditioning Program," *Journal of Health and Physical Education* 14, no. 4 (1943): 197.
29. Bank, 197.
30. Eli Ginzberg et al., *The Ineffective Soldier: Lessons for Management and the Nation—the Lost Divisions* (New York: Columbia University, 1959), 26–28.
31. War Department, *Field Manual 21-20: Basic Field Manual—Physical Training* (Washington, DC: Government Printing Office, 1941), 1.
32. War Department, 3.
33. War Department, 2.
34. War Department, 2.
35. War Department, 2–3.
36. War Department, 36.
37. Joseph E. Raycroft, *Mass Physical Training for Use in the Army and the Reserve Officers' Training Corps* (Washington, DC: United States Infantry Association, 1920), 38, 142–147; East, *A Historical Review and Analysis*, 86–87.
38. War Department, *Field Manual 21-20: Basic Field Manual*, 44–45.
39. War Department, 5.
40. Raycroft, *Mass Physical Training*, 148.
41. War Department, *Field Manual 21-20: Basic Field Manual*, 96.
42. War Department, 97.
43. Francis Keppel to Prof. A. A. Esslinger, 6 May 1942; Joint Army and Navy Committee on Welfare and Recreation, General Subject Files, 1941–1942, box 10; Joint Boards and Committees, Record Group (RG) 225, National Archives Building, College Park, MD (NACP).
44. Committee members included Frank Lloyd, Charles McCloy, T. Nelson Metcalf, Carl Schott, Seward Staley, and Joseph Raycroft. Report of the Special Survey Committee Made to the Chief, Bureau of Navigation, Navy Department, Subject: The Physical Fitness Program at the Naval Training Station at Norfolk, Virginia, 31 March 1942; Joint Army and Navy Committee on Welfare and Recreation, General Subject Files, 1941–1942, box 10; RG 225, NACP.
45. Report of the Special Survey Committee Made to the Chief, Bureau of Navigation, Navy Department, Subject: The Physical Fitness Program at the Naval Training Station at Norfolk, Virginia, 31 March 1942, p. 2; Physical Fitness Program Survey of Special Survey Committee; Joint Army and Navy Commit-

tee on Welfare and Recreation, General Subject Files, 1941–1942, box 10; Joint Boards and Committees, RG 225, NACP.

46. Report of the Special Survey Committee, 5.
47. Report of the Special Survey Committee, 17–21.
48. Report of the Special Survey Committee, 53.
49. Francis Keppel to Prof. A. A. Esslinger, 6 May 1942; Joint Army and Navy Committee on Welfare and Recreation, General Subject Files, 1941–1942, box 10; Joint Boards and Committees, RG 225, NACP.
50. Eleanor B. English, "Charles H. Mccloy: The Research Professor of Physical Education," *Journal of Physical Education, Recreation & Dance* 54, no. 4 (1983): 16.
51. Francis Keppel to Prof. Philip O. Badger, 8 April 1942; Joint Army and Navy Committee on Welfare and Recreation, General Subject Files, 1941–1942, box 10; Joint Boards and Committees, RG 225, NACP; Francis Keppel to Brig. General F. H. Osborn, 7 April 1942; Physical Fitness Program Survey of Special Survey Committee; Joint Army and Navy Committee on Welfare and Recreation, General Subject Files, 1941–1942, box 10; Joint Boards and Committees, RG 225, NACP.
52. Brig. General F. H. Osborn, Memorandum, Subject: Physical Conditioning and Physical Efficiency Tests, 13 April 1942; Joint Army and Navy Committee on Welfare and Recreation, General Subject Files, 1941–1942, box 10; Joint Boards and Committees, RG 225, NACP.
53. The Special Services Division is also sometimes referred to as the Special Services Branch. "Division" will be used in this chapter for the sake of consistency. John D. Millet, *The Organization and Role of the Army Service Forces* (Washington, DC: Center of Military History, 1998), 348.
54. Millet, 36–38.
55. East, *A Historical Review and Analysis*, 111.
56. East, 88–89.
57. Brig. General F. H. Osborn, Memorandum, Subject: Physical Conditioning and Physical Efficiency Tests, 13 April 1942; Joint Army and Navy Committee on Welfare and Recreation, General Subject Files, 1941–1942, box 10; Joint Boards and Committees, RG 225, NACP.
58. Francis Keppel to Mr. Harper, 17 April 1942; Joint Army and Navy Committee on Welfare and Recreation, General Subject Files, 1941–1942, box 10; Joint Boards and Committees, RG 225, NACP.
59. Francis Keppel to Mr. Harper, 17 April 1942, and Francis Keppel to Prof. A. A. Esslinger, 6 May 1942; Joint Army and Navy Committee on Welfare and Recre-

ation, General Subject Files, 1941–1942, box 10; Joint Boards and Committees, RG 225, NACP.

60. Charles McCloy to Francis Keppel, 25 June 1942; Joint Army and Navy Committee on Welfare and Recreation, General Subject Files, 1941–1942, box 10; Joint Boards and Committees, RG 225, NACP.
61. Francis Keppel to Lt. Col. Leon T. David, 17 April 1942; Joint Army and Navy Committee on Welfare and Recreation, General Subject Files, 1941–1942, box 10; Joint Boards and Committees, RG 225, NACP.
62. Theodore P. Bank to Francis Keppel, undated; Joint Army and Navy Committee on Welfare and Recreation, General Subject Files, 1941–1942, box 10; Joint Boards and Committees, RG 225, NACP.
63. Charles McCloy to Francis Keppel, 25 June 1942; Joint Army and Navy Committee on Welfare and Recreation, General Subject Files, 1941–1942, box 10; Joint Boards and Committees, RG 225, NACP.
64. East, *A Historical Review and Analysis*, 90. A decade later, Army officers responsible for physical training policy agreed. They hailed *TC 87* as a "radical departure from a century of formalism." Annex F—Training Literature and Training Aids, p. 1, enclosed in Physical Training Research and Development Studies—A Study of the Adequacy of the Present Army Physical Conditioning Program (Adequacy Study), October 1955; Research and Development Project Case Files—1955; R & D Case Files; U.S. Army Schools, Infantry School, Fort Benning, Georgia, box 67; Records of the United States Continental Army Command, RG 546, NACP.
65. War Department, *War Department Pamphlet No. 21-9: Physical Conditioning* (Washington, DC: Government Printing Office, 1944), cover page.
66. War Department, *Field Manual 21-20: Physical Training* (Washington, DC: Government Printing Office, 1946), i.
67. War Department, *Field Manual 21-20: Basic Field Manual—Physical Training* (Washington, DC: Government Printing Office, 1941), 2.
68. War Department, *Pamphlet No. 21-9: Physical Conditioning*, 2.
69. War Department, 2.
70. War Department, *Field Manual 21-20: Physical Training* (1946), 2–3.
71. Bank, "The Army Physical Conditioning Program," 195.
72. "What Combat Veterans Think of Army Training," *What the Soldier Thinks*, no. 4 (March 1944): 1–2.
73. War Department, *Field Manual 21-20: Physical Training* (1946), 4.
74. War Department, 4.
75. War Department, *Pamphlet No. 21-9: Physical Conditioning*, 15.

76. War Department, 6.

77. The test battery consisted of pull-ups, push-ups, sit-ups, broad jumps, twenty -second Burpee drills, a seventy-five-yard "pick-a-back" run, a three-hundred-yard run, and a "dodging run." War Department, 6.

78. War Department, 6.

79. War Department, 1.

80. War Department, 2.

81. War Department, *Field Manual 21-20: Physical Training* (1946), 3.

82. War Department, 1.

83. War Department, *Pamphlet No. 21-9: Physical Conditioning*, 1. Historians writing after the war endorsed this view. For instance, authors of one book in the Army's official history asserted that "the mobile tactics and open formations of World War II demanded the greatest possible physical vigor and mental alertness in individual combat soldiers and required strong powers of leadership in commanders, even in units as small as the squad. The intelligence, skill, and stamina of semi-isolated riflemen and small-unit commanders were to determine not only individual survival on the battlefield but also in many cases the outcome of battle." Palmer, Bell, and Keast, *The Army Ground Forces*, 3.

84. Antulio J. Echevarria, "The 'Cult of the Offensive' Revisited: Confronting Technological Change before the Great War," *Journal of Strategic Studies* 25, no. 1 (2002): 201.

85. War Department, *Field Manual 21-20: Physical Training* (1946), 1.

86. Bank, "The Army Physical Conditioning Program," 195.

87. War Department, *Field Manual 21-20: Physical Training* (1946), 2.

88. Bank, "The Army Physical Conditioning Program," 197.

89. War Department, *Pamphlet No. 21-9: Physical Conditioning*, 5.

90. Herman J. Koehler, "The Physical Training of Cadets, 1802–1902," in *The Centennial of the United States Military Academy at West Point, New York, 1802–1902* (Washington, DC: Government Printing Office, 1904), 893–908, quotation on 901–902.

91. Sargent's vertical jump test is still used today and commonly known as the "Sargent jump." Institute of Medicine, *Fitness Measures and Health Outcomes in Youth* (Washington, DC: National Academies Press, 2012), 24; Carolyn de la Pena, "Dudley Allen Sargent: Health Machines and the Energized Male Body," *Iron Game History* 8, no. 2 (2003): 11–16.

92. Raycroft, *Mass Physical Training*, viii.

93. Institute of Medicine, *Fitness Measures and Health Outcomes in Youth*, 24.

94. Institute of Medicine, 25.

95. Quantifying and standardizing fitness, then policing normalized "fit bodies,"

has also mirrored trends in US government advisory state actions designed to encourage citizens to become healthier since the early twentieth century. Rachel Louise Moran, *Governing Bodies: American Politics and the Shaping of the Modern Physique* (Philadelphia: University of Pennsylvania Press, 2018), 5–7.

96. War Department, *Pamphlet No. 21-9: Physical Conditioning*, 71.
97. War Department, *Field Manual 21-20: Physical Training* (1946), 333.
98. War Department, *Pamphlet No. 21-9: Physical Conditioning*, 71.
99. War Department, *Field Manual 21-20: Physical Training* (1946), 340–341.
100. Other alleged benefits included the instructor's reception of feedback about the efficacy of his program, the pointing out of specific deficiencies among a unit's men, provision of motivation to improve, and the ability to measure the effectiveness of different training programs. War Department, *Pamphlet No. 21-9: Physical Conditioning*, 69.
101. War Department, 69.
102. War Department, *Manual of Physical Training for Use in the United States Army* (New York: Military Publishing, 1914), 6.
103. No difference existed between *TC 87* (1942) and War Department, *Pamphlet 21-9* (1944), except for the addition of some supplemental guerrilla exercises. The latter was a graphic amplification of the former's system.
104. The calisthenic program as of 1944 included sets of the high jumper, Burpee, squad bender, rowers, push-up, sit-up, side bender, bank twist, squat jump, trunk twister, stationary run, eight-count push-up, straddle pull-up, mountain climber, woodchopper, and bridge exercises. In 1946, *FM 21-20* added a four-exercise warm-up drill and, for variety, a second twelve-exercise conditioning drill.
105. Movement toward functional fitness activities also seems to have bubbled up from below in the Army during World War II. For examples, see "Steeplechase for Soldiers," *Infantry Journal* 49, no. 1 (1941): 46–47; Avery Ashwood, "Building Brawn," *Infantry Journal* 53, no. 2 (1943): 47–50.
106. War Department, *No. 21-9: Physical Conditioning*, 7.
107. War Department, 7–8, 47–50.
108. Bank, "The Army Physical Conditioning Program," 195.
109. War Department, *Manual of Physical Training*, 30.
110. War Department, *Pamphlet No. 21-9: Physical Conditioning*, 62.
111. Quotation in War Department, *Manual of Physical Training*; Raycroft similarly urged progression without giving any detail. See Raycroft, *Mass Physical Training*, 3.
112. War Department, *Pamphlet No. 21-9: Physical Conditioning*, 61.

113. War Department, 63–68.
114. War Department, *Field Manual 21-20: Physical Training* (1946), 31–44.
115. Bank, "The Army Physical Conditioning Program," 195.
116. Bank, 195.
117. Palmer, Bell, and Keast, *The Army Ground Forces*, 326.
118. Palmer, Bell, and Keast, 338.
119. The Morale Branch had been a General Staff agency responsible for studying, devising, and implementing "psychological measures among the troops to produce and maintain good morale" in 1918. The Commission on Training Camp Activities (CTCA) had responsibility for providing the actual facilities and staff for recreation and welfare. The Morale Branch dissolved shortly after World War I, but some of its functions continued under the G-1. In March 1941, the Special Services Branch stood up under the G-1, combining the responsibilities of both the Morale Branch and CTCA. The Special Services Branch was later renamed the Special Service in 1942 and realigned under the new Army Service Force. War Department, *Technical Manual 21-205: Special Service Officer* (Washington, DC: United States Government Printing Office, 1942), 3.
120. War Department, 15–17; Bank, "The Army Physical Conditioning Program," 195.
121. War Department, *Field Manual 28–105: The Special Service Company* (Washington, DC: United States Government Printing Office, 1944), 1–3.
122. War Department, *Field Manual 28–105: The Special Service Company*, 5.
123. Bank, "The Army Physical Conditioning Program," 195.
124. Jeffery Allen Charlston, "From Indifference to Obsession: Origins of Athletic Programs in the United States Military, 1865–1935," (PhD diss., George Washington University, 2000).
125. Wanda Ellen Wakefield, *Playing to Win: Sports and the American Military, 1898–1945* (Albany: State University of New York Press, 1997), 110.
126. Wakefield, 110.
127. Bank, "The Army Physical Conditioning Program," 195.
128. War Department, *Pamphlet No. 21-9: Physical Conditioning*, 2.
129. War Department, 2.
130. Bank, "The Army Physical Conditioning Program," 238.
131. Bank, 238–239.
132. War Department, *Field Manual 21-20: Physical Training* (1946), 187.
133. War Department, *Pamphlet No. 21-9: Physical Conditioning*, 66; War Department, *Field Manual 21-20: Physical Training* (1946), 39.
134. War Department, *Field Manual 21-20: Physical Training* (1946), 187–188.

135. Bank, "The Army Physical Conditioning Program," 238.
136. Wakefield cites trophies, beer, and cigarettes as among the most common prizes used to incentivize participation and victory. Wakefield, *Playing to Win*, 86–87.
137. Examples of "practical courses" included Army administration, dealing with required reports and correspondence, Army mess, dealing with mess supplies and reports, and "Explanation of the Allied Cause." Mattie E. Treadwell, *The Women's Army Corps* (Washington, DC: Center of Military History, 1991), 635–638.
138. Treadwell, *The Women's Army Corps*, 638–639.
139. Van Rensselaer's background included training at Russell Sage College (a Progressive upstate New York college founded in 1916 to advance women's independence through liberal arts education and preparation for specific professional careers), as well as teaching experience at the Central School for Hygiene and Physical Education and at the American Woman's Association in New York. "Physical Training Planned for WAAC," *New York Times*, July 1, 1942.
140. The three assistant instructors were Mary Loomis from Syracuse University, Angela Kitzinger from Russell Sage, and Mary Foster from Stephens College. Public Relations Office, "The Physical Training Program of the W.A.A.C.," *Journal of Health and Physical Education* 14, no. 4 (1943): 209.
141. Public Relations Office, 209.
142. "Physical Training Planned for WAAC."
143. Treadwell, *The Women's Army Corps*, 639.
144. Treadwell, 639.
145. Public Relations Office, "The Physical Training Program of the W.A.A.C.," 240.
146. Public Relations Office, 209.
147. Donna I. Niles, "Physical Fitness and the W.A.C.," *Journal of Health and Physical Education* 14, no. 8:410.
148. War Department, *W.A.C. Field Manual: Physical Training* (Washington, DC: United States Government Printing Office, 1943), 4.
149. Niles, "Physical Fitness and the W.A.C.," 410; War Department, *W.A.C. Field Manual: Physical Training*, 1. The divide between these conceptions of fitness generally mirrored a similar divide in the civilian world over the value of strenuous exercise for women. Treadwell, *The Women's Army Corps*, 639–640.
150. War Department, *W.A.C. Field Manual: Physical Training*, 1.
151. War Department, 6.
152. War Department, 8.

153. Stability was defined as the ability to "be on the job all day, every day, as long as you are needed." Reliability, "regular" elimination, and "normal and easy" menstruation were all desired qualities. War Department, 8.

154. War Department, 12–14.

155. War Department, *Pamphlet No. 21-9: Physical Conditioning*, 1.

156. This is a change from the Army's Koehler-era physical culture, which had sought appearance-based outcomes such as symmetry and posture to a greater extent. War Department, 11.

157. War Department, *W.A.C. Field Manual: Physical Training*, 10, 14.

158. War Department, 24.

159. War Department, *War Department Pamphlet 35–3: WAC Life* (Washington, DC: United States Government Printing Office, 1943), 154.

160. War Department, *W.A.C. Field Manual: Physical Training*, 83.

161. War Department, 83.

162. Niles, "Physical Fitness and the W.A.C.," 409.

163. Niles, 408.

164. Niles, 409.

165. Basic and specialist training referred to the intitial entry training women underwent. First came a common basic training period, and then the more duty-specific specialist training. War Department, *W.A.C. Field Manual: Physical Training*, 117.

166. War Department, 123.

167. War Department, 123; War Department, *Pamphlet No. 21-9: Physical Conditioning*, 62.

168. War Department, *Pamphlet No. 21-9: Physical Conditioning*, 12–15; War Department, *Field Manual 21-20: Physical Training* (1946), 9–12.

169. War Department, *W.A.C. Field Manual: Physical Training*, 114.

170. War Department, 130.

171. Niles, "Physical Fitness and the W.A.C.," 450.

172. Treadwell, *The Women's Army Corps*, 640.

173. The Military Training Division test about which Culp and others complained was a four-event test, using the dip, sit-up, and wing-lift exercises from the WAC strength progressions, plus a squat-thrust event. For a "Good" rating, a woman of fifty had to do three to eight dips in a minute, twenty-eight to forty-eight sit-ups in a minute, sixty-nine to eight-five wing-lifts in a minute, and fifteen to eighteen squat thrusts in thirty seconds. Standards for younger women were higher. Treadwell, *The Women's Army Corps*, 664–665.

174. Treadwell, *The Women's Army Corps*, 666.

175. Treadwell, 666.

176. Director of the Service, Supply, and Procurement Division, *Logistics in World War II: Final Report of the Army Service Forces* (1948; Washington, DC: Center of Military History, 1993), 29.

177. Leisa D. Meyer, *Creating GI Jane: Sexuality and Power in the Women's Army Corps during World War II* (New York: Columbia University Press, 1996), 2.

178. Meyer, *Creating GI Jane*, 34–35.

179. Janann Sherman, "'They Either Need These Women or They Do Not': Margaret Chase Smith and the Fight for Regular Status for Women in the Military," *Journal of Military History* 54 (January 1990): 61.

180. Meyer, *Creating GI Jane*, 8.

181. Colonel Hobby's quotation in Treadwell, *The Women's Army Corps*, 665.

182. According to Christina Jarvis, American institutions shaped male bodies to "re-masculininze" the nation during World War II and to produce a "powerful male 'body politic'" to portray the United States' power and status. Improving American manhood by way of martial physical training thus remained very relevant in the 1940s. Jarvis, *The Male Body at War*, 4–5, 65.

183. This finding harmonizes with similar conclusions drawn by historian Wanda Wakefield about the role of sport in the Army during World War II. She argues that the Army's sporting culture created a hierarchy in which the "strongest and most courageous" athletes were valorized and those uninterested or less talented in athletics were disadvantaged. See Wakefield, *Playing to Win*, 110.

184. D'Ann Campbell, "Women in Combat: The World War II Experience in the United States, Great Britain, Germany, and the Soviet Union," *Journal of Military History* 57 (April 1993): 306.

185. Bank, "The Army Physical Conditioning Program," 196.

186. War Department, *Pamphlet No. 21-9: Physical Conditioning*, 2–5.

187. War Department, 15.

CHAPTER 6. HARD BODIES FOR A COLD WAR: CONDITIONING AND PREHABILITATION, 1945–1957

1. Maxwell D. Taylor, Memorandum Extract, Subject: Physical Fitness; vertical file, Office of Physical Education, USMA, September 1957, United States Military Academy Special Collections.
2. Taylor.
3. *Physical Fitness Seminar Report* (Fort Benning, GA: United States Army Infantry School, 1958), 4.
4. Ingo Trauschweizer, *The Cold War U.S. Army: Building Deterrence for Limited War* (Lawrence: University Press of Kansas, 2008), 18–19.
5. Trauschweizer, 19, 22.

6. War Department, *Field Manual 21-20: Physical Training* (Washington, DC: US Government Printing Office, 1946), 1–4; War Department, *War Department Pamphlet No. 21–9: Physical Conditioning* (Washington, DC: Government Printing Office, 1944), 1–5.
7. Annex F—Training Literature and Training Aids, p. 1, enclosed in Physical Training Research and Development Studies—A Study of the Adequacy of the Present Army Physical Conditioning Program (Adequacy Study), October 1955; Research and Development Project Case Files—1955; R & D Case Files; U.S. Army Schools, Infantry School, Fort Benning, Georgia, box 67; Records of the United States Continental Army Command, Record Group 546 (RG 546), National Archives Building, College Park, MD (NACP).
8. War Department, *Field Manual 21-20: Physical Training* (1946), 36–38, 43.
9. "Until it hurts" from War Department, *War Department Pamphlet No. 21-9: Physical Conditioning* (Washington, DC: Government Printing Office, 1944), 61. In terms of progression, *FM 21-20* recommended toughening for one to two weeks, slow improvement for six to ten weeks, and sustaining or maintaining beyond that. War Department, *Field Manual 21-20: Physical Training* (1946), 33–34.
10. War Department, 2–3.
11. War Department, 4.
12. War Department, 12.
13. For a description of "mass games," which were differentiated from organized athletics by their ease of organization and minimal equipment requirements, see Department of the Army, *Field Manual 21-20: Physical Training* (Washington: US Government Printing Office, 1950), 227.
14. Memorandum, Subject: A Study of the Adequacy of the Present Army Physical Conditioning Program, p. 3, 6 October 1955, enclosed in Adequacy Study, October 1955; Research and Development Project Case Files—1955; R & D Case Files; U.S. Army Schools, Infantry School, Fort Benning, Georgia, box 67; United States Continental Army Command, RG 546, NACP.
15. Quoted in *Staff Study: Institute of Physical Fitness* (Fort Benning, GA: United States Army, 1970), Appendix I to Annex B—1944 Conference on Physical Training.
16. Brian McAllister Linn, *Elvis's Army: Cold War GIs and the Atomic Battlefield* (Cambridge, MA: Harvard University Press, 2016), 28.
17. This corresponds well with a general "postwar lethargy" in the Eighth Army between 1945 and 1949 that historian Thomas Hanson found in his study. See Thomas E. Hanson, *Combat Ready? The Eighth U.S. Army on the Eve of the Korean War* (College Station: Texas A & M University Press, 2010), 14–15.

18. Colonel S. M. Prouty to the Quartermaster General, Subject: Establishment of Course for Directors of Physical Training and Athletics at the Quartermaster School, 30 November 1945; School Organization—Physical Training School, 1946–1953; General Orders and Organization Planning Files (GOOPF), 09/05/1946—07/28/1966; Fort Bragg, North Carolina/Physical Training School (PTS), box 1; United States Continental Army Command, RG 546, NACP.
19. Table of Distribution, Physical Training School; GOOPF, 09/05/1946—07/28/1966; PTS, box 1; United States Continental Army Command, RG 546, NACP.
20. General Jacob L. Devers to Major General Thomas B. Larkin, 20 September 1947; Physical Training and Athletic Director's Course, Schools Division—1947; Army Field Forces HQs, General Staff, G-3 Section, Training Group, Schools Division, Classified Decimal File, 1942–48, box 150; HQ Army Ground Forces, RG 337, NACP.
21. Ransom to Colonel Hendrix, 29 October 1947; Physical Training and Athletic Director's Course, Schools Division—1947; Army Field Forces HQs, General Staff, G-3 Section, Training Group, Schools Division, Classified Decimal File, 1942–48, box 150; HQ Army Ground Forces, RG 337, NACP.
22. In one example of many, First Corps's Maj. Gen. John "Iron Mike" O'Daniel ranked physical conditioning as a top priority alongside maintaining offensive mindedness and discipline in a September 1951 meeting with his subordinate commanders. HQ, I Corps, Corps and Army Unit Commanders Meeting, June 9, 13 June 1952; Folder 3—I U.S. Corps Commanders Notes, 1951–1953; Box 1—Correspondence, 1943–1953: North Africa, Italy, Korea; Lt. Gen. John W. O'Daniel Papers; Citadel Museum and Archives, Charleston SC.
23. Linn, *Elvis's Army*, 56–7, 69–72; Shelly McKenzie, *Getting Physical: The Rise of Fitness Culture in America* (Lawrence: University Press of Kansas, 2013), 44.
24. Charles S. Young, *Name, Rank, and Serial Number: Exploiting Korea War POWs at Home and Abroad* (Oxford: Oxford University Press, 2014), 3–5; McKenzie, *Getting Physical*, 44–46.
25. Hanson, *Combat Ready?*, 5.
26. McKenzie, *Getting Physical*, 46; for "give-it-upitis," see Linn, *Elvis's Army*, 11, 71; on the general political culture of the period characterized by an "excessive preoccupation" with masculinity and a "hard/soft dichotomy," see Kyle A. Cuordileone, "'Politics in an Age of Anxiety': Cold War Political Culture and the Crisis in American Masculinity, 1949–1960," *Journal of American History* 87, no. 2 (2000): 515–545.
27. Whitfield B. East, *A Historical Review and Analysis of Army Physical Readiness*

Training and Assessment (Fort Leavenworth, KS: Combat Studies Institute Press, 2013), 119.

28. Department of the Army, *Field Manual 21-20: Physical Training* (Washington, DC: US Government Printing Office, 1957), 10.
29. Department of the Army, *Field Manual 21-20: Physical Fitness Training* (Washington, DC: Headquarters, Department of the Army, 1998), iii.
30. *Infantry Instructors' Conference Report, 16–21 June 1952* (Fort Benning, GA: Infantry School, 1952), 36.
31. Linn, *Elvis's Army*, 194.
32. Annex G—Command Emphasis, p. 3, enclosed in Adequacy Study, October 1955; Research and Development Project Case Files—1955; R & D Case Files; U.S. Army Schools, Infantry School, Fort Benning, Georgia, box 67; United States Continental Army Command, RG 546, NACP. See also *Staff Study: Institute of Physical Fitness*, Appendix II to Annex B.
33. Department of the Army, *Field Manual 21-20: Physical Training* (1950), 227.
34. Annex F—Training Literature and Training Aids, p. 1, enclosed in Adequacy Study, October 1955; Research and Development Project Case Files—1955; R & D Case Files; U.S. Army Schools, Infantry School, Fort Benning, Georgia, box 67; United States Continental Army Command, RG 546, NACP.
35. Training Circular No. 27, Physical Training, 31 August 1951, enclosed in Adequacy Study, October 1955; Research and Development Project Case Files—1955; R & D Case Files; U.S. Army Schools, Infantry School, Fort Benning, Georgia, box 67; United States Continental Army Command, RG 546, NACP.
36. Specifically, *TC 27* called attention to *FM 21-20's* chapters 1–4 and 16. These chapters covered the definition of fitness, program planning, the set conditioning drills, and posture training. Exceptions to mandatory use of set drills with supplementary exercises such as guerrilla exercises were given to units finished with the unit training phase, those in postcycle training, in standby status, and in overseas commands, and those units not engaged in field exercises of maneuvers who "have attained a high degree of individual physical fitness" already. Those units could enter a sustaining phase that emphasized "highly competitive intracompany and intercompany athletics" so long as a "short intense warm-up" using one of the set drills preceded each period.
37. Army Ground Forces (AGF), referenced earlier, became the Army Field Forces in 1948.
38. Annex A—Authorization for Research Project, enclosed in Staff Study—The Army Physical Fitness Testing Program, August 1955; Research and Development Project Case Files—1955; R & D Case Files; U.S. Army Schools, Infantry

School, Fort Benning, Georgia, box 67; United States Continental Army Command, RG 546, NACP.

39. Memorandum, The Army Physical Fitness Testing Program, p. 1, enclosed in Staff Study—The Army Physical Fitness Testing Program, August 1955; Research and Development Project Case Files—1955; R & D Case Files; U.S. Army Schools, Infantry School, Fort Benning, Georgia, box 67; United States Continental Army Command, RG 546, NACP.

40. Different numbers are given in various documents. For the eight-thousand-range estimate, see Tab D, Annex A—Total Number of Cases Used to Determine Tables, enclosed in Staff Study—The Army Physical Fitness Testing Program, August 1955; Research and Development Project Case Files—1955; R & D Case Files; U.S. Army Schools, Infantry School, Fort Benning, Georgia, box 67; United States Continental Army Command, RG 546, NACP. The ten-thousand-result upper estimate comes from Memorandum—Projects Deemed Necessary by the Physical Training Department in Order to Fulfill the Mission of the Department; Research & Development Administrative Files—1954; U.S. Army Schools, Infantry School, Fort Benning, Georgia, box 67; United States Continental Army Command, RG 546, NACP. A wide variety of units produced these cards. OCAFF directed each training center and training division to test four companies each three times. The first two tests, conducted in the second and fourteenth weeks of training, used the existing assessment test. The third used a new "Physical Achievement Test" designed to measure skills and conditioning in events more closely aligned with combat requirements, such as a five-second rope climb and a 150-yard man carry. Additional data came from PTS classes, the Airborne School, Ranger Training Centers, and various units.

41. Colonel T. J. Smith to the Commandant, Physical Training School Fort Bragg, North Carolina, Subject: Research in Physical Fitness Tests, 29 April 1952, enclosed in Staff Study—The Army Physical Fitness Testing Program, August 1955; Research and Development Project Case Files—1955; R & D Case Files; U.S. Army Schools, Infantry School, Fort Benning, Georgia, box 67; United States Continental Army Command, RG 546, NACP.

42. Annex A—History of Study, enclosed in Staff Study—The Army Physical Fitness Testing Program, August 1955; Research and Development Project Case Files—1955; R & D Case Files; U.S. Army Schools, Infantry School, Fort Benning, Georgia, box 67; United States Continental Army Command, RG 546, NACP.

43. Captain Harold S. Tavzel to Commanding General, Third Army, 21 July 1953; School Organization—Physical Training School, 1946–53; General Orders

and Organization Planning Files, 09/05/1946—07/28/1966; Fort Bragg, North Carolina/Physical Training School, box 1; United States Continental Army Command, RG 546, NACP.

44. The Ground General School was organized in 1946 and outlived the PTS by only two years, closing in 1955. The school's mission included basic training for all officers, running an officer candidate school, and providing some instruction for intelligence officers. At the General School, the new Physical Training Department shrank to a mere two training officers, a single civilian physical education instructor, and two enlisted mathematical-statistical research assistants. Lt. Col. L. E. Barber to Commanding General, Fifth Army, Subject: Establishment of Physical Training Department at the Army General School, 28 October 1953; School Organization—Physical Training School, 1946–53; General Orders and Organization Planning Files, 09/05/1946—07/28/1966; Fort Bragg, North Carolina/Physical Training School, box 1; United States Continental Army Command, RG 546, NACP.

45. Lt. Col. Earl F. Klinck, Study for Continuation of Physical Training and Athletic Directors Course, undated; School Organization—Physical Training School, 1946–53; General Orders and Organization Planning Files, 09/05/1946—07/28/1966; Fort Bragg, North Carolina/Physical Training School, box 1; United States Continental Army Command, RG 546, NACP.

46. Staff Studies of Problems 1–4, 31 August 1953; School Organization—Physical Training School, 1946–53; General Orders and Organization Planning Files, 09/05/1946—07/28/1966; Fort Bragg, North Carolina/Physical Training School, box 1; United States Continental Army Command, RG 546, NACP.

47. Circular No. 72, Physical Training Proficiency, 19 August 1953; Research & Development Administration Files—1954; U.S. Army Schools, Infantry School, Fort Benning, Georgia, box 67; United States Continental Army Command, RG 546, NACP; Captain Harold S. Tavzel to Commandant, Physical Training School, Subject: Staff Study—Problem 1, 25 August 1953; School Organization—Physical Training School, 1946–53; General Orders and Organization Planning Files, 09/05/1946—07/28/1966; Fort Bragg, North Carolina/Physical Training School, box 1; United States Continental Army Command, RG 546, NACP.

48. A Study of the Adequacy of the Present Army Physical Conditioning Program, 6 October 1955, enclosed in Adequacy Study, p. 2, October 1955; Research and Development Project Case Files—1955; R & D Case Files; U.S. Army Schools, Infantry School, Fort Benning, Georgia, box 67; United States Continental Army Command, RG 546, NACP.

49. Memorandum—Projects Deemed Necessary by the Physical Training Depart-

ment in Order to Fulfill the Mission of the Department; Research & Development Administrative Files—1954; U.S. Army Schools, Infantry School, Fort Benning, Georgia, box 67; United States Continental Army Command, RG 546, NACP.

50. James Dawson became the sole human continuity between the PTS and its later reincarnation at the US Army Infantry School, working consecutively at Forts Bragg, Riley, and Benning. Lt. Col. L. E. Barber to Commandant, Army General School, Subject: Establishment of Physical Training Department at the Army General School, 28 October 1953; School Organization—Physical Training School, 1946–53; General Orders and Organization Planning Files, 09/05/1946—07/28/1966; Fort Bragg, North Carolina/Physical Training School, box 1; United States Continental Army Command, RG 546, NACP.
51. *Physical Fitness Seminar Report*, 25.
52. John Kelly, the former chairman of the World War II Committee on Physical Fitness who worried that America was becoming a "nation of weaklings," brought this report to Eisenhower's attention. John B. Kelly, "Are We Becoming a Nation of Weaklings?," *American Magazine* 161 (March 1956).
53. Col. James H. Kellers to Commanding General, Continental Army Command, Subject: Physical Conditioning Program, 13 August 1955, enclosed in Adequacy Study, October 1955; Research and Development Project Case Files—1955; R & D Case Files; U.S. Army Schools, Infantry School, Fort Benning, Georgia, box 67; United States Continental Army Command, RG 546, NACP.
54. Lt. Col. Samuel J. Chilk to Commanding Generals, First, Second, Third, Fourth, Fifth, and Sixth Armies, Subject: Physical Conditioning Program, 29 August 1955, enclosed in Adequacy Study, October 1955; Research and Development Project Case Files—1955; R & D Case Files; U.S. Army Schools, Infantry School, Fort Benning, Georgia, box 67; United States Continental Army Command, RG 546, NACP.
55. Those "certain modifications" primarily concerned increasing physical conditioning time allotments in the Specialized Assignment Phase of a soldier's training, adjusting the physical fitness test scoring tables based on new research, updating training literature, revising service school programs to provide more instruction on developing and leading physical training programs, and adopting the new physical achievement test for combat units. The study does not appear to have sought or used quantitative measures of physical demands in combat. Proper physical condition remained an absolute measure of physiological performance capacity, not a relative measure of an individual's ability to function effectively on the battlefield. Headquarters, the Infantry School to Commanding General, Continental Army Command, Subject: Phys-

ical Conditioning Program, Conclusions, p. 1, enclosed in Adequacy Study, October 1955; Research and Development Project Case Files—1955; R & D Case Files; U.S. Army Schools, Infantry School, Fort Benning, Georgia, box 67; United States Continental Army Command, RG 546, NACP.

56. Annex A—The Physical Training Program, p. 2, enclosed in Adequacy Study, October 1955; Research and Development Project Case Files—1955; R & D Case Files; U.S. Army Schools, Infantry School, Fort Benning, Georgia, box 67; United States Continental Army Command, RG 546, NACP.

57. A Study of the Adequacy of the Present Army Physical Conditioning Program, 6 October 1955, pp. 1–5, enclosed in Adequacy Study, October 1955; Research and Development Project Case Files—1955; R & D Case Files; U.S. Army Schools, Infantry School, Fort Benning, Georgia, box 67; United States Continental Army Command, RG 546, NACP.

58. Headquarters, the Infantry School to Commanding General, Continental Army Command, Subject: Physical Conditioning Program, Conclusions, p. 1, enclosed in Adequacy Study, October 1955; Research and Development Project Case Files—1955; R & D Case Files; U.S. Army Schools, Infantry School, Fort Benning, Georgia, box 67; United States Continental Army Command, RG 546, NACP.

59. A Study of the Adequacy of the Present Army Physical Conditioning Program, 6 October 1955, p. 7, enclosed in Adequacy Study, October 1955; Research and Development Project Case Files—1955; R & D Case Files; U.S. Army Schools, Infantry School, Fort Benning, Georgia, box 67; United States Continental Army Command, RG 546, NACP.

60. *Field Manual 21-20: Physical Training* (1950), 3; Training Circular No. 27, Physical Training, 31 August 1951, enclosed in Adequacy Study, October 1955; Research and Development Project Case Files—1955; R & D Case Files; U.S. Army Schools, Infantry School, Fort Benning, Georgia, box 67; United States Continental Army Command, RG 546, NACP.

61. Annex G—Command Emphasis, p. 2, enclosed in Adequacy Study, October 1955; Research and Development Project Case Files—1955; R & D Case Files; U.S. Army Schools, Infantry School, Fort Benning, Georgia, box 67; United States Continental Army Command, RG 546, NACP.

62. *Physical Fitness Seminar Report*, 11.

63. Annex G—Command Emphasis, pp. 1–2, enclosed in Adequacy Study, October 1955; Research and Development Project Case Files—1955; R & D Case Files; U.S. Army Schools, Infantry School, Fort Benning, Georgia, box 67; United States Continental Army Command, RG 546, NACP.

64. Annex A—The Physical Training Program, pp. 4–5, enclosed in Adequacy

Study, October 1955; Research and Development Project Case Files—1955; R & D Case Files; U.S. Army Schools, Infantry School, Fort Benning, Georgia, box 67; United States Continental Army Command, RG 546, NACP.

65. Linn, *Elvis's Army*, 293–294.

66. Annex H—Physical Training Leadership, p. 2, enclosed in Adequacy Study, October 1955; Research and Development Project Case Files—1955; R & D Case Files; U.S. Army Schools, Infantry School, Fort Benning, Georgia, box 67; United States Continental Army Command, RG 546, NACP.

67. A Study of the Adequacy of the Present Army Physical Conditioning Program, 6 October 1955, pp. 5–6, enclosed in Adequacy Study, October 1955; Research and Development Project Case Files—1955; R & D Case Files; U.S. Army Schools, Infantry School, Fort Benning, Georgia, box 67; United States Continental Army Command, RG 546, NACP.

68. Annex A—The Physical Training Program, p. 5, enclosed in Adequacy Study, October 1955; Research and Development Project Case Files—1955; R & D Case Files; U.S. Army Schools, Infantry School, Fort Benning, Georgia, box 67; United States Continental Army Command, RG 546, NACP.

69. Annex B—Activities Comprising the Physical Training Program, p. 3, enclosed in Adequacy Study, October 1955; Research and Development Project Case Files—1955; R & D Case Files; U.S. Army Schools, Infantry School, Fort Benning, Georgia, box 67; United States Continental Army Command, RG 546, NACP.

70. Annex G—Command Emphasis, pp. 1–3, enclosed in Adequacy Study, October 1955; Research and Development Project Case Files—1955; R & D Case Files; U.S. Army Schools, Infantry School, Fort Benning, Georgia, box 67; United States Continental Army Command, RG 546, NACP.

71. A Study of the Adequacy of the Present Army Physical Conditioning Program, 6 October 1955, p. 12, enclosed in Adequacy Study, October 1955; Research and Development Project Case Files—1955; R & D Case Files; U.S. Army Schools, Infantry School, Fort Benning, Georgia, box 67; United States Continental Army Command, RG 546, NACP.

72. United States Army Infantry School, *Infantry Instructors' Conference Report, 17–21 June 1957* (Fort Benning, GA: Infantry School, 1957), 132.

73. Specifically, the regulation required officers to spend one half day per work week, exclusive of Sundays and holidays, in physical exercise. The nature of that exercise was not prescribed. Department of the Army, *Army Regulations 600-160: Maintenance of Physical Fitness and Detecting and Correcting Physical Abnormalities among Officers* (Washington, DC: US Government Printing Office, 1955), 1–3. The regulation also reflected a growing concern about the

health of Army officers, especially their heart health, in encouraging them to take full advantage of their annual leave and to act to correct medical issues. These moves coincided with a growing awareness in America about the dangers of cholesterol that culminated in the "first cholesterol scare" of 1961. Harvey Levenstein, *Paradox of Plenty: A Social History of Eating in Modern America* (New York: Oxford University Press, 1993), 135–136.

74. A Study of the Adequacy of the Present Army Physical Conditioning Program, 6 October 1955, pp. 9–10, enclosed in Adequacy Study, October 1955; Research and Development Project Case Files—1955; R & D Case Files; U.S. Army Schools, Infantry School, Fort Benning, Georgia, box 67; United States Continental Army Command, RG 546, NACP.
75. A Study of the Adequacy of the Present Army Physical Conditioning Program, 10.
76. Annex H—Physical Training Leadership, p. 2, enclosed in Adequacy Study, October 1955; Research and Development Project Case Files—1955; R & D Case Files; U.S. Army Schools, Infantry School, Fort Benning, Georgia, box 67; United States Continental Army Command, RG 546, NACP.
77. East, *Historical Review and Analysis*, 158.
78. For a full explanation of changes, see Annex C—Physical Fitness Testing, enclosed in Adequacy Study, October 1955; Research and Development Project Case Files—1955; R & D Case Files; U.S. Army Schools, Infantry School, Fort Benning, Georgia, box 67; United States Continental Army Command, RG 546, NACP.
79. The PAT had been under study since at least 1952. A Study of the Adequacy of the Present Army Physical Conditioning Program, 6 October 1955, p. 6, enclosed in Adequacy Study, October 1955; Research and Development Project Case Files—1955; R & D Case Files; U.S. Army Schools, Infantry School, Fort Benning, Georgia, box 67; United States Continental Army Command, RG 546, NACP.
80. Annex C—Physical Fitness Testing, enclosed in Adequacy Study, October 1955, p. 7; Research and Development Project Case Files—1955; R & D Case Files; U.S. Army Schools, Infantry School, Fort Benning, Georgia, box 67; United States Continental Army Command, RG 546, NACP.
81. Physical training policy at this time did not stipulate any mandatory consequences for failing tests. The tests were explicitly intended to be assessment tools for commanders and thus did not include anything punitive. United States Army Infantry School, *Infantry Instructors' Conference Report, 17–21 June 1957*, 134.
82. Linn, *Elvis's Army*, 243–244.

83. Col. James H. Kellers to Commanding General, Continental Army Command, Subject: Physical Conditioning Program, 13 August 1955, enclosed in Adequacy Study, October 1955; Research and Development Project Case Files—1955; R & D Case Files; U.S. Army Schools, Infantry School, Fort Benning, Georgia, box 67; United States Continental Army Command, RG 546, NACP.
84. Albert E. Lockhart, "Overweight in Grade," *Infantry School Quarterly* 46, no. 3 (1956): 75–79.
85. Peter N. Stearns, *Fat History: Bodies and Beauty in the Modern West* (New York: New York University Press, 2002), 51–53, 60, 72, 100–22; Rachel Louise Moran, *Governing Bodies: American Politics and the Shaping of the Modern Physique* (Philadelphia: University of Pennsylvania Press, 2018), 87; Jesse Berrett, "Feeding the Organization Man: Diet and Masculinity in Postwar America," *Journal of Social History* 30, no. 4 (1997): 805–825; the first major cholesterol scare did not come until 1961, but reports linking cholesterol, obesity, and heart disease had been appearing since 1950. Levenstein, *Paradox of Plenty*, 135–137.
86. Annex E—Diet and Overweight, p. 1, enclosed in Adequacy Study, October 1955; Research and Development Project Case Files—1955; R & D Case Files; U.S. Army Schools, Infantry School, Fort Benning, Georgia, box 67; United States Continental Army Command, RG 546, NACP.
87. Annex E—Diet and Overweight, p. 1.
88. Tab A, Annex E—Weight Control Program of XVIII Airborne Corps, pp. 1–2, enclosed in Adequacy Study, October 1955; Research and Development Project Case Files—1955; R & D Case Files; U.S. Army Schools, Infantry School, Fort Benning, Georgia, box 67; United States Continental Army Command, RG 546, NACP.
89. Tab A, Annex E—Weight Control Program, 1.
90. Annex E—Diet and Overweight, p. 4, enclosed in Adequacy Study, October 1955; Research and Development Project Case Files—1955; R & D Case Files; U.S. Army Schools, Infantry School, Fort Benning, Georgia, box 67; United States Continental Army Command, RG 546, NACP.
91. The Army Weight Control Program (AWCP) became official policy in October 1963 through the publication of *Army Regulations 600-7*. The AWCP strongly resembled the Eighteenth Airborne Corps's program recommended in the adequacy study of 1955. For more on the AWCP program of 1963, see East, *Historical Review and Analysis*, 131–132.
92. The pentomic concept grew out of a "Pentana" study by CONARC in 1955. The pentomic experiment was problematic and short-lived. A second round of reorganization began in 1960 and culminated in the Reorganization Objectives

Army Divisions (ROAD) in 1963. Trauschweizer, *The Cold War U.S. Army,* 58–59; Linn, *Elvis's Army,* 84.

93. Historian Brian Linn has argued that the pentomic concept may also have been a scheme by Taylor to maintain or grow the number of Army divisions without additional manpower. Linn, *Echo of Battle: The Army's Way of War* (Cambridge, MA: Harvard University Press, 2007), 178.
94. Battlegroup headquarters also contained a heavy mortar battery, plus reconnaissance, signals intelligence, maintenance, and medical assets. Battlegroups remained reliant on the division for combat and combat service support, however. Richard W. Kedzior, *Evolution and Endurance: The U.S. Army Division in the Twentieth Century* (Arlington: RAND, 2000), 25–26; Linn, *Echo of Battle,* 87–89.
95. G. C. Reinhardt and W. R. Kintner, *Atomic Weapons in Land Combat,* 2nd ed. (Harrisburg, PA: Military Service Publishing, 1954), 72.
96. Kedzior, *Evolution and Endurance,* 25.
97. Trauschweizer, *The Cold War U.S. Army,* 33.
98. Carl F. Fritzsche, "Physical Fitness—a Must!," *Army Information Digest* 10, no. 7 (1955): 41–42.
99. Fritzsche, 41. Labeling soldiers "soft" carried meaning beyond battlefield endurance. It also suggested effeminacy, indolence, a lack of rugged individualism, and weakness in both mental and moral dimensions. See Berrett, "Feeding the Organization Man," 805–825; Cuordileone, "'Politics in an Age of Anxiety,'" 515–545; Kyle A. Cuordileone, *Manhood and American Political Culture in the Cold War* (New York: Routledge, 2005), 124–145.
100. *Physical Fitness Seminar Report,* 20.
101. Simon A. McNeely, "Physical Fitness in the Pentomic Age," *Journal of Health-Physical Education-Recreation* 29, no. 6 (1958): 21–22.
102. *TM 21-200*'s material was essentially just the middle chapters of earlier field manuals. *FM 21-20* expanded on guidance in earlier field manuals about how to construct a program and evaluate fitness. The new field manual also added synopsis of the human body's structure and functions.
103. Department of the Army, *Field Manual 21-20: Physical Training* (1957), 8.
104. Department of the Army, 8–11.
105. Department of the Army, 9.
106. Department of the Army, 12.
107. Department of the Army, 12–36.
108. Department of the Army, 39, 41, 45.
109. Department of the Army, *Technical Manual 21-200: Physical Conditioning*

(Washington, DC: US Government Printing Office, 1957), 5–7, 13–15; Department of the Army, *Field Manual 21-20: Physical Training* (1957), 5–7.

110. Department of the Army, *Field Manual 21-20: Physical Training* (1957), 5–7.
111. Department of the Army, 133.
112. Linn, *Echo of Battle*, 294–297.
113. Department of the Army, *Field Manual 21-20: Physical Training* (1957), 146.
114. Department of the Army, 72.
115. Department of the Army, *Technical Manual 21-200: Physical Conditioning*, 13–15.
116. Both the traditional physical fitness test and the PAT remained completely optional, except for two mandatory fitness tests during a new soldier's basic training phase.
117. United States Army Infantry School, *Infantry Instructors' Conference Report, 17–21 June 1957*, 133.
118. James E. Reilly and Robert M. Garrison, "Our Physical Unfitness," *Infantry* 49, no. 2 (1959): 20.
119. War Department, *Manual of Physical Training for Use in the United States Army* (New York: Military Publishing, 1914), 5.
120. Herman J. Koehler, "Letter from Captain Herman J. Koehler," *American Physical Education Review* 21, no. 3 (1916): 148–149.
121. Department of the Army, *Technical Manual 21-200: Physical Conditioning*, 44. Raycroft and his team had similarly articulated a greater focus on individual fitness between 1917 and 1920. Though submerged in the interwar years, the individual returned to the spotlight in 1942 and grew more prominent through 1957 and beyond.
122. *Physical Fitness Seminar Report*, i.
123. *Physical Fitness Seminar Report*, 5.
124. See, for instance, *Physical Fitness Seminar Report*, 18, 20.
125. *Physical Fitness Seminar Report*, 32, 34.
126. USAIS conducted this survey. The school sent one hundred questionnaires to division and Army headquarters, which in turn distributed copies to subordinate units. Of the one hundred questionnaires sent, eighty-three were returned. *Physical Fitness Seminar Report*, 11.
127. *Physical Fitness Seminar Report*, 11–12.
128. *Physical Fitness Seminar Report*, 26.
129. Specifically, the conferees recommended a central school like the defunct Physical Training School for training program managers and division- or post-level schools for producing unit instructors. *Physical Fitness Seminar Report*, 31–33.

130. *Physical Fitness Seminar Report*, 30.

131. *Physical Fitness Seminar Report*, 4.

132. Jeffrey Montez de Oca, "'As Our Muscles Get Softer, Our Missile Race Becomes Harder': Cultural Citizenship and the 'Muscle Gap,'" *Journal of Historical Sociology* 18, no. 3 (2005): 149.

133. Christina S. Jarvis, *The Male Body at War: American Masculinity during World War II* (DeKalb: Northern Illinois University Press, 2004), 21.

134. Michael M. Davis, "How Healthy Are We?," *New York Times*, February 22, 1942.

135. US Office of Civilian Defense Physical Fitness Committee, *Report on National Fitness: A Program through Schools and Colleges*, by Hiram A. Jones, Anne Schley Duggan, and August H. Pritzlaff, February 1942; Records of the Physical Fitness Committee, General Records, 1942–45, box 10; Records of the Community War Services, RG 215, NACP.

136. See chapter 5 for a more thorough discussion of John Kelly's organizations. Many physical educators from the American Association for Health, Physical Education, and Recreation eagerly participated and explained the goals of the program in their own publications. For contemporary explanations of this evolving organization's purpose, see "National Physical Fitness Program: A Statement by the Board of Directors," *Journal of Health and Physical Education* 12, no. 10 (1941): 547–548; Executive Office of the Committee on Physical Fitness, "Civilian Physical Fitness," *Journal of Health and Physical Education* 14, no. 10 (1943): 518. Several grassroots efforts also tapped into the groundswell of interest in prehabilitation. The authors of several new books advised boys on how to condition themselves for military service. Full "community physical fitness programs" crafted by physical educators aimed to improve citizenry's health generally. See Francois D'Eliscu, *How to Prepare for Military Fitness* (New York: W. W. Norton, 1943); Charles Ward Crampton, *Fighting Fitness: A Premilitary Training Guide* (New York: McGraw-Hill Book, 1944); Arthur H. Steinhaus et al., *How to Keep Fit and Like It: A Manual for Civilians and a Plan for a Community Approach to Physical Fitness* (Chicago: Consolidated Book Publishers, 1943). See also Physical Fitness Can Make the Difference in the Shops, Homes, Offices, Classrooms, Stores, Armed Forces, Just Living: A Community Plan for Physical Education, 8 October 1941; Com. On Physical Fitness, 1941, file 848; Records of the Physical Fitness Committee, General Records, 1942–45, box 1; Records of the Community War Services, RG 215, NACP.

137. Ethel Percy Andrus, "High School Victory Corps," *Journal of Educational Sociology* 16, no. 4 (1942): 231.

138. Richard M. Ugland, "'Education for Victory': The High School Victory Corps

and Curricular Adaptation during World War II," *History of Education Quarterly* 19, no. 4 (1979): 435, 438.

139. The five included the Air Service, Land Service, Sea Service, Production Service, and Community Service divisions.

140. *High-School Victory Corps, Pamphlet Number 1* (Washington, DC: US Government Printing Office, 1942), 7.

141. The manual was produced by the Federal Security Agency and US Office of Education, with considerable input from the armed forces.

142. "More Tarzans, Fewer Softies Needed for War," *Chicago Daily Tribune*, November 17, 1942; Bank regularly delivered this message in other forums too. For instance, see Theodore P. Bank, "The Army Physical Conditioning Program," *Journal of Health and Physical Education* 14, no. 4 (1943).

143. *Physical Fitness through Physical Education* (Washington, DC: US Government Printing Office, 1942), 4.

144. Of secondary interest were those destined for industrial work and girls responsible for maintaining the homefront. *Physical Fitness through Physical Education*, 25.

145. *Physical Fitness through Physical Education*, 26.

146. *Physical Fitness through Physical Education*, 30–46; Bank, "The Army Physical Conditioning Program," 197.

147. US Office of Education Committee on Wartime Physical Fitness for Colleges and Universities, *Handbook on Physical Fitness for Students in Colleges and Universities* (Washington, DC: US Government Printing Office, 1943).

148. Deobald B. Van Dalen and Bruce L. Bennett, *A World History of Physical Education: Cultural, Philosophical, Comparative*, 2nd ed. (Englewood Cliffs, NJ: Prentice Hall, 1971), 481–82; Rosalind Cassidy and Hilda Clute Kozman, "Trends in State Wartime Physical Fitness Programs," *Journal of Health and Physical Education* 14, no. 7 (1943): 357, 92–93.

149. Ugland, "'Education for Victory,'" 439.

150. Ugland, 441.

151. Stewart Atkinson, "What Holds Back the Victory Corps?," *Clearing House* 18, no. 3 (1943): 137–139.

152. E. B. White, "Victory Corps," *Bulletin of the American Association of University Professors (1915–1955)* 29, no. 2 (1943): 300.

153. Michael J. Hogan, *A Cross of Iron: Harry S. Truman and the Origins of the National Security State, 1945–1954* (Cambridge: Cambridge University Press, 1998), 122.

154. John Sager, "Universal Military Training and the Struggle to Define American Identity during the Cold War," *Federal History Journal*, no. 5 (2013): 57.

155. Hogan, *A Cross of Iron*, 125.
156. Lewis B. Hershey, "We Must Improve Our Youth," *New York Times*, February 10, 1946.
157. William A. Taylor, *Every Citizen a Soldier: The Campaign for Universal Military Training after World War II* (College Station: Texas A & M University Press, 2014), 99–100.
158. Harry S. Truman, "Remarks at the National Health Assembly Dinner," www.trumanlibrary.org/publicpapers/index.php?pid=1612.
159. Quotation from President Truman's guidance to his Advisory Commission on Universal Training in 1947 located in Taylor, *Every Citizen a Soldier*, 121.
160. Beyond generating some positive publicity, the experimental units did not generate much popular demand for the program, motivated too few attendees to enlist, and failed to "produce moral paragons." Linn, *Elvis's Army*, 31.
161. Sager, "Universal Military Training," 58–59, 73.
162. Sager, 64.
163. See, for instance, Charles F. Mourin, "Postwar Physical Education or Military Training?," *Journal of Health and Physical Education* 16, no. 4 (1945): 180, 220, 22; Harold K. Jack, "A Suggested Plan for Military Service," *Journal of Health and Physical Education* 19, no. 4 (1945): 181.
164. Jay B. Nash, "Is Compulsory Military Training the Answer? No!," *Journal of Health and Physical Education* 16, no. 2 (1945): 65.
165. Montez de Oca, "'As Our Muscles Get Softer,'" 147–148.
166. McKenzie, *Getting Physical*, 2–3, 41; Montez de Oca, "'As Our Muscles Get Softer,'" 149; Marc Richards, "The Cold War's 'Soft' Recruits," *Peace Review* 10, no. 3 (1998): 435. For a critique of this argument that suggests that a "general male panic" may not have been as universal as public intellectuals claimed, see James Gilbert, *Men in the Middle: Searching for Masculinity in the 1950s* (Chicago: University of Chicago Press, 2005), 3–9.
167. Kelly, "Are We Becoming a Nation of Weaklings?," 28.
168. Moran, *Governing Bodies*, 87; Richards, "The Cold War's 'Soft' Recruits," 437–438; Montez de Oca, "'As Our Muscles Get Softer,'" 150.
169. Quoted in Richards, "The Cold War's 'Soft' Recruits," 436.
170. James Gilbert, *A Cycle of Outrage: America's Reaction to the Juvenile Delinquent in the 1950s* (New York: Oxford University Press, 1986), 42. See also Leerom Medovoi, *Rebels: Youth and the Cold War Origins of Identity* (Durham, NC: Duke University Press, 2005), 26.
171. Gilbert, *Cycle of Outrage*, 66; Grace Palladino, *Teenagers: An American History* (New York: Basic, 1996), 81, 158.
172. Linn, *Elvis's Army*, 268–269.

173. McKenzie, *Getting Physical*, 44.
174. United States Army Infantry School, *Infantry Instructors' Conference Report, 16–21 June 1952*, 36.
175. McKenzie, *Getting Physical*, 44–45.
176. Richards, "The Cold War's 'Soft' Recruits," 437.
177. Moran, *Governing Bodies*, 88–89.
178. Robert H. Boyle, "The Report That Shocked the President," *Sports Illustrated*, 1955, 30.
179. Boyle, 73.
180. Moran, *Governing Bodies*, 90–94.
181. McKenzie, *Getting Physical*, 24; Moran, *Governing Bodies*, 87.
182. McKenzie, *Getting Physical*, 23.
183. For a more comprehensive overview of the PCYF's activities, see McKenzie, 24–40; Moran, *Governing Bodies*, 90–98.
184. *Physical Fitness Seminar Report*, 6–7.
185. *Physical Fitness Seminar Report*, 6.
186. *Physical Fitness Seminar Report*, 8.
187. For more on Kennedy's Council on Physical Fitness and Lyndon Johnson's Council on Physical Fitness and Sports, during which the greatest changes to this program occurred, see Moran, *Governing Bodies*, 98–111.
188. *Physical Fitness Seminar Report*, 20.
189. Reilly and Garrison, "Our Physical Unfitness," 21.
190. On the "advisory state," see Reilly and Garrison, 2–9.

CONCLUSION: FASHIONING THAT "CERTAIN STRENGTH OF BODY AND SOUL," 1885–1957

1. The ACFT comprises six events: a three-repetition maximum deadlift, a standing power throw, a hand release push-up, a "spring-drag-carry" shuttle run, a hanging leg tuck, and a two-mile run. In contrast, the APFT was comprised of three events: push-ups, sit-ups, and a two-mile run. The APFT also used an age- and gender-based scoring system, whereas the ACFT's scoring is neutral, but with three different performance thresholds aligned with duty positions.
2. Meghann Myers, "A New Army PT Test Is on Its Way: This Is Not a Drill," July 9, 2018, www.armytimes.com/news/your-army/2018/07/09/a-new-army-pt-test-is-o n-its-way-this-is-not-a-drill/.
3. David Barno and Nora Bensahel, "Dumb and Dumber: The Army's New PT Test," October 16, 2018, https://warontherocks.com/2018/10/dumb-and-dumber-the-armys-new-pt-test/; Emma Moore, "The ACFT and the Problems with the Military's Cult of Physical Fitness," December 16, 2019, www.military.com

/daily-news/2019/12/16/acft-and-problems-militarys-cult-physical-fitness.html.

4. Scott McDonald, "U.S. Army Aims for Tougher Fitness Standards Despite Amount of Overweight Recruits," December 4, 2018, www.newsweek.com/us-army-aims-tougher-fitness-standards-despite-amount-overweight-recruits-1244644.
5. Miranda Summers Lowe, "'Swat the Kaiser' and Stork Stands: The History of Army Physical Fitness," *New York Times*, March 28, 2019, www.nytimes.com/2019/03/28/magazine/army-physical-fitness-test.html.
6. Herman J. Koehler, "Letter from Captain Herman J. Koehler," *American Physical Education Review* 21, no. 3 (1916): 148.
7. Koehler, 150.
8. Lewis shows that this deep-rooted cultural belief has been at odds since World War II with another trend—the substitution of technology for manpower. Adrian R. Lewis, *The American Culture of War: The History of U.S. Military Force from World War II to Operation Enduring Freedom*, 2nd ed. (New York: Routledge, 2012), 41.
9. Historian Shelly McKenzie arrives at a similar conclusion in her study of American fitness culture since the 1950s. See Shelly McKenzie, *Getting Physical: The Rise of Fitness Culture in America* (Lawrence: University Press of Kansas, 2013), 178.
10. For an entry to this literature, see Anthony Kellett, *Combat Motivation: The Behavior of Soldiers in Battle* (Boston: Kluwer, Nijhoff, 1982); John Ellis, *Sharp End: The Fighting Man in World War II* (New York: Scribner's, 1980); Samuel A. Stouffer et al., *The American Soldier: Combat and Its Aftermath*, vol. 2 (New York: John Wiley & Sons, 1949); J. Glenn Gray, *The Warriors: Reflections on Men in Battle* (Lincoln: University of Nebraska Press, 1998); Gerald F. Linderman, *The World within War: America's Combat Experience in World War II* (Cambridge, MA: Harvard University Press, 1999); Richard Holmes, *Acts of War: The Behavior of Men in Battle* (London: Weidenfeld & Nicholson, 2003); S. L. A. Marshall, *Men against Fire: The Problem of Battle Command* (Norman: University of Oklahoma Press, 2000); Rune Henrikson, "Warriors in Combat—What Makes People Actively Fight in Combat?," *Journal of Strategic Studies* 30, no. 2 (2007).
11. Lewis, *The American Culture of War*, 35.
12. For an overview of doctrinal and policy developments since 1958, see Whitfield B. East, *A Historical Review and Analysis of Army Physical Readiness Training and Assessment* (Fort Leavenworth, KS: Combat Studies Institute Press, 2013).

13. "Soldier Athlete Initiative," US Army, August 16, 2010, www.army.mil/article/43820/soldier_athlete_initiative.
14. As an example, a twenty-two-year-old male soldier needs to complete forty pushups in two minutes and run two miles in less than 16:36 to achieve a passing score. A twenty-two-year-old female soldier needs to complete seventeen pushups in two minutes and run two miles in less than 19:36.
15. Early ACFT trials as of 2019 showed an overall 84 percent fail rate for women and a 30 percent fail rate for men, chiefly due to the leg tuck exercise. Men and women passed the other events at similar rates. Moore, "The ACFT and the Problems with the Military's Cult of Physical Fitness," www.military.com/daily-news/2019/12/16/acft-and-problems-militarys-cult-physical-fitness.html.
16. Mission: Readiness, Council for a Strong America, www.strongnation.org/missionreadiness; and "Citadel-Led Study Reveals Threat to U.S. Military Readiness Due to Unfit Recruits," January 11, 2018, https://today.citadel.edu/citadel-led-study-reveals-threat-to-u-s-military-readiness-due-to-unfit-recruits/. One of the three leading disqualifiers for service is obesity. See "Unfit to Serve: Obesity is Impacting National Security," March 2019, www.cdc.gov/physicalactivity/downloads/unfit-to-serve.pdf.
17. James E. Pilcher, "The Building of the Soldier," *United Service* 7, no. 4 (1892): 323.

BIBLIOGRAPHY

BIBLIOGRAPHIC AND METHODOLOGICAL NOTE

Capt. James Pilcher once contrasted the attention military historians paid to developments in weapons technology, the "apparatus of war," with how little attention they paid to the "most important portion of the military *matériel*, the soldier himself" (Pilcher, "The Building of the Soldier," *United Service* 7, no. 4 [1892]: 22). Although Pilcher wrote in 1892, he could find a modern audience, especially as a reactionary against the technological determinism and triumphalism of the 1980s and 1990s. (See Jeremy Black, *War and the Cultural Turn* [Cambridge: Polity, 2012], viii–ix.) This study follows Pilcher's lead and addresses the existing historiography in two ways. First, it fills a gap similar to the one Pilcher identified. Army leaders since the turn of the twentieth century have had only a limited ability to sculpt the contours and character of a battlefield, but they felt able to sculpt a man's contours and character. The means developed to do so reflected understandings of the battlefield on which bodies would be deployed for combat. Second, this study investigates the rich connectedness between making men, soldiers, and citizens, especially in an era of warfare that demanded mass conscription. Physical training links all three, just as its practice has linked the experiences of millions of soldiers over time.

Historians have rarely addressed physical fitness in war in a sustained way. When fitness does appear, it is usually as a vaguely conceived factor in the outcome of a campaign or battle, or perhaps in the performance of a particular officer. However, two recent works put physical fitness front and center. James Campbell's *"The Army Isn't All Work": Physical Culture in the Evolution of the British Army, 1860–1920* (Burlington, VT: Ashgate, 2012) examines sport and physical training practices in the British Army. Whitfield East's *A Historical Review and Analysis of Army Physical Readiness Training and Assessment* (Fort Leavenworth, KS: Combat Studies Institute Press, 2013) analyzes physical training practices throughout the US Army's entire history. These books highlight crucial differences in the development of British and American martial physical cultures. The former evolved in a relatively coherent, linear form and was "inextricably tied" to the story of reform and modernization in the late Victorian and Edwardian Army (p. 4). The latter evolved in a "sinusoidal pattern of surge and consolidation through multiple force mobilizations and times of peace" (p. 197). British physical culture (and Campbell's study) benefited from a central proponent agency, the Army Gymnastic Staff. East shows that the creative sources of American physical training practices were more diffuse. Campbell moves outside the military to consider the reciprocal impact of British civilian and military physical cultures on one another. East limits his analysis to practices within the US Army, which tends to mask the cultural aspects of those practices.

Historians of sport have been more sensitive to the larger implications of physical activity. Donald Mrozek (in *Sport and American Mentality, 1880–1910* [Knoxville: University of Tennessee Press, 1983], xiv–xx), for instance, considers military sport in the context of wider American culture. He perceives a rising moral tone in sport at the turn of the century based on sport's seeming social utility. In the military, this utility manifested in understanding the athletic field as a site for cultivating "primitive combativeness" and the "experience of victory" (p. 46). Sports helped shape character, and character improved combat effectiveness. This complex of beliefs is still alive and well in the Army's culture. Wanda *Wakefield* (in *Playing to Win: Sports and the American Military, 1898–1945* [Albany: State University of New York Press, 1997], 137–140) charts the US military's embrace of sports and finds interconnectedness between war, sports, nationalism, and masculinity. Steven Pope (in *Patriotic Games: Sporting Traditions in the American Imagination, 1876–1926* [New York: Oxford University Press, 1997], 15–17) goes further in arguing that the military helped forge an invented national sporting culture at the turn of the twentieth century. See also Pope, "An Army of Athletes: Playing Fields, Battlefields, and the American Military Sporting Experience, 1890–1920," *Journal of Military History* 59, no. 3 (1995): 435–437.

Sport was one means by which Army leaders sought to sculpt bodies, but too tight a focus on sport obscures the significance of systematic physical training and the contingency in its adoption and development. Like sport, physical training reflected the ways in which Army leaders imagined the battlefield of the future and the soldier's role on it. Like sport, physical training was a tool for shaping individuals. Unlike sport, physical training promised a more scientific, rational, and precise way of sculpting bodies in line with Progressive impulses, technological systems, and industrial engineering. Army leaders therefore invested more intention when crafting physical training systems than when enabling athletic competition. Army leaders thought and acted within a cultural context when developing those systems. Historians have filled out our understanding of that cultural context through studies of fitness and health trends, movements, and thought in America: James C. Whorton, *Crusaders for Fitness: The History of American Health Reformers; Harvey Green, Fit for America: Health, Fitness, Sport, and American Society* (New York: Pantheon, 1986); Kathryn Grover, *Fitness in American Culture: Images of Health, Sport, and the Body, 1830–1940* (Rochester: University of Massachusetts Press, 1989); Shelly McKenzie, *Getting Physical: The Rise of Fitness Culture in America* (Lawrence: University Press of Kansas, 2013). Yet rarely have they addressed the linkages between the battlefield and gymnasium. This study traces linkages, and demonstrates in doing so the two-way flow of ideas and practices between the military and civilian society.

Physical training connected more than the battlefield and gymnasium. Army leaders in the first half of the twentieth century claimed a role in three related projects: making men, making soldiers, and making citizens. Those projects converged on the male body. Army leaders saw potential in using physical training as a tool to sculpt people along ideal lines in all three categories. Scholars have addressed each project individually, and occasionally in pairs. A vast literature exists on manhood and masculinity at the turn of the twentieth century, and many of those works specifically address relationships between masculinity and war. Works on masculinity that have most influenced this study include E. Anthony Rotundo, *American Manhood: Transformations in Masculinity from the Revolution to the Modern Era* (New York: Basic, 1993); Gail Bederman, *Manliness & Civilization: A Cultural History of Gender and Race in the United States, 1880–1917* (Chicago: University of Chicago Press, 1994); Kristin L. Hoganson, *Fighting for American Manhood: How Gender Politics Provoked the Spanish-American and Philippine-American Wars* (New Haven, CT: Yale University Press, 1998); John F. Kasson, *Houdini, Tarzan, and the Perfect Man: The White Male Body and the Challenge of Modernity in America* (New York: Hill and Wang, 2001); Michael S. Kimmel, *The History of Men* (Albany: State University of New York Press, 2005); John Pettegrew, *Brutes in Suits: Male Sensibility in America, 1890–1920* (Baltimore: Johns Hopkins University Press, 2007); Elliott J. Gorn, *The Manly Art: Bare-Knuckle Prize Fighting in America*, updated ed. (Ithaca, NY: Cornell University Press, 2010). For a useful overview, see Robert A. Nye, "Western Masculinities in War and Peace," *American Historical Review* 112, no. 2 (2007).

Scholars have also thoroughly explored relationships between soldiering and citizenship, and their ability to generate militarization. For a concise introduction, see Eliot A. Cohen, *Citizens and Soldiers: The Dilemmas of Military Service* (Ithaca, NY: Cornell University Press, 1985). This study primarily engages the citizen/soldier relationship through arguments for Universal Military Training. On that topic, see also Michael J. Hogan, *A Cross of Iron: Harry S. Truman and the Origins of the National Security State, 1945–1954* (Cambridge: Cambridge University Press, 1998); John Sager, "Universal Military Training and the Struggle to Define American Identity during the Cold War." *Federal History Journal*, no. 5 (2013): 57–74; William A. Taylor, *Every Citizen a Soldier: The Campaign for Universal Military Training after World War II* (College Station: Texas A & M University Press, 2014).

Much less has been done to articulate just what it means to make an American soldier, or on the methods employed to do so. Christina Jarvis is an exception in that she links all three projects in her book *The Male Body at War*, though only between the late Depression and the end of World War II: Christina S. Jarvis, *The Male Body at War: American Masculinity during World War II* (DeKalb: Northern Illinois University Press, 2004). Historian Rachel Moran's recent book complements Jarvis's work on federal efforts to shape citizens' bodies, although it deals less with the soldier-making project. See Rachel Louise Moran, *Governing Bodies: American Politics and the Shaping of the Modern Physique* (Philadelphia: University of Pennsylvania Press, 2018). This study similarly links all three, but through analysis of a longer period that is grounded more in policy and practice than in discourse. Physical training hardened, toughened, and improved men's bodies. Army leaders intended it to do the same for the body politic. To understand that approach's varied effectiveness over time, we need to understand the fundamental connectedness between making men, soldiers, and citizens.

For all its potential, physical culture is a new and understudied pathway in military history. Exercise is ubiquitous in military life today, and even those unfamiliar with military matters tend to intuitively associate combat and physical fitness. Since the late 1960s, military historians have expanded the scope of military history while incorporating fresh methodologies in their investigations of subjects both old and new. See John Whiteclay Chambers, "The New Military History: Myth and Reality," *Journal of Military History* 55, no. 3 (1991). Though this movement's "new military history" moniker is of dubious value half a century later, the method of examining interfaces between war and society is still alive and well. See Robert Citino, "Military Histories Old and New: A Reintroduction," *American Historical Review* 112, no. 4 (2007). Centering physical culture as an object of historical analysis fits within this conceptual framework. A military's physical culture is itself an interface between war and society. Military physical cultures grow out of civilian society, but they are mediated through the demands of the battlefield as perceived by military leaders and institutions. By analyzing a military's exercise systems as cultural expressions, historians can find evidence of beliefs within a military organization and its society on topics as diverse as combat, soldier ideals, relationships between man and machine, race, gender, citizenship, and more. Because physical cultures also exist outside the military, the concept should likewise be of interest to the wider scholarly community. The ways people exercise, use their leisure time, and define fitness reveal other beliefs and values. Studying these issues, especially the interaction between civilian and military physical cultures, will enrich the ever-expanding literatures on weight and physique culture, biopolitics, food and eating history, state development, and federal policy-making, among others.

The amount of work left to be done on the Army's physical culture between 1885 and 1957 alone suggests the potential in physical culture studies. This project primarily examines the official culture created by elite producers, captured in articles, doctrine, and policy, and propagated downward with varying degrees of effectiveness throughout the rest of the organization. However, evidence suggests that the official culture did not penetrate everywhere and that not everyone bought in to it. Journal articles bemoaning an undue focus on field days at the turn of the century, reports of custom-made obstacle courses at Fort Belvoir in 1941, and complaints in the 1950s about the recreational tail wagging the conditioning dog after World War II all show that the Army's official physical culture had competition. Future work might explore these subcultures and their divergence from the official culture. Historians may also find an examination of the physical cultures developing in other branches of the armed forces during the same period productive, especially in their interactions with the Army's culture. Future work might also explore the lived experience of soldiers. Men toiling through the Army Dozen on parade grounds around the world may not have understood fitness or exercise in the same way as Koehler, Raycroft, Bank, McCloy, or other cultural producers. There is more of this story to be told beyond 1957 as well. For instance, future researchers might usefully apply the concept of physical cultures to learn more about the US Army's development and its relationship to American society in the latter half of the twentieth century.

Cultural history inspired this project's approach to exploring the creation and development of the US Army's physical training philosophies and practices in the first half of the twentieth century. Physical training policy, doctrine, and practice are loaded with meaning. They simultaneously represent and construct values, assumptions, and beliefs widely held within the Army. This draws on historian Joan Burbick's observation that "language about the body is saturated with culture": Joan Burbick, *Healing the Republic: The Language of Health and the Culture of Nationalism in Nineteenth-Century America* (Cambridge: Cambridge University Press, 1994), 3. Together, these values, assumptions, and beliefs constitute a physical culture, but they did not arise spontaneously. Rather, they emerged and developed in a specific context that was discursively constructed. Discourses about the decline of white manhood in the West, perfectible bodies, and the criticality of discipline, high morale, and resilience to victory in modern war created a perceived need for systematic exercise in the Army. These discourses also inclined the organization to embrace certain solutions, namely, Koehler's Turner-based system. Activities included in that system came laden with meaning, and in practicing them members of the Army layered atop the exercises new and different meanings. The actual practice of physical training inculcated assumptions, values, and beliefs in participants. This made physical training a deployable tool for shaping people in ways beyond bodily strength and endurance. This study therefore considers both the discourse on and the practice of physical training in the period because both contributed to the development of the Army's physical culture.

Influence vectors and agency also bear mentioning because of their relevance to this study's methodology. External sources of influence dominated the Army physical culture's initial period of development. They were resources upon which members of the Army drew that both enabled and constrained their imaginations. After the core of the Army's systematic training-based physical culture coalesced, it also became a resource upon which individuals and organizations external to the Army could draw. Influence eventually moved in both directions. This study is sensitive to the changing magnitude and direction of influence as it relates to exercise and its meanings. Also, individual actors decisively shaped the Army physical culture's character and path of development at various inflection points. This was not an abstract, amorphous culture that emerged solely from the accretion of popular thought and practice. The tremendous influence of a select few people such as Herman Koehler, Joseph Raycroft, and Charles McCloy must therefore be acknowledged.

Because physical training philosophy and practice each influence the other, two overlapping types of sources provided the basis for research. First were actual Army physical training practices. The Army first published standardized, universal training guidance in 1914. Before that, many related systems published by several officers were in use. After 1914, doctrine began standardizing unit-training practices. Published manuals supplemented by memoirs and articles in newspapers, periodicals, and professional journals enable a close study of the means employed to sculpt bodies. Except for East's monograph on Army physical readiness training, no focused study of these practices exists. Second, this study accesses the philosophy underlying and bound up in training practices through the forums in which cultural producers proposed and debated practices. Professional journals are especially useful here. Within the military, key journals include the *Journal of the Military Service Institute* and the *Infantry Journal* (later *Army*). Journals serving the combat arms, especially the infantry, and the medical corps proved most sensitive to physical training issues. Outside the military, the *American Physical Education Review* (1896–1929) and its successors, the *Journal of Health and Physical Education* (1930–1948) and the *Journal of the American Association for Health, Physical Education, and Recreation* (1949–1954), reveal discussions among physical educators. These professionals are important because they influenced the Army's philosophies and practices, sometimes through direct involvement, but often by setting the intellectual and cultural context for military practice. Physical educators also transmitted Army ideas and systems into wider American society, sometimes as promoters, and sometimes as opponents.

While many of these sources are published, unpublished sources chiefly reside in three locations: the United States Military Academy (USMA), Princeton University's library, and the National Archives. The USMA and its Department of Physical Education exerted an enormous influence on physical training philosophy and practice throughout most of the period under study. Historians have made little use of the Academy's files on physical training, except in exploring sport at the USMA. Princeton University's library holds the papers of Dr. Joseph Raycroft, a Princeton faculty member and leader in the Commission on Training Camp Activities who played a deeply influential role in Army physical training during and after World War I. The National Archives hold files pertaining to wartime practices, physical training schools, Army boards responsible for writing and approving physical training policies, and extramilitary spaces such as the Citizens' Military Training Camps, the Victory Corps, the post–World War II Universal Military Training initiative, and President Eisenhower's President's Council on Youth Fitness.

Pilcher's implied pathway for research remains valid and wide open for continued study by historians. Alternative and subcultures deserve investigation. The lived experience of the official physical culture awaits exploration. Application of this study's methodology to other times and places will yield insights into military culture writ large, interactions between militaries and societies, changing gender norms, and more. The practical relevance of these studies should also be obvious, given current concerns in the United States and elsewhere over the military preparedness of citizenries and the gender integration of combat units. If this study points the way for others, then it has achieved success.

PRIMARY SOURCES

Archives

National Archives at College Park, MD

Record Group 165: Records of the War Department General and Special Staffs
Record Group 215: Records of the Community War Services
Record Group 225: Joint Boards and Committees
Record Group 337: HQ Army Ground Forces
Record Group 546: Records of the United States Continental Army Command

Department of Rare Books and Special Collections, Princeton University Library, Princeton, NJ

Joseph Edward Raycroft Papers

Citadel Museum and Archives, Charleston, SC

Lt. Gen. John W. O'Daniel Papers

Newspapers and Magazines

Chicago Daily Tribune
The Independent
New York Times
New York Tribune

The Sporting Goods Dealer
Sports Illustrated
The Washington Post

Unpublished

West Point, NY, US Military Academy Library, Special Collections and Archives Division, Record Group 404.

Published

Allen, Edward Frank. *Keeping Our Fighters Fit for War and After*. Edited by Raymond B. Fosdick. New York: Century, 1918.

Allen, R. H. "Athletics and the Infantry Spirit." *Infantry Journal* 28, no. 1 (1926): 24–26.

Andrus, Ethel Percy. "High School Victory Corps." *Journal of Educational Sociology* 16, no. 4 (1942): 231–240.

Annual Report of the Board of Visitors to the United States Military Academy for the Year 1881. Washington, DC: Government Printing Office, 1881.

"The Army Builds Men." *Infantry Journal* 18, no. 1 (1921): 80–81.

Army War College. *Infantry Training*. Washington, DC: Government Printing Office, 1917.

———. *Notes on Bayonet Training Compiled from Foreign Reports*. Washington, DC: Government Printing Office, 1917.

Ashwood, Avery. "Building Brawn." *Infantry Journal* 53, no. 2 (1943): 47–50.

Atkinson, Stewart. "What Holds Back the Victory Corps?" *Clearing House* 18, no. 3 (1943): 137–139.

Balck, Wilhelm. *Tactics*. Translated by Walter Krueger. 4th ed. Vol. 1. Fort Leavenworth, KS: US Cavalry Association, 1911.

Bank, Theodore P. "The Army Physical Conditioning Program." *Journal of Health and Physical Education* 14, no. 4 (1943): 195–197, 238–240.

Barrows, Isabel C., ed. *Physical Training: A Full Report of the Papers and Discussions of the Conference Held in Boston in November, 1889*. Boston: Press of George H. Ellis, 1890.

Beard, George M. *American Nervousness: Its Causes and Consequences*. New York: Putnam, 1881.

Becke, Archibald F. *An Introduction to the History of Tactics, 1740–1905*. London: Hugh Rees, 1909.

Besson, Frank S. "Physical Training in the Army." *Journal of the Military Service Institution of the United States* 55 (1914): 37–51.

Beyer, Henry G. "Military Physical Training." In *Proceedings of the Seventh Annual Meeting of the Association of Military Surgeons of the United States*, edited by James E. Pilcher, 265–310. Columbus: Berlin Printing, 1897.

Bjornstad, A. W. "Athletic Policy of Infantry School." *Infantry Journal* 26, no. 1 (1925): 44–46.

Bolin, Jakob. *What Is Gymnastics?* New York: Willett, 1902.

Bond, P. S. *Your Boy & the Other in Universal Training: The Nation's School for Citizenship*. Edited by Charles Fletcher Martin. Washington, DC: Press of the Military Engineer, 1920.

Bond, P. S., O. O. Ellis, E. B. Garey, and T. L. McMurray. *The Red, White and Blue Manual: A Text Book for the Citizens' Military Training Camp*. Vol. 1, *Red Course*. Baltimore, MD: Johns Hopkins Press, 1921.

Braun, G. J. "Physical Training at Infantry School." *Infantry Journal* 25, no. 2 (1924).

Britt, Albert. "From Playing Field to Battle Field." *Outing* 73 (1919).

Browne, A. D. "Physical Education in the Light of the Present National Situation." *American Physical Education Review* 24, no. 2 (1919): 69–74.

Bullard, Robert L., and H. S. Hawkins. "Athletics in the Army." *Journal of the Military Service Institution of the United States* 37 (1905): 399–409.

Butts, Edmund L. "Athletic Training." *Infantry Journal* 2, no. 1 (1905): 3–25.

———. *Manual of Physical Drill, United States Army*. New York: D. Appleton, 1900.

———. "Military Athletics." *Harper's Weekly*, no. 41 (January 9, 1897): 39–41.

———. "Physical Training of the American Soldier." *Journal of the Military Service Institution of the United States* 61, no. 75 (1895): 499–512.

———. "Soldierly Bearing, Health and Athletics." *Outing*, March 1904, 707.

Camp, Walter. *Keeping Fit All the Way: How to Obtain and Maintain Health, Strength, and Efficiency*. New York: Harper, 1919. Kindle.

Carter, W. H. "A Meet in the Philippines: A Rational Plan of Athletic Training." *Journal of the Military Service Institution of the United States* 36, no. 135 (1905): 455–466.

Cassidy, Rosalind, and Hilda Clute Kozman. "Trends in State Wartime Physical Fitness Programs." *Journal of Health and Physical Education* 14, no. 7 (1943): 357, 92–93.

Coteau, Marc Bellin du. "The Physical Education of the Fighting Man: Method in Use in the National Military School of St. Cyr, France." *American Physical Education Review* 22, no. 9 (1917): 521–524.

Crampton, Charles Ward. *Fighting Fitness: A Premilitary Training Guide*. New York: McGraw-Hill, 1944.

Davis, Bowers. "A System for Army Athletics." *Infantry Journal* 3, no. 2 (1906): 79–83.

D'Eliscu, Francois. *How to Prepare for Military Fitness*. New York: W. W. Norton, 1943.

Department of the Army. *Army Regulations 600-160: Maintenance of Physical Fitness and Detecting and Correcting Physical Abnormalities among Officers.* Washington, DC: US Government Printing Office, 1955.

———. *Field Manual 21-20: Physical Training.* Washington, DC: US Government Printing Office, 1950.

———. *Field Manual 21-20: Physical Training.* Washington, DC: US Government Printing Office, 1957.

———. *Field Manual 21-20: Physical Fitness Training.* Washington, DC: Headquarters, Department of the Army, 1998.

———. *Technical Manual 21-200: Physical Conditioning.* Washington, DC: US Government Printing Office, 1957.

Donworth, A. B. "Gymnasium Training in the Army." *Journal of the Military Service Institution of the United States* 21 (1897): 508–515.

Dougherty, J. H. *Indian Clubs and Dumb Bells.* New York: American Sports, 1911.

Drain, J. C. "New Physical and Bayonet Training Course." *Infantry Journal* 16, no. 6 (1919): 474–484.

Elliott, F. Haws. *Trench Fighting.* Boston, MA: Houghton Mifflin, 1917.

Executive Office of the Committee on Physical Fitness. "Civilian Physical Fitness." *Journal of Health and Physical Education* 14, no. 10 (1943): 518–519, 53–54.

"Extracts from Occasional Letters from Physical Directors in Army Camps to Dr. George J. Fisher, Director, War Work Council, Young Men's Christian Association." *American Physical Education Review* 22, no. 9 (1917): 558–566.

Farrow, Edward Samuel. *A Military System of Gymnastic Exercises and a System of Swimming.* New York: Metropolitan, 1881.

Fisher, George J. "Physical Training in the Army." *American Physical Education Review* 23, no. 2 (1918): 65–76.

———. "Points of Emphasis in a Post-War Program of Physical Training." *American Physical Education Review* 24, no. 3 (1919): 125–136.

Fleet, H. W. "Citizens' Military Training Camps." *Infantry Journal* 32, no. 5 (1928): 492–499.

Fosdick, Raymond B. "The Commission on Training Camp Activities." *Proceedings of the Academy of Political Science in the City of New York* 7, no. 4 (1918): 163–170.

Francis, R. J. "Toward a Philosophy of Physical Education." *Journal of Health and Physical Education* 10, no. 4 (1939): 216–217, 58–59.

Fritzsche, Carl F. "Physical Fitness—a Must!" *Army Information Digest* 10, no. 7 (1955): 41–43.

Garey, Enoch B. *Manual of Physical Drill.* Kansas City: Franklin Hudson, 1911.

Gentz, T. "Gymnastics as a Branch of Military Education." *Army and Navy Journal* 9, no. 35 (1872): 562–565.

Greenleaf, Charles R. "Physical Training in the U.S. Army." In *Proceedings of the American Association for the Advancement of Physical Education at Its Sixth Annual Meeting*, 58–80. Ithaca: Andrus & Church, 1891.

Gulick, Luther H. "Physical Fitness in the Fighting Armies." *American Physical Education Review* 23, no. 6 (1918): 341–354.

Hagedorn, Hermann. *That Human Being, Leonard Wood*. New York: Harcourt, Brace, and Howe, 1920.

Hall, G. Stanley. "Feminization in School and Home." *World's Work* 16 (1908): 10237–10244.

———. "Some Relations between Physical and Mental Training." In *Report of the Ninth Annual Meeting of the American Association for the Advancement of Physical Education*, 30–37. New Haven, CT: Press of Clarence H. Ryder, 1894.

Harrison, Roy S. *Physical Training and Games as Used in the Canadian Forces*. New York: US Marine Corps Mobilization Bureau, 1918.

Hartwell, Edward Mussey. "The Nature of Physical Training, and the Best Means of Securing Its Ends." In *Physical Training: A Full Report of the Papers and Discussions of the Conference Held in Boston in November, 1889*, edited by Isabel C. Barrows, 5–22. Boston: Press of George H. Ellis, 1890.

———. "Physical Training in American Colleges and Universities." In *Circulars of Information of the Bureau of Education*. Washington, DC: Bureau of Education, 1886.

———. *Physical Training Treated from American and European Points of View*. Boston: G. H. Ellis, 1890.

"Health of the Youth of the Nation (Editorial)." *Journal of American Medical Association* 114, no. 5 (1940): 414–415.

Henderson, G. F. R. *The Science of War: A Collection of Essays and Lectures, 1891–1903*. London: Longmans, Green, 1906.

Hershey, Lewis B., and Thomas M. Watlington. "The Man Selected for Service." *Infantry Journal* 47, no. 6 (1940): 530–535.

High-School Victory Corps, Pamphlet Number 1. Washington, DC: US Government Printing Office, 1942.

Hinman, George Wheeler. "Citizens Military Training Camps." *Infantry Journal* 18, no. 6 (1921): 579–583.

Hobbs, Percy. "Bayonet Fighting and Physical Training." *Infantry Journal* 14, no. 2 (1917): 79–85.

Hughes, William L. "The Civilian Defense Physical Fitness Program." *Journal of Health and Physical Education* 13, no. 2 (1942): 71–73, 106–108.

Jack, Harold K. "A Suggested Plan for Military Service." *Journal of Health and Physical Education* 19, no. 4 (1945): 181.

Jones, Hiram A. "Report on National Fitness: A Program through Schools and Colleges." *Journal of Health and Physical Education* 13, no. 3 (1942): 133–135, 93–95.

———. "The Revised Preparedness Bill: The Status of the Physical Preparedness Legislation." *Journal of Health and Physical Education* 12, no. 2 (1941): 67–73, 117, 19.

Kahn, Ely J. *Army Life*. Washington, DC: Infantry Journal, 1943.

Kelly, John B. "Are We Becoming a Nation of Weaklings?" *American Magazine* 161 (March 1956).

Kilbourne, Henry S. "The Physical Proportions of the American Soldier." In *Proceedings of the Seventh Annual Meeting of the Association of Military Surgeons of the United States*, edited by James E. Pilcher, 328–39. Columbus: Berlin, 1897.

King, Edward L. "Athletics for the Physical Betterment of the Enlisted Men in the Army." *Outing*, January 1902, 432.

Koehler, Herman J. "Competitive Athletics at the United States Military Academy." *Pointer* (September 29, 1923): 8–11.

———. "General Remarks on Physical Training in the Service." *Infantry Journal* 3, no. 4 (1907): 103–121.

———. *Koehler's West Point Manual of Disciplinary Physical Training*. New York: E. P. Dutton, 1919.

———. "Letter from Captain Herman J. Koehler." *American Physical Education Review* 21, no. 3 (1916): 148–152.

———. *Manual of Calisthenic Exercises*. Washington, DC: Government Printing Office, 1892.

———. *Manual of Gymnastic Exercises: Prepared for Use in Service Gymnasiums*. Washington, DC: Government Printing Office, 1904.

———. "Military Drill Vs. Gymnastics." *Mind and Body* 3, no. 28 (1896): 79–80.

———. "Physical Training in the Army." *Infantry Journal* 1, no. 1 (1904): 8–13.

———. "The Physical Training of Cadets, 1802–1902." In *The Centennial of the United States Military Academy at West Point, New York, 1802–1902*, 893–908. Washington, DC: Government Printing Office, 1904.

———. *The Theory and Practice of Athletics at the Military Academy*. West Point, NY: Military Academy Printing Office, 1909.

Kulp, John Stewart. "What to Avoid in Army Athletics." In *Proceedings of the Seventh Annual Meeting of the Association of Military Surgeons of the United States*, edited by James E. Pilcher, 311–320. Columbus: Berlin, 1897.

Lamb, A. S. "On Physical Education." *Canadian Medical Association Journal* 16, no. 1 (1926): 67–69.

Leonard, Fred Eugene. *Pioneers of Modern Physical Training*. New York: Association Press, 1919.

Lockhart, Albert E. "Overweight in Grade." *Infantry School Quarterly* 46, no. 3 (1956): 75–79.

Love, Albert G., and Charles B. Davenport. *Defects Found in Drafted Men*. Washington, DC: Government Printing Office, 1920.

———. "Defects Found in Drafted Men." *Scientific Monthly* 10, no. 1 (1920): 5–25.

———. "Defects Found in Drafted Men, II." *Scientific Monthly* 10, no. 2 (1920): 125–141.

MacDonald, Charles B. "The Qualities of a Soldier." *Army Information Digest* 5, no. 12 (1950): 7–13.

Maroney, F. W. "Physical Education Looks Ahead." *Journal of Health and Physical Education* 5, no. 8 (1933).

Maude, Frederic N. *Notes on the Evolution of Infantry Tactics*. London: William Clowes and Sons, 1905.

McClellan, George B. *Report of the Secretary of War Communicating the Report of Captain George B. McClellan, One of the Officers Sent to the Seat of War in Europe in 1855 and 1856*. Washington, DC: A.O.P. Nicholson, 1857.

McCurdy, James Huff. *The Objectives of the American Physical Education Association*. Springfield, MA: American Physical Education Association, 1927.

———. "Physical Efficiency as a National Asset." *American Physical Education Review* 25, no. 3 (1920): 101–106.

McEntee, James J. *Now They Are Men: The Story of the CCC*. Washington, DC: National Home Library Foundation, 1940.

McNeely, Simon A. "Physical Fitness in the Pentomic Age." *Journal of Health-Physical Education-Recreation* 29, no. 6 (1958): 21–23, 30.

Merriam, Charles Edward. *The Making of Citizens: A Comparative Study of Methods of Civic Training*. Chicago: University of Chicago Press, 1931.

"Military Training in Foreign Countries." *American Physical Education Review* 22, no. 8 (1917): 508–509.

Morrow, F. J. "Military Preparedness." *American Physical Education Review* 24, no. 5 (1919): 80–81.

Mourin, Charles F. "Postwar Physical Education or Military Training?" *Journal of Health and Physical Education* 16, no. 4 (1945): 180, 220, 22.

Nash, Jay B. "Is Compulsory Military Training the Answer? No!" *Journal of Health and Physical Education* 16, no. 2 (1945): 65, 94.

"National Physical Fitness Program: A Statement by the Board of Directors." *Journal of Health and Physical Education* 12, no. 10 (1941): 547–548.

"The Need in the Army and Navy." *American Physical Education Review* 23, no. 4 (1918): 251.

Niles, Donna I. "Physical Fitness and the W.A.C." *Journal of Health and Physical Education* 14, no. 8 (1943): 408–411, 48–50.

Palmer, Guy G. "Physical Culture and Training in the Army." *Journal of the United States Infantry Association* 2, no. 4 (1906): 119–126.

Paxson, Frederic L. "The Rise of Sport." *Mississippi Valley Historical Review* 4, no. 2 (1917): 143–168.

Perrott, G. St. J. "Selective Service Rejection Statistics and Some of Their Implications." *American Journal of Public Health* 36 (April 1946): 336–342.

Photographs of Gymnastic Apparatus in United States Army Post Plattsburg, N.Y.: Arranged to List and Plans of Lieut. Herman J. Koehler, U.S.A. Providence, RI: Narragansett Machine, 1903.

"Physical and Bayonet Training (Editorial)." *Infantry Journal* 16, no. 6 (1919): 515–516.

"Physical Fitness." *Military Engineer* 14, no. 75 (1922): 163–164.

Physical Fitness through Physical Education. Washington, DC: US Government Printing Office, 1942.

Picq, Charles Ardant du. *Battle Studies: Ancient and Modern Battle.* Translated by John N. Greely and Robert C. Cotton. 8th ed. New York: Macmillan, 1921.

Pilcher, James E. "The Building of the Soldier." *United Service* 7, no. 4 (1892): 321–337.

———. "The Place of Physical Training in the Military Service." In *The Proceedings of the Fourth Annual Meeting of the Association of Military Surgeons of the United States*, 170–78. St. Louis, MO: Suxton & Skinner Stationary, 1894.

"Proceedings of the Society of Directors of Physical Education in Colleges." *American Physical Education Review* 22, no. 4 (1917): 189–197.

Public Relations Office. "The Physical Training Program of the W.A.A.C." *Journal of Health and Physical Education* 14, no. 4 (1943): 209, 40–41.

Raycroft, Joseph E. "The Educational Value of Athletics in Schools and Colleges." *School and Society* 3, no. 61 (1915): 295–300.

———. *Mass Physical Training for Use in the Army and the Reserve Officers' Training Corps.* Washington, DC: United States Infantry Association, 1920.

———. "Safeguarding the Health of College Students." *Science* 39, no. 1011 (1914): 707–711.

———. "Training Camp Activities." *American Physical Education Review* 23, no. 3 (1918): 143–150.

Reilly, James E., and Robert M. Garrison. "Our Physical Unfitness." *Infantry* 49, no. 2 (1959): 20–22.

Reinhardt, G. C., and W. R. Kintner. *Atomic Weapons in Land Combat.* 2nd ed. Harrisburg: Military Service Publishing, 1954.

Report of the Board of Visitors to the United States Military Academy for the Year 1889. Washington, DC: Government Printing Office, 1889.

Rogers, James Edward. "Trends in Physical Education." *Journal of Health and Physical Education* 2, no. 8 (1931): 18–19, 47.

Roosevelt, Theodore. *The Strenuous Life: Essays and Addresses.* New York: Century, 1903.

Rowntree, Leonard G. "National Program for Physical Fitness." *Journal of American Medical Association* 125, no. 12 (1944): 821–827.

Sargent, Dudley A. "Taking Account of Stock." *American Physical Education Review* 27, no. 2 (1922): 47–50.

Select Committee on Expenditures in the War Department, House of Representatives. *War Expenditures: Hearings before the Select Committee on Expenditures in the War Department.* Washington, DC: Government Printing Office, 1919.

Sharpe, A. C. "Comment & Criticism: Athletics in the Army." *Journal of the Military Service Institution of the United States* 38, no. 141 (1906): 538–540.

Shaw, John H. "American Physical Fitness." *Phi Delta Kappan* 24, no. 7 (1942): 284–285.

Sherff, Wilhelm Karl Friedrich Gustav von. *The New Tactics of Infantry.* Translated by Lumley Graham. Leavenworth, KS: C. J. Smith, 1891.

Small, Willard S. "The Nation's Need of Physical Education." *American Journal of Public Health* 8, no. 11 (1918): 830–832.

Smart, Robert. "The Physical Development of the Recruit." In *Proceedings of the Association of Military Surgeons of the United States at Its Tenth Annual Meeting,* 572–576. Carlisle, PA: Association of Military Surgeons, 1901.

"Steeplechase for Soldiers." *Infantry Journal* 49, no. 1 (1941): 46–47.

Steinhaus, Arthur H., Alma M. Hawkins, Charles D. Giauque, and Edward C. Thomas. *How to Keep Fit and Like It: A Manual for Civilians and a Plan for a Community Approach to Physical Fitness.* Chicago: Consolidated Book, 1943.

Stewart, Merch B. *The Physical Development of the Infantry Soldier.* Menasha, WI: George Banta, 1913.

———. "A Thirty-Minute Talk: Military Discipline." *Infantry Journal* 16, no. 6 (1919): 491–499.

Storey, Thomas A. "War-Time Revelations in Physical Education." *American Physical Education Review* 25, no. 2 (1920): 47–52.

Sundwall, John. "Health Education and Activities in Colleges and Universities." *American Physical Education Review* 26, no. 4 (1921): 164–171.

Tupes, Herschel. "Annual Athletic and Gymnastic Tests for the Army." *Infantry Journal* 2, no. 2 (1905): 103–109.

Turner, Frederick Jackson. *The Frontier in American History.* New York: Henry Holt, 1920.

United States Army Infantry School. *Infantry Instructors' Conference Report, 16–21 June 1952.* Fort Benning, GA: Infantry School, 1952.

———. *Infantry Instructors' Conference Report, 17–21 June 1957.* Fort Benning, GA: Infantry School, 1957.

———. *Physical Fitness Seminar Report*. Fort Benning, GA: United States Army Infantry School, 1958.

———. *Staff Study: Institute of Physical Fitness*. Fort Benning, GA: United States Army, 1970.

United States Military Academy. *Annual Report of the Superintendent*. West Point, NY: United States Military Academy Press, 1922.

Upton, L. S. "Physical Training in the Army." *Infantry Journal* 2, no. 2 (1905): 110–115.

US Office of Education Committee on Wartime Physical Fitness for Colleges and Universities. *Handbook on Physical Fitness for Students in Colleges and Universities*. Washington, DC: US Government Printing Office, 1943.

Waldron, William H. *Army Physical Training*. New York: H. Holt, 1919.

War Department. *Army Regulations No. 850–120: Athletics*. Washington, DC: War Department, 1928.

———. *Army Training Develops Essentials of Success in Life*. Washington, DC: Department of the Adjutant General Publications, 1924.

———. *Basic Field Manual*. Vol. 1, chap. 4, *Physical Training*. Washington, DC: Government Printing Office, 1936.

———. *Commission on Training Camp Activities*. Washington, DC: Government Printing Office, 1917.

———. *Field Manual 21-20: Basic Field Manual—Physical Training*. Washington, DC: Government Printing Office, 1941.

———. *Field Manual 21-20: Physical Training*. Washington, DC: US Government Printing Office, 1946.

———. *Field Manual 28-105: The Special Service Company*. Washington, DC: United States Government Printing Office, 1944.

———. *General Order, No. 44*. Washington, DC: War Department, March 1, 1906.

———. *Manual of Physical Training for Use in the United States Army*. New York: Military Publishing, 1914.

———. *Special Regulations, No. 23: Field Physical Training of the Soldier*. Washington, DC: Government Printing Office, 1917.

———. *Technical Manual 21-205: Special Service Officer*. Washington, DC: United States Government Printing Office, 1942.

———. *Training Regulations No. 115-5: Physical Training*. Washington, DC: Government Printing Office, 1928.

———. *W.A.C. Field Manual: Physical Training*. Washington, DC: United States Government Printing Office, 1943.

———. *War Department Pamphlet No. 21-9: Physical Conditioning*. Washington, DC: Government Printing Office, 1944.

———. *War Department Pamphlet 35–3: WAC Life*. Washington, DC: United States Government Printing Office, 1943.

War Department Commission on Training Camp Activities. *Outline of Plan for Military Training in Public Schools of the United States*. Washington, DC: Government Printing Office, 1916.

———. *Rules for Boxing*. Washington, DC: Government Printing Office, 1918.

War Plans Division. *Training Circular No. 19: Organization of Physical and Bayonet Training*. Washington, DC: War Department, 1918.

"What Combat Veterans Think of Army Training." *What the Soldier Thinks*, no. 4 (March 1944): 1–5.

White, E. B. "Victory Corps." *Bulletin of the American Association of University Professors (1915–1955)* 29, no. 2 (1943): 299–301.

Wood, Thomas D. "Schools Hold Health Key for All Future Citizens." *Journal of Health and Physical Education* 1, no. 3 (1930): 3–5, 60.

SECONDARY SOURCES

Adams, Mark. *Mr. America: How Muscular Millionaire Bernarr Macfadden Transformed the Nation through Sex, Salad, and the Ultimate Starvation Diet*. New York: Harper, 2009.

Ambrose, Stephen E. *Duty, Honor, Country: A History of West Point*. Baltimore, MD: Johns Hopkins University Press, 1999.

Baker, Anni. "The Abolition of the U.S. Army Canteen, 1898–1914." *Journal of Military History* 80, no. 3 (2016): 697–724.

Barrow, Harold M., and Janie P. Brown. *Man and Movement: Principles of Physical Education*. 4th ed. Philadelphia: Lea & Febiger, 1988.

Baumer, William H. *West Point: Molder of Men*. New York: D. Appleton-Century, 1942.

Becquemont, Daniel. "Social Darwinism: From Reality to Myth and from Myth to Reality." *Studies in History and Philosophy of Science* 42, no. 1 (2011): 12–19.

Bederman, Gail. *Manliness & Civilization: A Cultural History of Gender and Race in the United States, 1880–1917*. Chicago: University of Chicago Press, 1995.

Berrett, Jesse. "Feeding the Organization Man: Diet and Masculinity in Postwar America." *Journal of Social History* 30, no. 4 (1997): 805–825.

Betros, Lance. *Carved from Granite: West Point since 1902*. College Station: Texas A & M University Press, 2012.

Black, Jeremy. *War and the Cultural Turn*. Cambridge: Polity, 2012.

Bourke, Joanna. *Dismembering the Male: Men's Bodies, Britain and the Great War*. Chicago: University of Chicago Press, 1996.

Bowen, William G., and James Lawrence Schulman. *The Game of Life: College Sports and Educational Values.* Princeton, NJ: Princeton University Press, 2001.

Bowers, Matthew T., and Thomas M. Hunt. "The President's Council on Physical Fitness and the Systematisation of Children's Play in America." *International Journal of the History of Sport* 28, no. 11 (2011): 1496–1511.

Bristow, Nancy K. *Making Men Moral: Social Engineering during the Great War.* New York: New York University Press, 1996.

Brosius, George. *Fifty Years Devoted to the Cause of Physical Culture, 1864–1914.* Milwaukee, WI: Germania, 1914.

Budd, Michael Anton. *The Sculpture Machine: Physical Culture and Body Politics in the Age of Empire.* New York: New York University Press, 1997.

Burbick, Joan. *Healing the Republic: The Language of Health and the Culture of Nationalism in Nineteenth-Century America.* Cambridge: Cambridge University Press, 1994.

Campbell, D'Ann. "Women in Combat: The World War II Experience in the United States, Great Britain, Germany, and the Soviet Union." *Journal of Military History* 57 (April 1993): 301–323.

Campbell, James D. *"The Army Isn't All Work": Physical Culture in the Evolution of the British Army, 1860–1920.* Burlington, VT: Ashgate, 2012.

Cavallo, Dominick. *Muscles and Morals: Organized Playgrounds and Urban Reform, 1880–1920.* Philadelphia: University of Pennsylvania Press, 1981.

Chambers, John Whiteclay. "Conscripting for Colossus: The Progressive Era and the Origin of the Modern Military Draft in the United States in World War I." In *The Military in America from the Colonial Era to the Present,* edited by Peter Karsten, 275–296. New York: Free Press, 1980.

———. "The New Military History: Myth and Reality." *Journal of Military History* 55, no. 3 (1991): 395–406.

Chapman, David L. *Sandow the Magnificent: Eugen Sandow and the Beginnings of Bodybuilding.* Urbana: University of Illinois Press, 1994.

Charlston, Jeffery Allen. "Disorganized and Quasi-Official but Eventually Successful: Sport in the U.S. Military, 1814–1914." *International Journal of the History of Sport* 19, no. 4 (2002): 70–88.

———. "From Indifference to Obsession: Origins of Athletic Programs in the United States Military, 1865–1935." PhD diss., George Washington University, 2000.

Citino, Robert. "Military Histories Old and New: A Reintroduction." *American Historical Review* 112, no. 4 (2007): 1070–1090.

———. *Quest for Decisive Victory: From Stalemate to Blitzkrieg in Europe, 1899–1940.* Lawrence: University Press of Kansas, 2002.

Clausewitz, Carl von. *On War.* Translated by Michael Howard and Peter Paret. Indexed ed. Princeton, NJ: Princeton University Press, 1989.

Clifford, John Garry. *The Citizen Soldiers: The Plattsburg Training Camp Movement, 1913–1920.* Lexington: University Press of Kentucky, 1972.

Coffman, Edward M. *The Old Army: A Portrait of the American Army in Peacetime, 1784–1898.* New York: Oxford University Press, 1986.

Cohen, Eliot A. *Citizens and Soldiers: The Dilemmas of Military Service.* Ithaca, NY: Cornell University Press, 1985.

———. *The Regulars: The American Army, 1898–1941.* Cambridge: Belknap Press of Harvard University Press, 2004.

Cuordileone, Kyle A. *Manhood and American Political Culture in the Cold War.* New York: Routledge, 2005.

———. "'Politics in an Age of Anxiety': Cold War Political Culture and the Crisis in American Masculinity, 1949–1960." *Journal of American History* 87, no. 2 (2000): 515–545.

Cutler, Elliott C. "Lt. Col. Herman J. Koehler, Master of the Sword: An Account of His Service and Influence." *Assembly* 39, no. 3 (1980): 20–23, 48–50.

Degen, Robert. "The Evolution of Physical Education at the United States Military Academy." Master's thesis, University of Wisconsin, 1966.

Degler, Carl N. *In Search of Human Nature: The Decline and Revival of Darwinism in American Social Thought.* New York: Oxford University Press, 1991.

Director of the Service, Supply, and Procurement Division. *Logistics in World War II: Final Report of the Army Service Forces.* Washington, DC: Center of Military History, 1993 (originally published 1948).

East, Whitfield B. *A Historical Review and Analysis of Army Physical Readiness Training and Assessment.* Fort Leavenworth, KS: Combat Studies Institute Press, 2013.

Echevarria, Antulio J. "The 'Cult of the Offensive' Revisited: Confronting Technological Change before the Great War." *Journal of Strategic Studies* 25, no. 1 (2002): 199–214.

Edwards, William H. *Football Days: Memories of the Game and of the Men behind the Ball.* New York: Moffat, Yard, 1916.

Ellis, John. *Sharp End: The Fighting Man in World War II.* New York: Scribner's, 1980.

English, Eleanor B. "Charles H. Mccloy: The Research Professor of Physical Education." *Journal of Physical Education, Recreation & Dance* 54, no. 4 (1983): 16–18.

English, John A. *On Infantry.* Rev. ed. Westport, CT: Praeger, 1994.

Ernst, Robert. *Weakness Is a Crime: The Life of Bernarr Macfadden.* Garden City, NY: Syracuse University Press, 1991.

Faulkner, Richard S. *The School of Hard Knocks: Combat Leadership in the American Expeditionary Forces.* College Station: Texas A & M University Press, 2012.

Faulks, Keith. *Citizenship*. New York: Routledge, 2000.

Fielding, Lawrence W. "War and Trifles: Sport in the Shadows of Civil War Army Life." *Journal of Sport History* 4, no. 2 (Summer 1977): 151–168.

Flynn, George Q. *The Draft, 1940–1973*. Lawrence: University Press of Kansas, 1993.

Forth, Christopher E. *Masculinity in the Modern West: Gender, Civilization and the Body*. New York: Palgrave Macmillan, 2008.

———. "Surviving Our Paradoxes? Masculinity, Modernity, and the Body." *Culture, Society, and Masculinities* 1, no. 1 (Spring 2009): 6–32.

Foster, William B., Ida Levin Hellman, Douglas Hesford, and Darrell G. McPherson. *Physical Standards in World War II*. Washington, DC: Office of the Surgeon General, Department of the Army, 1967.

Fussell, Paul. *Wartime: Understanding and Behavior in the Second World War*. New York: Oxford University Press, 1988.

Gat, Azar. *The Development of Military Thought: The Nineteenth Century*. Oxford: Clarendon, 1992.

Gibbs, Marilyn J., and Claudius W. Griffin. "Physical Fitness." In *Handbook of American Popular Culture*, edited by M. Thomas Inge, vol. 2, 925–955. New York: Greenwood, 1989.

Gilbert, James. *A Cycle of Outrage: America's Reaction to the Juvenile Delinquent in the 1950s*. New York: Oxford University Press, 1986.

———. *Men in the Middle: Searching for Masculinity in the 1950s*. Chicago: University of Chicago Press, 2005.

Gilmore, Russell. "'The New Courage': Rifles and Soldier Individualism, 1876–1918." *Military Affairs* 40 (October 1976): 97–102.

Ginzberg, Eli, James K. Anderson, Sol Ginsburg, and John L. Herma. *The Ineffective Soldier: Lessons for Management and the Nation—the Lost Divisions*. New York: Columbia University Press, 1959.

Gorn, Elliott J. *The Manly Art: Bare-Knuckle Prize Fighting in America*. Updated ed. Ithaca, NY: Cornell University Press, 2010.

Gray, J. Glenn. *The Warriors: Reflections on Men in Battle*. Lincoln: University of Nebraska Press, 1998.

Green, Harvey. *Fit for America: Health, Fitness, Sport, and American Society*. New York: Pantheon, 1986.

———. "Introduction." In *Fitness in American Culture: Images of Health, Sport, and the Body, 1830–1940*, edited by Kathryn Grover, 3–17. Amherst: University of Massachusetts Press, 1989.

Grover, Kathryn. *Fitness in American Culture: Images of Health, Sport, and the Body, 1830–1940*. Rochester: University of Massachusetts Press, 1989.

Grunberger, Lisa Robin. "Bernarr Macfadden's 'Physical Culture': Muscles, Morals, and the Millenium." PhD diss., University of Chicago, 1997.

Gruneau, Richard. "The Politics and Ideology of Active Living in Historical Experience." In *Physical Activity in Human Experience: Interdisciplinary Perspectives,* edited by James E. Curtis and Storm J. Russell, 191–228. Champaign, IL: Human Kinetics, 1997.

Hanson, Thomas E. *Combat Ready? The Eighth U.S. Army on the Eve of the Korean War.* College Station: Texas A & M University Press, 2010.

Heater, Derek. *A Brief History of Citizenship.* Edinburgh: Edinburgh University Press, 2004.

Heller, Charles E. "The U.S. Army, the Civilian Conservation Corps, and Leadership for World War II, 1933–1942." *Armed Forces & Society* 36, no. 3 (2010): 439–453.

Henrikson, Rune. "Warriors in Combat—What Makes People Actively Fight in Combat?" *Journal of Strategic Studies* 30, no. 2 (2007): 187–223.

Hofmann, Annette R. "The American Turners: Their Past and Present." *Revista Brasileira de Ciencias do Esporte* 37, no. 2 (2015): 119–127.

Hogan, Michael J. *A Cross of Iron: Harry S. Truman and the Origins of the National Security State, 1945–1954.* Cambridge: Cambridge University Press, 1998.

Hoganson, Kristin L. *Fighting for American Manhood: How Gender Politics Provoked the Spanish-American and Philippine-American Wars.* New Haven, CT: Yale University Press, 1998.

Holmes, Richard. *Acts of War: The Behavior of Men in Battle.* London: Weidenfeld & Nicholson, 2003.

Howard, Michael. "Men against Fire: The Doctrine of the Offensive in 1914." In *Makers of Modern Strategy from Machiavelli to the Nuclear Age,* edited by Peter Paret, 510–526. Princeton, NJ: Princeton University Press, 1986.

Hughes, Thomas Parke. *American Genesis: A Century of Invention and Technological Enthusiasm, 1870–1970.* New York: Viking, 1989.

Hunt, William R. *Body Love: The Amazing Career of Bernarr Macfadden.* Bowling Green, OH: Bowling Green State University Popular Press, 1989.

Institute of Medicine. *Fitness Measures and Health Outcomes in Youth.* Washington, DC: National Academies Press, 2012.

Jamieson, Perry D. *Crossing the Deadly Ground: United States Army Tactics, 1865–1899.* Tuscaloosa: University of Alabama Press, 1994.

Jardins, Julie des. *Walter Camp: Football and the Modern Man.* New York: Oxford University Press, 2015.

Jarvis, Christina S. *The Male Body at War: American Masculinity during World War II.* DeKalb: Northern Illinois University Press, 2004.

Karsten, Peter. "Armed Progressives: The Military Reorganizes for the American Century." In *The Military in America from the Colonial Era to the Present*, edited by Peter Karsten, 229–271. New York: Free Press, 1980.

Kasson, John F. *Houdini, Tarzan, and the Perfect Man: The White Male Body and the Challenge of Modernity in America*. New York: Hill and Wang, 2001.

Katzenbach, Edward L. "The Mechanization of War, 1880–1919." In *Technology in Western Civilization*, edited by Melvin Kranzberg and Carroll W. Pursell, 548–561. New York: Oxford University Press, 1967.

Kedzior, Richard W. *Evolution and Endurance: The U.S. Army Division in the Twentieth Century*. Arlington, VA: RAND, 2000.

Keegan, John. *The Face of Battle*. New York: Penguin, 1978.

Keene, Jennifer D. *Doughboys, the Great War, and the Remaking of America*. Baltimore, MD: Johns Hopkins University Press, 2001.

Kellett, Anthony. *Combat Motivation: The Behavior of Soldiers in Battle*. Boston: Kluwer, Nijhoff, 1982.

Kimmel, Michael S. *The History of Men*. Albany: State University of New York Press, 2005.

———. *Manhood in America: A Cultural History*. 3rd ed. New York: Oxford University Press, 2012.

Kington, Donald M. *Forgotten Summers: The Story of the Citizens' Military Training Camps, 1921–1940*. San Francisco: Two Decades, 1995.

Krause, Michael D. "History of U.S. Army Soldier Physical Fitness." In *National Conference on Military Physical Fitness: Proceedings Report*, edited by Lois A. Hale, 20–23. Washington, DC: US Department of Health and Human Services in cooperation with the National Defense University, 1990.

Kretchik, Walter E. *U.S. Army Doctrine from the American Revolution to the War on Terror*. Lawrence: University Press of Kansas, 2011.

Lears, T. J. Jackson. "American Advertising and the Reconstruction of the Body, 1880–1930." In *Fitness in American Culture: Images of Health, Sport, and the Body, 1830–1940*, edited by Kathryn Grover, 47–66. Amherst: University of Massachusetts Press, 1989.

Leonard, Fred Eugene. *A Guide to the History of Physical Education*. Edited by George Baird Affleck. 3rd ed. Philadelphia: Lea & Febiger, 1947.

Levenstein, Harvey. *Paradox of Plenty: A Social History of Eating in Modern America*. New York: Oxford University Press, 1993.

Lewis, Adrian R. *The American Culture of War: The History of U.S. Military Force from World War II to Operation Enduring Freedom*. 2nd ed. New York: Routledge, 2012.

Linderman, Gerald F. *The World within War: America's Combat Experience in World War II*. Cambridge, MA: Harvard University Press, 1999.

Linn, Brian McAllister. *Echo of Battle: The Army's Way of War*. Cambridge, MA: Harvard University Press, 2007.

———. *Elvis's Army: Cold War GIs and the Atomic Battlefield*. Cambridge, MA: Harvard University Press, 2016.

Mandell, Richard D. *Sport, a Cultural History*. New York: Columbia University Press, 1984.

Mansoor, Peter R. *The GI Offensive in Europe: The Triumph of American Infantry Divisions, 1941–1945*. Lawrence: University Press of Kansas, 2002.

Markula, Pirkko, and Richard Pringle. *Foucault, Sport and Exercise: Power, Knowledge, and Transforming the Self*. London: Routledge, 2006.

Marshall, S. L. A. *Men against Fire: The Problem of Battle Command*. 1947; Norman: University of Oklahoma Press, 2000.

———. *The Soldier's Load and the Mobility of a Nation*. Quantico, VA: Marine Corps Association, 1980.

McGerr, Michael. *A Fierce Discontent: The Rise and Fall of the Progressive Movement in America*. Oxford: Oxford University Press, 2003.

McKenzie, Shelly. *Getting Physical: The Rise of Fitness Culture in America*. Lawrence: University Press of Kansas, 2013.

Medovoi, Leerom. *Rebels: Youth and the Cold War Origins of Identity*. Durham, NC: Duke University Press, 2005.

Mennell, James. "The Service Football Program of World War I: Its Impact on the Popularity of the Game." *Journal of Sport History* 16, no. 3 (1989): 248–260.

Meyer, Leisa D. *Creating GI Jane: Sexuality and Power in the Women's Army Corps during World War II*. New York: Columbia University Press, 1996.

Millet, John D. *The Organization and Role of the Army Service Forces*. Washington, DC: Center of Military History, 1998.

Montez de Oca, Jeffrey. "'As Our Muscles Get Softer, Our Missile Race Becomes Harder': Cultural Citizenship and the 'Muscle Gap.'" *Journal of Historical Sociology* 18, no. 3 (2005): 145–172.

Moran, Rachel Louise. *Governing Bodies: American Politics and the Shaping of the Modern Physique*. Philadelphia: University of Pennsylvania Press, 2018.

Mosse, George L. *The Image of Man the Creation of Modern Masculinity*. Oxford: Oxford University Press, 1998.

Mrozek, Donald J. "The Habit of Victory: The American Military and the Cult of Manliness." In *Manliness and Morality: Middle-Class Masculinity in Britain and America, 1800–1940*, edited by J. A. Mangan and James Walvin, 220–241. Oxford: Manchester University Press, 1987.

———. *Sport and American Mentality, 1880–1910*. Knoxville: University of Tennessee Press, 1983.

Murray, Williamson, and Allan R. Millett. *A War to Be Won: Fighting the Second World War.* Cambridge, MA: Harvard University Press, 2000.

Noverr, Douglas A., and Lawrence E. Ziewacz. *The Games They Played: Sports in American History, 1865–1980*. Chicago: Nelson-Hall, 1983.

Nye, Robert A. "Western Masculinities in War and Peace." *American Historical Review* 112, no. 2 (2007): 417–438.

Official Register of the Officers and Cadets United States Military Academy. West Point, NY: United States Military Academy Printing Office, 1913.

Overy, Richard. *Why the Allies Won*. New York: W. W. Norton, 1997.

Ozolins, John. "The Body and the Place of Physical Activity in Education: Some Classical Perspectives." *Educational Philosophy and Theory* 45, no. 9 (2013): 892–907.

Palladino, Grace. *Teenagers: An American History*. New York: Basic, 1996.

Palmer, Robert R. "Manpower for the Army: How the Physical Profile System Affected the Infantry." *Infantry Journal* 41, no. 6 (1947): 38–45.

Palmer, Robert R., I. Wiley Bell, and William R. Keast. *The Army Ground Forces: The Procurement and Training of Ground Combat Troops*. Washington, DC: Center of Military History, 1991.

Park, Roberta J. "Healthy, Moral, and Strong: Educational Views of Exercise and Athletics in Nineteenth-Century America." In *Fitness in American Culture: Images of Health, Sport, and the Body, 1830–1940*, edited by Kathryn Grover, 123–168. Amherst: University of Massachusetts Press, 1989.

———. *Measurement of Physical Fitness: A Historical Perspective*. Washington, DC: US Dept of Human Services, Public Health Service, 1989.

———. "Physiologists, Physicians, and Physical Educators: Nineteenth-Century Biology and Exercise, *Hygienic* and *Educative*." In *Sport and Exercise Science: Essays in the History of Sports Medicine*, edited by Jack W. Berryman and Roberta J. Park, 137–181. Urbana: University of Illinois Press, 1992.

Pena, Carolyn de la. "Dudley Allen Sargent: Health Machines and the Energized Male Body." *Iron Game History* 8, no. 2 (2003): 3–19.

Pettegrew, John. *Brutes in Suits: Male Sensibility in America, 1890–1920*. Baltimore, MD: Johns Hopkins University Press, 2007.

Pfister, Gertrud. "The Role of German Turners in American Physical Education." *International Journal of the History of Sport* 26, no. 13 (October 2009): 1893–1925.

Pick, Daniel. *War Machine: The Rationalisation of Slaughter in the Modern Age*. New Haven, CT: Yale University Press, 1993.

Pope, Steven. "An Army of Athletes: Playing Fields, Battlefields, and the American Military Sporting Experience, 1890–1920." *Journal of Military History* 59, no. 3 (1995): 435–456.

———. *Patriotic Games: Sporting Traditions in the American Imagination, 1876–1926*. New York: Oxford University Press, 1997.

Putney, Clifford. *Muscular Christianity: Manhood and Sports in Protestant America, 1880–1920*. Cambridge, MA: Harvard University Press, 2001.

Ready, Marie M. *Physical Education in American Colleges and Universities*. Washington, DC: Government Printing Office, 1927.

Reagor, Michael J. "Herman J. Koehler: The Father of West Point Physical Education." *Assembly* 51, no. 3 (1993): 16–19.

Rice, Emmett A. *A Brief History of Physical Education*. Edited by John L. Hutchinson. 3rd ed. New York: A. S. Barnes, 1952.

Richards, Marc. "The Cold War's 'Soft' Recruits." *Peace Review* 10, no. 3 (1998): 435–441.

Rodgers, Daniel T. *Atlantic Crossings: Social Politics in a Progressive Age*. Cambridge, MA: Belknap Press of Harvard University Press, 1998.

Rotundo, E. Anthony. *American Manhood: Transformations in Masculinity from the Revolution to the Modern Era*. New York: Basic, 1993.

Sager, John. "Universal Military Training and the Struggle to Define American Identity during the Cold War." *Federal History Journal*, no. 5 (2013): 57–74.

Salmond, John A. *The Civilian Conservation Corps, 1933–1942: A New Deal Case Study*. Durham, NC: Duke University Press, 1967.

Schneider, James J. "The Theory of the Empty Battlefield." *Royal United Services Institute for Defence Studies Journal* 132, no. 3 (1987): 37–44.

Schwartz, Hillel. "Torque: The New Kinaesthetic of the Twentieth Century." In *Incorporations*, edited by Jonathan Crary and Sanford Kwinter, 71–127. New York: Zone, 1992.

Scott, Joan W. "Gender: A Useful Category of Historical Analysis." *American Historical Review* 91, no. 5 (1986): 1053–1075.

Sherman, Janann. "'They Either Need These Women or They Do Not': Margaret Chase Smith and the Fight for Regular Status for Women in the Military." *Journal of Military History* 54 (January 1990): 47–78.

Stearns, Peter N. *Fat History: Bodies and Beauty in the Modern West*. New York: New York University Press, 2002.

Stouffer, Samuel A., Arthur A. Lumsdaine, Marion H. Lumsdaine, Robin M. Williams, M. Brewster Smith, Ivring L. Janis, Shirley A. Star, and Leonard S. Cottrell. *The American Soldier: Combat and Its Aftermath*. Vol. 2. New York: John Wiley & Sons, 1949.

Strachan, Hew. "Training, Morale and Modern War." *Journal of Contemporary History* 41, no. 2 (2006): 211–227.

Taylor, William A. *Every Citizen a Soldier: The Campaign for Universal Military Training after World War II*. College Station: Texas A & M University Press, 2014.

Terret, Thierry, and J. A. Mangan, eds. *Sport, Militarism and the Great War: Martial Manliness and Armageddon*. London: Routledge, 2012.

Thelin, John R. *A History of American Higher Education*. Baltimore, MD: Johns Hopkins University Press, 2011.

Trauschweizer, Ingo. *The Cold War U.S. Army: Building Deterrence for Limited War*. Lawrence: University Press of Kansas, 2008.

Treadwell, Mattie E. *The Women's Army Corps*. Washington, DC: Center of Military History, 1991.

Ugland, Richard M. "'Education for Victory': The High School Victory Corps and Curricular Adaptation during World War II." *History of Education Quarterly* 19, no. 4 (1979): 435–451.

Van Dalen, Deobald B., and Bruce L. Bennett. *A World History of Physical Education: Cultural, Philosophical, Comparative*. 2nd ed. Englewood Cliffs, NJ: Prentice Hall, 1971.

Van Evera, Stephen. "The Cult of the Offensive and the Origins of the First World War." *International Security* 9, no. 1 (1984): 58–107.

Veit, Helen Zoe. *Modern Food, Moral Food: Self-Control, Science, and the Rise of Modern American Eating in the Early Twentieth Century*. Chapel Hill: University of North Carolina Press, 2013.

Wakefield, Wanda Ellen. *Playing to Win: Sports and the American Military, 1898–1945*. Albany: State University of New York Press, 1997.

Welch, Paula D. *History of American Physical Education and Sport*. 3rd ed. Springfield, IL: Charles C. Thomas, 2004.

Whorton, James C. *Crusaders for Fitness: The History of American Health Reformers*. Princeton, NJ: Princeton University Press, 1982.

Young, Charles S. *Name, Rank, and Serial Number: Exploiting Korea War POWs at Home and Abroad*. Oxford: Oxford University Press, 2014.

Zeigler, Earle F. *History of Physical Education and Sport*. Rev. ed. Champaign: Stipes, 1988.

Zweiniger-Bargielowska, Ina. "Building a British Superman: Physical Culture in Interwar Britain." *Journal of Contemporary History* 41, no. 4 (2006): 595–610.

INDEX

Page numbers in italics refer to figures.